Evaluation and Management of Cleft Lip and Palate

A Developmental Perspective

Evaluation and Management of Cleft Lip and Palate

A Developmental Perspective

David J. Zajac, PhD, CCC-SLP
Linda D. Vallino, PhD, CCC-SLP/A

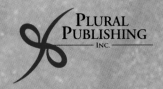

PLURAL
PUBLISHING
INC.

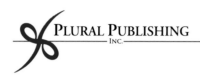

5521 Ruffin Road
San Diego, CA 92123

e-mail: info@pluralpublishing.com
Website: http://www.pluralpublishing.com

Typeset in 10.5/13 Palatino by Flanagan's Publishing Services, Inc.
Printed in Korea by Four Colour Print Group
20 19 18   2 3 4 5

Names: Zajac, David J., author. | Vallino, Linda D., author.
Title: Evaluation and management of cleft lip and palate : a developmental
   perspective / David J. Zajac, Linda D. Vallino.
Description: San Diego : Plural, [2017] | Includes bibliographical references
   and index.
Identifiers: LCCN 2015042352 | ISBN 9781597565516 (alk. paper) | ISBN
   1597565512 (alk. paper)
Subjects: | MESH: Cleft Lip. | Cleft Palate. | Speech Disorders—prevention &
   control. | Velopharyngeal Insufficiency.
Classification: LCC RD525 | NLM WV 440 | DDC 617.5/22—dc23
LC record available at http://lccn.loc.gov/2015042352

Contents

Preface

This book is intended to be a concise, practical, and evidence-based text on cleft lip and palate and related craniofacial disorders for advanced undergraduate students, graduate students, and professionals in speech-language pathology. Students and professionals in related disciplines such as dentistry, medicine, psychology, and social work also may find this book useful in providing information on individuals with craniofacial conditions. Cleft palate with or without cleft lip is a congenital defect that varies both in its severity and impact on facial and oral structures and communication. Treatment of individuals is typically a long and often-complicated process, extending into early adulthood and beyond, that is best accomplished in a team setting. In addition to the speech-language pathologist, other team members typically include a plastic surgeon, dentist, orthodontist, oral and maxillofacial surgeon, otolaryngologist, audiologist, geneticist, social worker, and psychologist. Even though all members of the team contribute to the habilitation of the individual througout his or her life span, certain team members assume critical roles at specific times of life. The purpose of the book is to provide the student and professional in speech-language pathology the information needed to (a) evaluate and treat communication disorders associated with cleft palate regardless of their primary place of employment (i.e., craniofacial team, hospital, school, or private practice), and (b) understand the complex—and sometimes controversial— surgical and dental management of individuals across the life span.

To help achieve these goals, the material in the book is presented in a developmental framework that emphasizes the most critical needs of the individual from birth to adulthood. This organizational approach has both practical and conceptual advantages. Practically, it allows the reader to access information more readily according to the age and presenting condition of the individual (i.e., birth, lip repair, palate repair, alveolar cleft repair or bone grafting, maxillary advancement). Conceptually, it chronicles the lifelong impact of craniofacial birth defects on the individual and elucidates the timing and rationale of surgical, dental, and behavioral interventions.

Part I provides necessary fundamentals for the student and professional. Chapter 1 reviews anatomy and physiology of the facial, oral, and velopharyngeal structures that are affected by clefts. Chapter 2 describes the types and causes of clefts with an emphasis on embryological development and classification. The controversy regarding timing of palate repair is discussed from the perspective of speech and language development. Chapter 3 provides an overview of genetics and the terminology used to categorize and identify congenital anomalies. A select group of craniofacial anomalies most likely to be encountered by the professional is reviewed.

Part II focuses on evaluation and management of the individual from birth to 3 years of age. Chapter 4 describes normal feeding physiology, feeding problems associated with cleft palate, and approaches to facilitate feeding prior to palate repair. Chapter 5 describes presurgical and surgical management of cleft lip and palate. Chapter 6 covers the almost universal occurrence of otitis media with effusion and conductive hearing loss that occurs in infants with cleft palate and current methods of management. Chapter 7 reviews early linguistic development in infants with cleft palate and intervention strategies before and after palate repair.

Part III focuses on evaluation and management of the individual from age 3 throughout the middle school years. Chapter 8 describes the resonance, nasal emission, articulation, voice, fluency, and intelligibility characteristics of children with repaired cleft palate. Chapter 9 provides detailed coverage of perceptual assessment and an overview of instrumental assessment techniques. Chapter 10 describes practical approaches to treating children with articulation problems in the school setting. Chapter 11 presents an overview of behavioral, surgical, and prosthetic options to manage velopharyngeal inadequacy that persists following initial palate surgery. Chapter 12 describes the orthodontic preparation and surgical correction of clefts of the alveolus.

Part IV focuses on evaluation and management of adolescents and adults with cleft palate. Chapter 13 describes the rationale and timing of maxillary advancement in adolescents to improve facial aesthetics, dental occlusion, and articulation. Chapter 14 discusses issues facing adult patients.

Although clefts of the lip and palate are among the most frequently occurring birth defects, the actual number of individuals affected in the United States is relatively low. It is not unusual, therefore, for speech-language pathologists working in the schools to infrequently see children with clefts. It is our hope that the materials in this book will be a valuable resource for school-based clinicians when they do encounter children with clefts. Some material traditionally covered in other texts is, unfortunately, omitted in the book. Due to a goal to be concise and follow a developmental framework, separate chapters on craniofacial team function and psychosocial aspects of individuals with craniofacial anomalies are not included. These are obviously important areas. We have, however, interweaved these materials in various chapters throughout the book. Maternal reactions to an infant born with a cleft are covered in Chapter 4, learning disabilities of children with cleft palate and treatment collaboration models with teams are reviewed in Chapter 10, and the last chapter deals exclusively with quality of life issues facing the adult.

Finally, the book has been written with a goal to be concise and cite evidence-based sources to support intervention approaches. In some areas, there is little objective evidence available to guide clinical decision making. In those areas, we note the lack of evidence and suggest directions for future research. It is our hope that this book will not only inform but also challenge clinicians in speech-language pathology to provide the best evidence-based evaluation and management of individuals with craniofacial anomalies as possible.

Acknowledgments

I am indebted to many who have contributed either directly or indirectly to this book. While at the University of Pittsburgh, I was fortunate to have Betty Jane McWilliams as an early mentor. Dr. McWilliams, the first and longtime director of the Cleft Palate Center, was an inexhaustible clinician and researcher who first and foremost put the welfare of the patient above all else. I have been truly influenced by her wisdom, knowledge, and caring. Campbell C. Yates and Raymond Linville also were mentors at Pittsburgh. Professor Yates, chair and emeritus professor of mechanical engineering, volunteered his time to establish aerodynamic assessment procedures at the center. Professor Yates helped me to understand and appreciate the nuances of fluid dynamics when applied to the complex geometry of the human upper airways. Raymond Linville, a mentor and friend, was influential in guiding my early research endeavors.

Many colleagues have been influential during the past 20 years at the University of North Carolina at Chapel Hill. Donald W. Warren, the Craniofacial Center's first director, was a prolific researcher who applied aerodynamic techniques to the evaluation of nasal and palatal function. Don was a role model whom I strived to emulate relative to scholarship and research productivity. Others at the University of North Carolina at Chapel Hill who have been influential include Amelia Drake, Tim Turvey, Gerald Sloan, Wolf Losken (also at Pittsburgh), and John van Aalst. They were instrumental in helping me understand surgical treatment of patients.

I am most appreciative of Linda Vallino, co-author of the book, and Jamie Perry, Nancy Scherer, Dennis Ruscello, and Joseph Napoli, contributors to the book. They are outstanding clinicians and researchers in their respective areas. This book would not be what it is without their input. A special thanks is also due to Marziye Eshghi, Jacqueline Dorry, and Ramona Hutton-Howe for their help with figures, tables, and photography.

On a personal note, I am indebted to my family for their support and encouragement. They graciously endured countless dinnertime book conversations—and dinners without me—during the writing of the book. I am grateful to my loving wife, Robin, children, Jared and Rachel, daughter-in-law Elizabeth, son-in-law, Matt, and grandson, William, for their encouragement. The thought of William's wonderful smile was the best inspiration.

—David J. Zajac
Chapel Hill, North Carolina

This book would not have been possible without the encouragement, mentorship, and friendship of some very special people. Like David, I received my training and doctoral degree at the University of Pittsburgh, under the direction of Dr. Betty Jane McWilliams. Dr. McWilliams was the quintessential teacher, researcher and clinician. She cared deeply for her patients and their families. I value all that she has taught me.

I would like to express my gratitude to Drs. William Garret (University of Pittsburgh), John B. Mulliken (Boston Children's Hospital), Ronald R. Zuker (Hospital for Sick Children), and Joseph A. Napoli (Nemours/Alfred I. DuPont Hospital for Children) for teaching me about cleft and craniofacial surgery and enhancing my education. They are talented and compassionate surgeons.

I am appreciative of David Zajac, my colleague and friend, who graciously invited me to coauthor this book with him, and our contributors, Jamie Perry, Nancy Scherer, Dennis Ruscello, and Joseph Napoli. They are among the best at what they do.

My patients and their caregivers have also been my teachers. I have learned much from all of them. Over the years, these families allowed me the opportunity to be a part of their children's care, and trusted that I would always do the best I could for them. I hope I have served them well.

Thanks to Cindy Brodoway and Brad Gelman, medical photographers at Nemours, for capturing the beautiful smiles of some of the children shown in this book.

My father always thought I should write a book, my mother agreed, and so I wrote one. This book is for both of you. To my sister Rita, and brother-in-law, Boyd—thank you always for caring about me. A special thank you to my wonderful family, Nicholas, Caroline, John, and Eleanor. You four are the best ever. Above all, my heartfelt thanks to my husband, Joe for his endless love and support for everything I do. It means the world to me.

—Linda D. Vallino
Wilmington, Delaware

Contributors

Joseph A. Napoli, MD, DDS
Associate Professor of Surgery
Sidney Kimmel Medical College
Thomas Jefferson University
Chief, Division of Plastic and
  Maxillofacial Surgery
Nemours Children's Clinic
Director, Cleft Lip and Palate/
  Craniofacial Anomalies Program
Alfred I. duPont Hospital for Children
Wilmington, Delaware
Chapters 12 and 13

Jamie Perry, PhD
Associate Professor
Department of Communication Sciences
  and Disorders
East Carolina University
Greenville, North Carolina
Chapter 1

Dennis M. Ruscello, PhD
Professor of Communication Sciences
  and Disorders
Adjunct Professor of Otolaryngology
West Virginia University
Morgantown, West Virginia
Chapter 10

Nancy J. Scherer, PhD, CCC-SLP
ASHA Fellow

Professor and Chair
Department of Speech and Hearing
  Sciences
Arizona State University
Tempe, Arizona
Chapter 7

Linda D. Vallino, PhD, CCC-SLP/A
Head of the Craniofacial Outcomes
  Research Laboratory
Center for Pediatric Auditory and Speech
  Sciences
Alfred I. duPont Hospital for Children
Wilmington, Delaware
Professor of Pediatrics
Sidney Kimmel Medical College
Thomas Jefferson University
Philadelphia, PA
Adjunct Associate Professor
University of Delaware
Newark, Delaware

David J. Zajac, PhD, CCC-SLP
Professor, Department of Dental
  Ecology
Adjunct Associate Professor, Division
  of Speech and Hearing Sciences,
  Department of Allied Health Sciences
University of North Carolina at Chapel
  Hill
Chapel Hill, North Carolina

PART I

Fundamentals

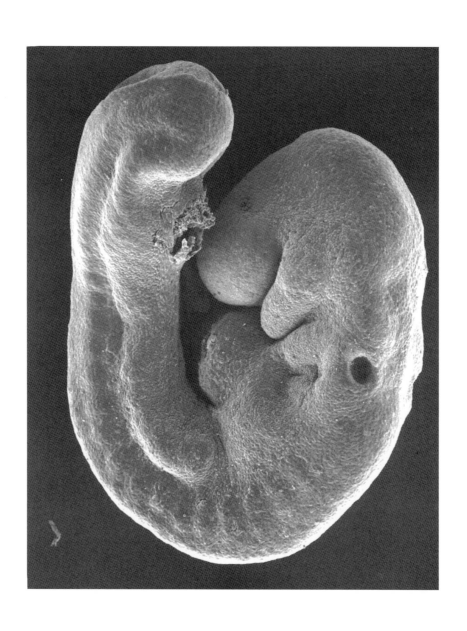

We intend this book to serve as a roadmap to the diagnosis and care of individuals with orofacial clefts and other craniofacial conditions from birth through adulthood. To do so, the speech-language pathologist (SLP) and other health care providers must know certain fundamentals. Chapter 1, Orofacial and Velopharyngeal Structure and Function, provides information on normal anatomy and physiology. Major landmarks of the face, nose, and oral cavity are identified, and detailed descriptions of the velopharyngeal muscles and functions are provided. Chapter 2, Clefts of the Lip and Palate, describes the types of clefts that are commonly encountered in the clinic. Special attention is given to submucous clefts as these may be subtle and difficult to identify. Causes of clefts and epidemiology relative to prevalence and recurrence are reviewed. Finally, Chapter 3, Syndromes and Associated Anomalies, provides an overview of genetics and the terminology used to categorize and identify congenital anomalies. A select group of craniofacial anomalies that impact communication is presented. The information in Part I sets the stage for the remainder of the book.

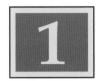

Orofacial and Velopharyngeal Structure and Function

Jamie Perry and David J. Zajac

INTRODUCTION

Orofacial clefts can involve structural anomalies of the upper lip and gum ridge, nose, hard palate, and soft palate to various degrees. If a cleft is part of a syndrome or sequence, then additional craniofacial anomalies may be present involving the lower jaw, face, ears, and skull. In order to understand the nature and management of clefts—including embryological development, anomalies at birth, impact on feeding, hearing and speech, and surgical repair—the speech-language pathologist must have a fundamental understanding of orofacial and velopharyngeal structures and function. The purpose of this chapter is to review (a) structures of the face, nasal cavity, oral cavity, pharynx, and velopharynx that may be affected by clefts, and (b) velopharyngeal function of normal speech production.

THE FACE

The face is part of the skull that contains the forehead and bony framework for the eyes, nose, and mouth. Facial landmarks of the nose and upper lip can be seen in Figure 1–1. The nasion is the bony structure at the root of the nose between the eyes. The nasal columella consists of skin and underlying tissue that separates the nose into two nostrils. It courses from the anterior nasal spine (shown in Figure 1–3) to the nasal tip. Nostrils, also called nares, are openings bounded laterally by a cartilaginous ala nasi (curved lateral portion of the nose) and alar rim (outer rim). The alar base connects the alar rim to the upper lip. The philtrum, also called philtral dimple or groove, is a midline indentation that courses from the nose to the upper lip and is bounded laterally by the philtral ridges, also called philtral

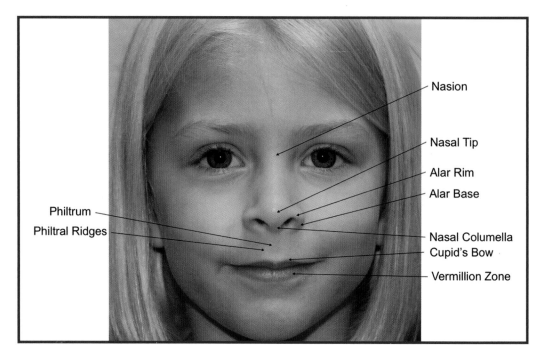

Figure 1–1. Facial landmarks.

columns. The philtral ridges are created by fusion of the maxillary, medial nasal, and lateral nasal processes during embryological development (see Chapter 2). The vermilion zone is the pigmented portion of the lips. The Cupid's bow is defined by a double curve along the superior edge of the upper lip. The white roll is a distinctive landmark that surrounds the vermilion zone. When a cleft of the lip occurs, symmetrical reconstruction of the Cupid's bow presents a particular challenge for the surgeon (see Chapter 5).

Nasal Cavity

The nasal cavity consists of the airway from the nares to the nasopharynx (Figure 1–2). The nasal cavity is the first and last point of airflow to and from the lungs and provides important physiologic func-

tions such as filtering, humidification, and temperature regulation of inspired air. During speech production, the nasal cavity also functions as an air-filled resonator for nasal consonants (see Chapter 8). The smallest cross-sectional area of the nasal cavity is called the internal nasal valve (Hixon, Weismer, & Hoit, 2008; Proctor, 1982). This valve is located approximately 1 cm from the vestibule (entrance) of the nose and is bounded by the upper lateral cartilage, the medial wall of the septum, and the anterior part of the inferior turbinate. The internal nasal valve provides the greatest resistance to inspired airflow, accounting for approximately two-thirds of the total resistance of the nasal airway (Foster, 1962). Just before entering the nasopharynx, the nasal airway narrows again into a funnel-like structure called the choanae.

The nasal cavity is lined with mucous membrane that is continuous with the

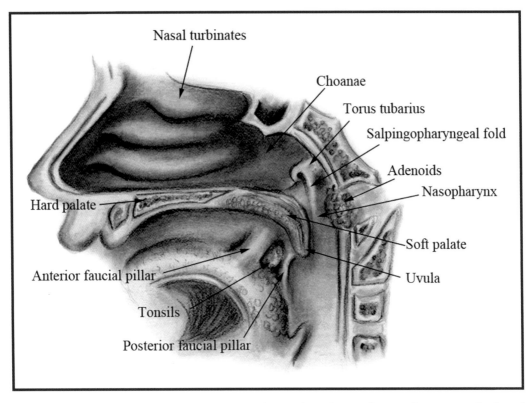

Figure 1–2. Lateral view of the nasal cavity, oral cavity, and nasopharynx and related structures.

pharynx and oral cavity. The lateral walls of the nasal cavity are made up of three bones called nasal turbinates or nasal conchae (see Figure 1–2). The superior and middle nasal turbinates are part of the ethmoid bone and the inferior turbinate articulates with the maxilla anteriorly and the palatine bone posteriorly. The mucous-covered turbinates function to warm and moisten incoming air. The grooves formed under each turbinate are called nasal meatuses. Proctor (1982) refers to the middle and inferior meatuses and turbinates as the "main nasal airway" and the area above the middle turbinate as the "olfactory airway." As discussed in Chapter 9, clinicians attempt to pass a nasal endoscope over the inferior turbi-nate and through the middle nasal meatus to obtain a view of the nasal surface of the velum.

The midline nasal septum consists of cartilage and bone. Specifically, the sep-tum contains the single unpaired vomer bone, perpendicular plate of the ethmoid bone, and septal (quadrangular) cartilage (Figure 1–3). The septal cartilage connects to the nasal columella forming the ante-rior portion of the nasal septum. In an unrepaired cleft palate, the vomer bone can be visualized during oral inspection (Figure 1–4).

The floor of the nasal cavity—which also forms the roof of the mouth—is made up of the bones of the hard palate. A bony ridge, called the nasal crest, runs the

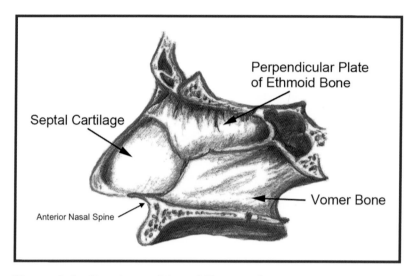

Figure 1–3. Structures of the midline nasal septum.

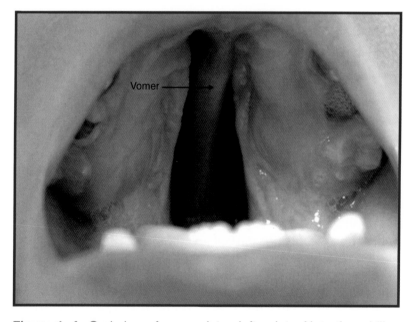

Figure 1–4. Oral view of a complete cleft palate. Note the midline nasal septum visible through oral inspection.

length of the superior nasal surface of the hard palate and serves as the attachment of the nasal septum (vomer bone) to the nasal floor. As shown in Figure 1–4, how- ever, the vomer bone does not attach to the hard palate when a complete bilateral cleft of the secondary palate occurs (see Chapter 2).

Oral Structures

Figure 1–5 shows structures of the oral cavity. The palate consists of hard bony and soft muscular parts. The soft palate, also called the velum, extends beyond the hard palate and terminates at the uvula. As seen in Figures 1–2 and 1–5, the anterior and posterior faucial pillars attach the soft palate to the tongue and pharynx, respectively. The palatoglossus muscle courses inferiorly through the anterior faucial pillar, while the palatopharyngeus muscle courses inferiorly through the posterior faucial pillar (see Figure 1–8). Between the two pillars is the faucial isthmus, where the palatine tonsils can be found. Lingual tonsils are located on the base of the tongue (not visible in Figure 1–5). The alveolar ridge is the raised portion of the upper and lower dental arches, which provides support for the teeth.

Hard Palate

The hard palate is the bony structure that forms the floor of the nasal cavity and roof of the oral cavity. During embryological development, the hard palate evolves from two vertical shelves of bone that elevate and fuse in the midline (see Chapter 2, Figure 2–12). The line of fusion is called the median palatine suture, or the intermaxillary suture (Figure 1–6). The bony hard palate is divided into the premaxilla, palatine processes, and palatine bones. The premaxilla is anterior to the incisive foramen and contains the central and lateral incisors. The incisive foramen is a small opening that passes nerves (nasopalatine nerve) and blood vessels (sphenopalatine artery) to the oral mucosa of the hard palate. The premaxilla is separated from the palatine processes by the incisive sutures. As discussed in Chapter 2, the premaxilla fuses to the palatine processes along

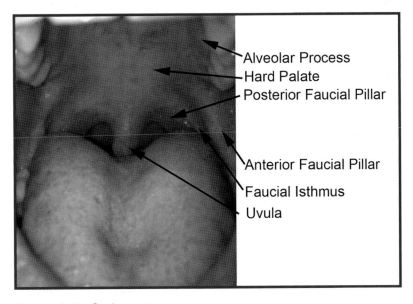

Figure 1–5. Oral structures.

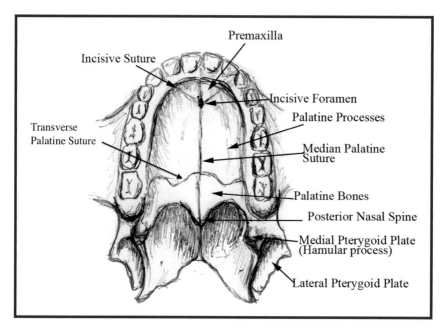

Figure 1–6. Hard palate.

the incisive sutures during embryological development.

The paired palatine processes form most of the hard palate, approximately three-fourths of its length. The transverse palatine sutures separate the palatine processes from the horizontal plates of the palatine bones. The palatine bones are directly behind the palatine processes and form the posterior one-fourth of the hard palate. The bony hard palate terminates at the posterior nasal spine. Posterior to the palatine bones is the palatine aponeurosis, an extension of the tensor veli palatini muscle (see Figure 1–8). The palatine aponeurosis is a broad, flat tendinous sheath that provides friction-free motion between a highly movable velum and rigid hard palate.

Soft Palate

The soft palate or velum extends beyond the hard palate via the palatine aponeu-

rosis. The velum is continuous with the uvula proper (uvula), which is the pendulous structure at the end of the velum (see Figure 1–5). When the mouth is closed, a minimal negative pressure keeps the oral surface of the velum at rest against the base of the tongue. During production of oral speech sounds, the velum elevates with the nasal surface contacting the pharyngeal walls and adenoids or both. During production of nasal sounds, the velum lowers but is not at rest position. Although the uvula takes the same movement path as the velum, it is not considered to have any contribution to velopharyngeal closure.

Histology studies show that the velum contains tendinous, muscular, adipose, glandular, and connective tissues (Ettema & Kuehn, 1994; Kuehn & Kahane, 1990). The anterior two thirds of the velum is structurally consistent in organization compared to the posterior one third. The anterior segment of the velum contains little to no muscle fibers (Perry & Kuehn, 2014). Rather, the anterior portion of the velum is predominantly glandular and adipose tissue (Pruzansky & Mason, 1969; Simpson & Austin, 1972). This velar composition is likely what gives way to the velar stretch, described later in the chapter. The middle portion of the velum is largely muscular tissue from the levator veli palatini and musculus uvulae fibers. The posterior-inferior portion of the velum and the uvula are irregular across individuals but consist primarily of connective, glandular, adipose, and vascular tissue (Kuehn & Moon, 2005).

Pharynx

The pharynx is a muscular tube that extends from the base of the skull to the level of the sixth cervical vertebrae (C6) (Zemlin, 1998). It is divided into the laryngopharynx, oropharynx, and nasopharynx (Figure 1–7). The laryngopharynx is the most inferior part of the pharynx extending from the hyoid bone inferiorly to C6, where it communicates with the larynx (Zemlin, 1998). The oropharynx is the middle part that extends superiorly from the level of the hyoid bone to the nasal surface of the velum. The nasopharynx is

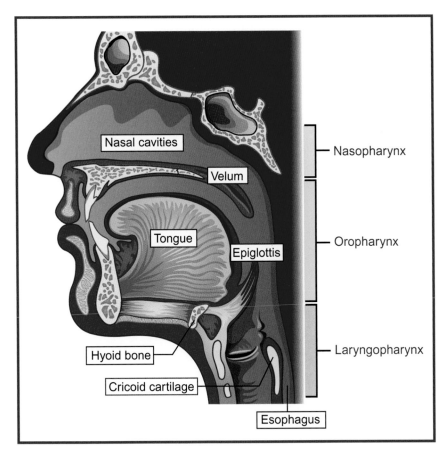

Figure 1–7. Pharynx and subdivisions. (Hixon, Weismer, and Hoit. *Preclinical Speech Science* (2nd ed.), 2014, Plural Publishing, Inc. Reprinted with permission.)

the most superior part of the pharyngeal tube. It extends from the velum to the cranial base. Velopharyngeal closure occurs at the level of the nasopharynx and is described later in the chapter. The pharynx functions as both an aero-digestive pathway and as an air-filled resonator during phonation.

Velopharyngeal Muscles

The bulk of the velum consists of five pairs of muscles—levator veli palatini, tensor veli palatini, palatopharyngeus, palatoglossus, and musculus uvulae (Figure 1–8 and Table 1–1). It is well accepted that the muscle responsible for elevation and retraction of the velum is the levator veli palatini. The coordinated control of the velum, however, is facilitated by additional muscles such as palatopharyngeus and palatoglossus that assist in positioning the velum within the velopharyngeal port (Moon, Smith, Folkins, Lemke, & Gartlan, 1994). There is a sixth, smaller velar muscle, salpingopharyngeus, that may assist swallowing function. With the exception of the musculus uvulae, all velar muscles are paired, having a muscle bundle on the right and left sides. The musculus uvulae has been observed to be both paired and unpaired among individuals with normal anatomy (Azzam & Kuehn, 1977; Dickson, 1975; Kuehn & Moon, 2005; Langdon & Klueber, 1978). This variability, however, is likely not functionally significant.

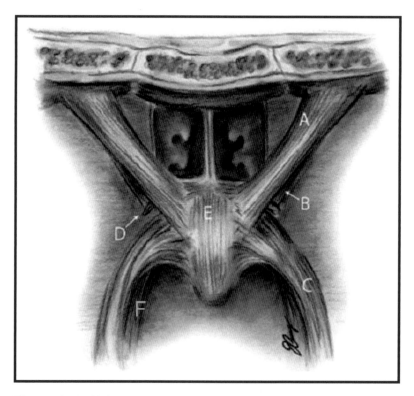

Figure 1–8. Velar muscles, posterior view. *A*, levator veli palatini; *B*, tensor veli palatini; *C*, palatopharyngeus; *D*, hamular process; *E*, musculus uvulae; *F*, palatoglossus.

Table 1–1. Summary of Velopharyngeal Muscles

Muscle	Origin	Insertion	Motor Nerve Supply	Primary Function
Levator veli palatini	Apex of petrous part of temporal bone and cartilaginous eustachian tube	Soft palate	IX, X	Elevates and retracts velum
Tensor veli palatini	Scaphoid fossa of sphenoid, eustachian tube	Aponeurosis of velum	V	Dilates eustachian tubes
Musculus uvulae	Palatal aponeurosis	Mucous membrane of uvula	IX, X	Adds bulk and stiffness to velum; may provide firm contact to posterior pharyngeal wall
Palatopharyngeus	Posterior border of aponeurosis	Lateral pharynx and larynx	IX, X	Horizontal fibers provide sphincter action to pull lateral pharyngeal walls medially; vertical fibers may lower velum and elevate pharynx/larynx during deglutition
Palatoglossus	Lateral aspects of velum	Lateral aspects of tongue	IX, X Possibly XII	Antagonistic to levator; lowers velum; lifts tongue and propels food
Salpingopharyngeus	Inferior segment of the torus tubarius	Lateral pharyngeal walls	IX, X	Vestigial
Superior constrictor	Pterygoimandibular raphe, mylohyoid line of the mandible, medial pterygoid plate, hamulus, lateral aspects of the tongue, and lateral margins of the velum	Median pharyngeal raphe	IX, X	Medial displacement of lateral pharynx

11

Levator Veli Palatini

The levator veli palatini muscle originates at the anterior petrous portion of the temporal bone. Huang, Lee, and Rajendran (1997) documented a possible origin of levator veli palatini fibers along the medial cartilaginous portion of the auditory (eustachian) tube. From the muscle origin, levator fibers course medially, inferiorly, and anteriorly to enter the body of the velum. The muscle bundles insert into the middle 40% of the velum (Boorman & Sommerlad, 1985), where the fibers converge and become more irregular (Perry, Kuehn, & Sutton, 2013). The muscle fibers inside the velum fan out and intermingle with the opposing levator veli palatini muscle bundle (Kuehn & Moon, 2005; Perry et al., 2013). Kuehn and Moon (2005) demonstrated no septum or separation between the two levator veli palatini muscle bundles in the velar midline. As seen in Figure 1–8, the levator veli palatini muscle forms a cohesive sling coursing from the base of the skull into the body of the velum. Because of the muscle course and fiber arrangement, the levator veli palatini is in the most favorable position for elevating and retracting the velum during velopharyngeal closure.

In infants born with cleft palate, levator veli palatini fibers attach abnormally to the posterior margin of the bony hard palate. This bone-to-bone attachment causes isometric contraction of the muscle, inhibiting elevation and retraction of the velum. As discussed in Chapter 5, the primary aim of cleft palate surgery is to remove the anterior lateral fiber attachment from the hard palate and retrodisplace the fibers into the cohesive sling through the body of the velum.

Tensor Veli Palatini

The tensor veli palatini muscle runs parallel but anterior to the levator veli palatini muscle. Abe et al. (2004) described the muscle as having two origins including the cartilaginous and membranous portions of the eustachian tube and the pterygoid plate of the sphenoid bone. Barsoumain, Kuehn, Moon, and Canady (1998) identified an attachment of the anterior muscle segment, referred to as the tensor veli palatini proper to the hamulus. Based on the fixed osseous attachments of the anterior segment, it may serve to secure, support, and function synergistically with the tensor tympani muscle to influence movements of the malleus (Barsoumain et al., 1998). The posterior belly, referred to as the dilator tubae, has been identified as the primary segment responsible for opening the eustachian tube (Barsoumain et al., 1998; Goss, 1973; Rood & Doyle, 1978). Barsoumain et al. (1998) suggested the integration of anterior segment fibers with those of the dilator tubae may also reinforce the anterior attachment of the dilator tubae. The tensor veli palatini muscle terminates near the junction between the hard and soft palate where it becomes tendinous as it winds around the hamulus of the medial pterygoid plate (see Figure 1–8). The tensor tendon converges toward the midline of the velum where it contributes to the palatal aponeurosis. The palatal aponeurosis, as previously mentioned, is a broad flat tendinous sheath that functions to provide friction-free movement between the hard and soft palates.

As indicated above, the primary function of the tensor veli palatini muscle is to open the eustachian tube (Barsoumain et al., 1998; Dickson & Maue-Dickson, 1982; Goss, 1973; Rood & Doyle, 1978).

The eustachian tube consists of an osseous portion, a membranous portion, and a cartilaginous portion. The osseous portion is the bony and most lateral segment of the eustachian tube that leads toward the outer ear. The membranous portion includes the tympanic membrane, which divides the outer and middle ear cavities. The cartilaginous portion is the most medial segment of the eustachian tube that leads into the nasopharynx. A ring of cartilage called the torus tubarius surrounds the opening (also called orifice or ostia) of the eustachian tube (see Figure 1–2). A fold of tissue called the salpingopharyngeal fold extends inferiorly below the torus tubarius. The region posterior to the torus tubarius and salpingopharyngeal fold is called the fossa of Rosenmüller (also called pharyngeal recess).

Contraction of the tensor veli palatini muscle dilates and opens the eustachian tube, causing equalization of middle ear pressure and drainage of unwanted middle ear fluid. Based on their observations of consistent hamular insertion of the tensor tendon, Barsoumain et al. (1998) suggested tensor veli palatini contraction could not cause lateral displacement to tense the velum. Instead, the authors proposed muscle contraction may serve as a bridge between the hard and soft palates that acts as a buffer to provide stiffness to the anterior portion of the velum. Due to the position of the tensor veli palatini muscle fibers and tendon in the body of the velum, it is unlikely that the tensor veli palatini muscle contributes to velopharyngeal closure during speech (Fritzell, 1969; Kuehn & Kahane, 1990; Perry & Kuehn, 2014).

In infants born with cleft palate, the tensor veli palatini demonstrates a lateral insertion onto the bony aspects of the cleft. Specifically, fibers may end at the maxillary tuber or hamulus, or may terminate in bundles along with the levator veli palatini (Punjabi & Hardesty, 2006). Contraction of the muscles, therefore, does not dilate the eustachian tube. As discussed in Chapter 6, this anomaly causes almost universal eustachian tube dysfunction and conductive hearing loss in infants with unrepaired cleft palate.

Musculus Uvulae

The musculus uvulae, also called uvular muscle, is the only intrinsic velar muscle, meaning both attachments are contained entirely within the body of the velum. The musculus uvulae lies along the midline of the dorsal (nasal) surface of the velum and is cradled by the levator veli palatini muscle sling (see Figure 1–8). Through histology, Kuehn and Moon (2005) observed variability in the musculus uvulae across velar specimens and within individuals with normal anatomy. The authors noted the existence of a septum and surrounding sheath in the majority of specimens, even in those in which paired musculus uvulae fibers were not identified. Fibers of the musculus uvulae originate at the palatal aponeurosis but do not attach to the hard palate (Kuehn & Kahane, 1990). The muscle fibers are enclosed within a thin connective tissue capsule that extends the length of the velum into the uvula proper. The musculus uvulae show the greatest bulk at the level of the levator veli palatini sling. As the muscle courses along the length of the velum, it becomes diffuse and, in some cases, is void as it approximates the uvula proper (Azzam & Kuehn, 1977; Kuehn & Moon, 2005).

During speech, contraction of the musculus uvulae adds bulk to the nasal surface of the velum. It is suggested that the bulge created by the musculus uvulae functions to add stiffness to the velum to help fill the velopharyngeal gap (Azzam & Kuehn, 1977; Croft, Shprintzen, Daniller, & Lewin, 1978; Dickson, 1975; Langdon & Klueber, 1978). The added bulk along the nasal velar surface provides the convex appearance to the velar knee during elevation. Kuehn, Folkins, and Cutting (1982) proposed a second function of the musculus uvulae fibers. The authors described the velum as a double-layered beam. Contraction of the upper beam, containing the musculus uvulae, causes the posterior and superior extension of the lower beam (velum) that provides the firm contact of the velum against the posterior pharyngeal wall. This extensor action may serve to provide an extra seal between the velum and the posterior pharyngeal wall during velopharyngeal closure.

Nasoendoscopy studies have shown some individuals with repaired cleft palate to have abnormalities in the musculus uvulae. Pigott (1969) described the bulge of the musculus uvulae along the nasal surface of the velum in subjects with normal anatomy. Later, Pigott, Bensen, and White (1969) suggested insufficient musculus uvulae fibers as a potential cause of lasting velopharyngeal insufficiency in individuals with repaired cleft palate. Croft, Shprintzen, and Rakoff (1981) documented absent musculus uvulae fiber bulging on the nasal surface of the velum in 100% of subjects with hypernasal speech but observed its presence in all subjects with normal anatomy/resonance. Lewin, Croft, and Shprintzen (1980) observed unusual musculus uvulae bulge in 100% of subjects with velopharyngeal insufficiency related to overt or occult submucous cleft palate and neurological and functional disorders. More spe-

cifically, the authors suggested absent or hypoplastic musculus uvulae fibers based on visualization of a concave nasal velar surface and midline indentation along the full length of the velum. Muscle imaging studies in vivo, however, have yet to confirm the lack of musculus uvulae fibers in individuals born with cleft palate.

Palatopharyngeus

The palatopharyngeus muscle consists of vertically and horizontally oriented fibers. The vertical fibers (called palatothyroideus) course through the posterior faucial pillar and inferiorly insert into the greater horns of the thyroid cartilage (Cassell & Elkadi, 1995). The transverse (horizontal) fibers (called palatopharyngeus proper) course posteriorly from the velum to the lateral and posterior pharyngeal walls (Cassell & Elkadi, 1995). Because of the variation in the muscle bundles' direction and course, the palatopharyngeus likely has different functions. Vertical fibers may function to elevate the pharynx and depress the velum during deglutition (Sumida, Yamashita, & Kitamura, 2012). Transverse fibers function to provide inward movement of the lateral pharyngeal walls to assist with velopharyngeal closure and may contribute to a Passavant's ridge, when present (described later in the chapter).

Palatoglossus

The palatoglossus muscle courses inferiorly from the lateral aspects of the soft palate to insert into the lateral aspects of the tongue. The palatoglossus muscle courses through the anterior faucial pillar. Because both attachment sites of the palatoglossus are highly movable structures, the muscle has multiple functions depending on the task. The muscle can function to draw the tongue posteriorly and superiorly. This movement along with a narrowing of the faucial isthmus has been shown to function in the transit of a bolus from the oral to pharyngeal cavity (Tachimura, Ojima, Nohara, & Wada, 2005). Studies do not agree on the function of the palatoglossus muscle for speech. Electromyographic studies demonstrated activation of the palatoglossus in lowering the velum during nasalized production for three out of five subjects, suggesting functional differences between individuals (Kuehn et al., 1982). Kuehn and Azzam (1978) identified a more anterior vertical position of the muscle fibers in some individuals, while others displayed a more posterior oblique muscle course. Vertical anterior fibers would most likely function for tongue elevation. A more posterior oblique fiber direction would function as an antagonist to the levator veli palatini muscle to lower the velum. This lowering of the velum may also serve to create a patent and open nasopharyngeal airway for nasal breathing (Kuehn & Azzam, 1978).

Salpingopharyngeus

This muscle originates at the inferior segment of the torus tubarius, which is the ring of cartilage that surrounds the mouth or opening of the eustachian tube at the level of the nasopharynx. The muscle courses through the salpingopharyngeus fold along the lateral pharyngeal walls where it terminates around the level of the palatopharyngeus fibers. Due to variability in size and presence, salpingopharyngeus is thought to have little if any significant impact on speech (Dickson & Dickson, 1972; Fritzell, 1969; Trigos, Ysunza, Vargas, & Vazquez, 1988). During swallowing, the salpingopharyngeus muscle may function to elevate the pha-

ryngeal walls to assist in movement of the bolus through the pharyngeal cavity.

Pharyngeal Constrictors

The pharyngeal constrictors (inferior, medial, and superior) collectively form the muscular tube of the pharyngeal wall (Figure 1–9). The superior, middle, and inferior pharyngeal constrictors are stacked together with overlapping segments along the length of the pharynx. The constrictor muscle fibers have bipinnate muscle architecture in that they diverge away from a central tendon called the median pharyngeal raphe. The median pharyngeal raphe is located on the posterior aspect of the pharynx. The inferior pharyngeal constrictor courses from the median pharyngeal raphe to the thyroid and cricoid cartilages of the laryngeal system. The middle pharyngeal constrictor extends from the median pharyngeal raphe to the hyoid bone. The inferior and middle pharyngeal constrictors are important during deglutition through pharyngeal constriction and posterior and superior movements of the larynx.

The superior pharyngeal constrictor is the segment of the pharyngeal tube that is involved in velopharyngeal closure due to its location at the level of the nasopharynx. The superior pharyngeal constrictor functions to narrow the pharyngeal airway through medial movements of the lateral pharyngeal walls and, in some cases, anterior movement of the posterior pharyngeal wall (Iglesias, Kuehn, & Morris, 1980; Shprintzen, McCall, Skolnick, & Lencione, 1975). From the median pharyngeal raphe, muscle fibers from the superior pharyngeal constrictor course around the pharyngeal tube and attach to several structures including the pterygomandibular raphe, mylohyoid line of the mandible,

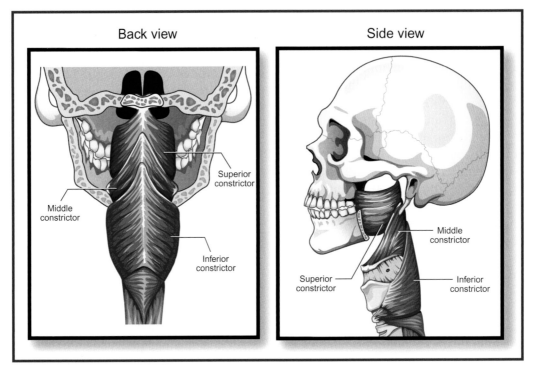

Figure 1–9. Pharyngeal constrictor muscles, posterior and lateral views. (Hixon, Weismer, and Hoit. *Preclinical Speech Science* (2nd ed.), 2014, Plural Publishing, Inc. Reprinted with permission.)

medial pterygoid plate, hamulus, lateral aspects of the tongue, and lateral margins of the velum.

Fibers from the pharyngeal constrictor and horizontal fibers from the palatopharyngeus likely contribute to the formation of a Passavant's ridge, when present. A Passavant's ridge is a shelf-like muscular band that protrudes anteriorly from the posterior pharyngeal wall upon phonation (see Chapter 9, Figure 9–25). At rest, the muscular ridge is not present. At times, instructing an individual with repaired cleft palate to widely open the mouth and protrude the tongue during phonation of a low vowel may elicit Passavant's ridge. In such cases, the ridge may be triggered by mechanical linkage between the protruded tongue and superior constrictor

muscle as noted above. Zim et al. (2003) reported that individuals with velocardiofacial syndrome (also known as 22q11.2 deletion syndrome) have a hypoplastic superior pharyngeal constrictor muscle. Along with cranial base and levator veli palatini muscle variations, this places the individual at risk of pharyngeal hypotonia and hypernasal speech (see Chapter 3).

Velopharyngeal Motor and Sensory Innervation

With the exception of the tensor veli palatini muscles, motor innervation to velopharyngeal muscles arises from the pharyngeal plexus. The pharyngeal plexus is a network of branches of the glossopharyngeal (CN IX), vagus (CN X), and accessory (CN XI) cranial nerves. Cassell and Elkadi (1995) described additional motor innervation to the palatoglossus via the hypoglossal nerve (CN XII). The tensor veli palatini muscle is innervated by the motor root of the mandibular branch of the trigeminal cranial nerve (CN V). Shimokawa, Yi, and Tanaka (2005) studied 15 specimens through histology and suggested a possible double innervation of the levator veli palatini muscle through the lesser palatine nerve in addition to the pharyngeal plexus. The lesser palatine nerve also provides innervation to fibers of the palatopharyngeus and musculus uvulae.

Although there is disagreement, the role of the facial nerve (through the lesser palatine branch) has been suggested as a possible source of motor innervation to muscles of the velopharyngeal mechanism (Bosma, 1986; Dickson & Dickson, 1980; Nishio, Matsuya, Machida, & Miyazaki, 1976a; Sedlackova, Lastovia, & Sram, 1973). Nishio et al. (1976a) suggested possible involvement of the facial nerve (CN VII) in addition to branches from the pharyngeal plexus in motor innervation to the levator veli palatini muscle, uvula, and superior pharyngeal constrictor muscle. A later study by Nishio, Matsuya, Machida, and Miyazaki (1976b) used electrical stimulation to examine responses of the facial, glossopharyngeal, and vagus nerves. The authors reported varied degrees of muscle activation across the cranial nerves examined. It was suggested that these data demonstrate a potential specificity of the facial nerve in controlling finer movements compared to glossopharyngeal and vagal nerve stimulation.

Sensory innervation to the palatal and pharyngeal mucosa is provided by branches of the trigeminal (V), facial (VII), glossopharyngeal (IX), and vagus (X) cranial nerves (Shimokawa et al., 2005). Sensory innervation to the pharynx and soft palate is via the pharyngeal branch of the vagus nerve (Bass & Morrell, 1992). Sensory fibers terminate in the spinal nucleus of the trigeminal nerve (Cassell & Elkadi, 1995).

VELOPHARYNGEAL FUNCTION

The velopharyngeal mechanism creates a tight seal between the soft palate and pharyngeal walls to separate the oral and nasal cavities. The tight seal directs acoustic energy and airflow into the oral cavity instead of the nasal cavity during speech. During production of non-nasal sounds, contraction of the levator veli palatini muscle elevates and retracts the velum, while contraction of the superior pharyngeal constrictor muscle—and likely transverse fibers from the palatopharyngeus—causes medial displacement of the lateral pharyngeal walls around the velum, creating sphincter-like closure. Although less common, anterior movement of the posterior pharyngeal wall can also assist in velopharyngeal closure (Iglesias et al., 1980). During elevation, the velum forms an eminence (called the velar knee) that makes contact against the pharyngeal wall (Figure 1–10). Velar contact can also be made against an enlarged adenoid pad. Adenoids are a lymphatic tissue located along the posterior wall of the nasopharynx (see Figure 1–2). The adenoids grow rapidly during the first year of life, fill most of the nasopharynx by four years of age, peak in size around 12 years of age, and then begin to involute during adolescence (Mason & Warren, 1980).

A Passavant's ridge may serve as a place of velar contact in some individuals (Casey & Emrich, 1988; Croft, Shprintzen,

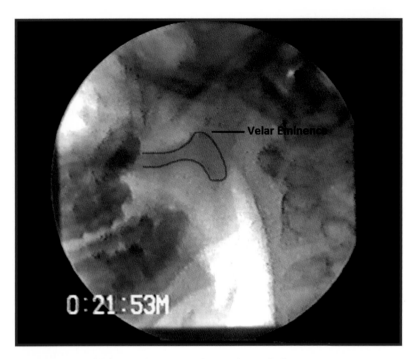

Figure 1–10. Velar eminence or knee, lateral view.

& Rakoff, 1981; Glaser, Skolnick, McWilliams, & Shprintzen, 1979). As described previously, a Passavant's ridge is a localized projection of the posterior pharyngeal wall. Croft et al. (1981) reported the occurrence of Passavant's ridge in 19% of normal speakers and in 24% of speakers with velopharyngeal inadequacy. The location of a Passavant's ridge along the posterior pharyngeal wall and its orientation to the velum are quite variable. Glaser et al. (1979) reported that the position of Passavant's ridge was below the uvula and provided no functional benefit in approximately 12% of speakers. As described in Chapter 9, imaging procedures such as lateral view videofluoroscopy—and perhaps nasoendoscopy—can be used to determine the functional role of a Passavant's ridge during speech, when present.

There are several patterns associated with velopharyngeal closure—coronal, sagittal, and circular. Coronal closure is achieved primarily by elevation and retraction of the velum and, in some cases, anterior movement of the posterior pharyngeal wall. Sagittal closure involves primarily medial movement of the lateral pharyngeal walls to approximate the posterior margin of the velum. Circular closure involves a sphincter-like closure through velar, lateral pharyngeal wall, and posterior pharyngeal wall movement. Circular closure can also occur against a Passavant's ridge in both individuals with normal anatomy and those with cleft palate.

Croft et al. (1981) reported that coronal was the most common velopharyngeal closure pattern, occurring in 55% of individuals with normal anatomy and 45% of individuals with velopharyngeal inadequacy. They reported that sagittal closure patterns were observed among 16% of individuals with normal anatomy and 11% of individuals with velopharyngeal inadequacy; circular closure patterns were found in 10% of individuals with normal anatomy and 20% of those with velopharyngeal inadequacy.

Closure force of the velum against the posterior pharyngeal wall varies based on the type of sound produced (Kuehn, 1976; Kuehn & Moon, 1998; McKerns & Bzoch, 1970; Moon Kuehn, & Huisman, 1994). Closure force is greater for high vowels compared to low vowels (Kuehn & Moon, 1998). Stops, affricates, and fricatives show greater closure force compared to vowels (Kuehn & Moon, 1998). Velar height also varies based on the phoneme produced. In general, high-pressure consonants have the greatest velar height. High vowels are produced with a greater velar height compared to low vowels (Moon, Kuehn, & Huisman, 1994). It is not clear if the greater closure force and velar height associated with obstruent consonants are due to the need for increased closure during high-pressure segments or as a result of high pressure in the oral cavity, or both.

CHAPTER SUMMARY

The speech-language pathologist needs to have fundamental knowledge of orofacial and velopharyngeal structure and function that may be affected by clefts. This chapter reviewed the nose and nasal passage, oral cavity, pharynx, and velopharynx relative to major anatomical structures and function. Velopharyngeal muscles were described in detail, and the velopharyngeal mechanism was presented as a complex three-dimensional muscular structure that functions in a sphincter-like manner to separate the oral and nasal cavities during non-nasal speech segments. As described in subsequent chapters, clefts can significantly disrupt the structural and functional integrity of the oral and nasal cavities and velopharyngeal mechanism with the potential for lifelong impact on aesthetics, respiration, hearing, and speech production.

REFERENCES

Abe, M., Murakami, G., Noguchi, M., Kitamura, S., Shimada, K., & Kohama, G. I. (2004). Variations in the tensor veli palatini muscle with special reference to its origin and insertion. *Cleft Palate Craniofacial Journal, 41*, 474–484.

Azzam, N. A., & Kuehn, D. P. (1977). The morphology of musculus uvulae. *Cleft Palate Journal, 14*(1), 78–87.

Barsoumain, R., Kuehn, D. P., Moon, J. B., & Canady, J. W. (1998). An anatomic study of the tensor veli palatini and dilator tubae muscles in relation to Eustachian tube and velar function. *Cleft Palate-Craniofacial Journal, 35*, 101–110.

Bass, N. H., & Morrell, R. M. (1992). The neurology of swallowing. In M. E. Groher (Ed.), *Dysphagia: Diagnosis and management* (3rd ed., pp. 7–35). Newton, MA: Butterworth-Heinemann.

Boorman, J. G., & Sommerlad, B. C. (1985). Levator palati and palatal dimples: Their anatomy, relationship and clinical significance. *British Journal of Plastic Surgery, 38*, 326–332.

Bosma, J. F. (1986). *Anatomy of the infant head*. Baltimore, MD: Johns Hopkins University Press.

Casey, D. M., & Emrich, L. J. (1988). Passavant's ridge in patients with soft palatectomy. *Cleft Palate Journal, 25*(1), 72–77.

Cassell, M. D., & Elkadi, H. (1995). Anatomy and physiology of the palate and velopharyngeal structures. In R. J. Shprintzen & J.

Bardach (Eds.), *Cleft palate speech management: A multidisciplinary approach* (pp. 45–62). St. Louis, MO: Mosby.

Croft, C. B., Shprintzen, R. J., Daniller, A., & Lewin, M. L. (1978). The occult submucous cleft palate and the musculus uvulae. *Cleft Palate Journal, 15*, 150–154.

Croft, C. B., Shprintzen, R. J., & Rakoff, S. J. (1981). Patterns of velopharyngeal valving in normal and cleft palate subjects: A multiview videofluoroscopic and nasendoscopic study. *Laryngoscope, 91*(2), 265–271.

Dickson, D. R. (1975). Anatomy of the normal velopharyngeal mechanism. *Clinics in Plastic Surgery, 2*, 235–247.

Dickson, D. R., & Dickson, W. M. (1972). Velopharyngeal anatomy. *Journal of Speech and Hearing Research, 15*, 372–381.

Dickson, D. R., & Dickson, W. M. (1980). Velopharyngeal structure and function: A model for biomechanical analysis. In N. J. Lass (Ed.), *Speech and Language: Advances in Basic Research and Practice* (pp. 168–222). New York, NY: Academic Press.

Dickson, D. R., & Maue-Dickson, W. (1982). *Anatomical and physiological bases of speech.* Boston, MA: Little, Brown and Co.

Ettema, S. L., & Kuehn, D. P. (1994). A quantitative histologic study of the normal human adult soft palate. *Journal of Speech and Hearing Research, 37*, 303–313.

Foster, T. (1962). Maxillary deformities in repaired clefts of the lip and palate. *British Journal of Plastic Surgery, 15*, 182–190.

Fritzell, B. (1969). The velopharyngeal muscles in speech. *Acta Oto-Laryngologica, 250* (Suppl.), 1–81.

Glaser, E. R., Skolnick, M. L., McWilliams, B. J., & Shprintzen, R. J. (1979). The dynamics of Passavant's ridge in subjects with and without velopharyngeal insufficiency— A multiview videofluoroscopic study. *Cleft Palate Journal, 16*, 24.

Goss, C. M. (1973). *Gray's anatomy of the human body.* Philadelphia, PA: Lea and Febiger.

Hixon, T. J., Weismer, G., & Hoit, J. D. (2008). *Preclinical speech science: Anatomy, physiology, acoustics, perception.* San Diego, CA: Plural.

Huang, M. H., Lee, S. T., & Rajendran, K. (1997). A fresh cadaveric study of the paratubal muscles: Implications for Eustachian tube function in cleft palate. *Plastic and Reconstructive Surgery, 100*, 833–842.

Iglesias, A., Kuehn, D. P., & Morris, H. L. (1980). Simultaneous assessment of pharyngeal wall and velar displacement for selected speech sounds. *Journal of Speech and Hearing Research, 23*, 429–446.

Kuehn, D. P. (1976). A cineradiographic investigation of velar movement variables in two normals. *Cleft Palate Journal, 13*, 88–103.

Kuehn, D. P., & Azzam, N. A. (1978). Anatomical characteristics of palatoglossus and the anterior falanucial pillar. *Cleft Palate Journal, 15*, 349–359.

Kuehn, D. P., Folkins, J. W., & Cutting, C. B. (1982). Relationships between muscle activity and velar positioning. *Cleft Palate Journal, 19*, 25–35.

Kuehn, D. P., & Kahane, J. C. (1990). Histologic study of the normal human adult soft palate. *Cleft Palate Journal, 27*, 26–34.

Kuehn, D. P., & Moon, J. B. (1998). Velopharyngeal closure force and levator veli palatini activation levels in varying phonetic contexts. *Journal of Speech, Language, and Hearing Research, 41*, 51–62.

Kuehn, D. P., & Moon, J. B. (2005). Histologic study of intravelar structures in normal human adult specimens. *Cleft Palate-Craniofacial Journal, 42*(5), 481–489.

Langdon, H. L., & Klueber, K. (1978). The longitudinal fibromuscular component of the soft palate in the fifteen-week human fetus: Musculus uvulae and palatine raphe. *Cleft Palate Journal, 15*, 337–348.

Lewin, M. L., Croft, C. B., & Shprintzen, R. J. (1980). Velopharyngeal insufficiency due to hypoplasia of the musculus uvulae and occult submucous cleft palate. *Plastic and Reconstructive Surgery, 65*(5), 585–591.

Mason, R. M., & Warren, D. W. (1980). Adenoid involution and developing hypernasality in cleft palate. *Journal of Speech and Hearing Disorders, 45*(4), 469–480.

McKerns, D., & Bzoch, K. R. (1970). Variations in velopharyngeal valving: The factor of sex. *Cleft Palate Journal, 7*, 652–662.

Moon, J. B., Kuehn, D. P., & Huisman, J. (1994). Measurement of velopharyngeal closure force during vowel production. *Cleft Palate-Craniofacial Journal, 31*(5), 356–363.

Moon, J. B., Smith, A. E., Folkins, J. W., Lemke, J. H., & Gartlan, M. (1994). Coordination of velopharyngeal muscle activity during positioning of the soft palate. *Cleft Palate-Craniofacial Journal, 31*(1), 45–55.

Nishio, J., Matsuya, T., Machida, J., & Miyazaki, T. (1976a). The motor supply of the velopharyngeal muscles. *Cleft Palate Journal, 13*, 20–30.

Nishio, J., Matsuya, T., Machida, J., & Miyazaki, T. (1976b). Roles of the facial, glossopharyngeal and vagus nerves in velopharyngeal movement. *Cleft Palate Journal, 13*, 201–214.

Perry, J. L., & Kuehn, D. P. (2014). Anatomy and physiology of the velopharynx. In J. Losee & R. E. Kirschner (Eds.), *Comprehensive cleft care* (2nd ed.). New York, NY: McGraw-Hill.

Perry, J. L., Kuehn, D. P., & Sutton, B. P. (2013). Morphology of the levator veli palatini muscle using magnetic resonance imaging. *Cleft Palate-Craniofacial Journal, 50*(1), 64–75.

Pigott, R. W. (1969). The nasendoscopic appearance of the normal palato-pharyngeal valve. *Plastic and Reconstructive Surgery, 43*(1), 19–24.

Pigott, R. W., Bensen, J. F., & White, F. D. (1969). Nasendoscopy in the diagnosis of velopharyngeal incompetence. *Plastic and Reconstructive Surgery, 43*(2), 141–147.

Proctor, D. F. (1982). The upper airway. In D. F. Proctor & I. B. Anderson (Eds.), *The nose: Upper airway physiology and the atmospheric environment*. New York, NY: Elsevier Biomedical Press.

Pruzansky, S., & Mason, R. (1969). The stretch factor in soft palate function. *Journal of Dental Research, 48*, 972.

Punjabi, A. P., & Hardesty, R. A. (2006). Classification and anatomy of cleft palate. In S. J. Mathes (Ed.), *Plastic surgery. Volume 4: Pediatric plastic surgery* (pp. 55–68). Philadelphia, PA: Saunders Elsevier.

Rood, S. R., & Doyle, W. J. (1978). Morphology of the tensor veli palatini, tensor tympani, and dilatator tubae muscles. *Annals of Otolaryngology, 87*, 202–210.

Sedlackova, E., Lastovia, N., & Sram, F. (1973). Contribution to knowledge of soft palate innervation. *Folia Phoniatrica, 25*, 434–441.

Shimokawa, T., Yi, S., & Tanaka, S. (2005). Nerve supply to the soft palate muscles with special reference to the distribution of the lesser palatine nerve. *Cleft Palate-Craniofacial Journal, 42*(5), 495–500.

Shprintzen, R. J., McCall, G. N., Skolnick, M. L., & Lencione, R. M. (1975). Selective movements of the lateral aspects of the pharyngeal walls during velopharyngeal closure for speech, blowing, and whistling in normals. *Cleft Palate Journal, 12*(1), 51–58.

Simpson, R. K., & Austin, A. A. (1972). A cephalometric investigation of velar stretch. *Cleft Palate Journal, 9*, 341–351.

Sumida, K., Yamashita, K., & Kitamura, S. (2012). Gross anatomical study of the human palatopharyngeus muscle throughout its entire course from origin to insertion. *Clinical Anatomy, 25*(3), 314–323.

Tachimura, T., Ojima, M., Nohara, K., & Wada, T. (2005). Change in palatoglossus muscle activity in relation to swallowing volume during the transition from the oral phase to the pharyngeal phase. *Dysphagia, 20*, 32–39.

Trigos, I., Ysunza, A., Vargas, D., & Vazquez, M. C. (1988). The San Venero Roselli pharyngoplasty: An electromyographic study of the palatopharyngeus muscle. *Cleft Palate Journal, 25*, 385–388.

Zemlin, W. R. (1998). *Speech and hearing science: Anatomy and physiology* (4th ed.). London, UK: Pearson.

Zim, S., Schelper, R., Kellman, R., Tatum, S., Ploutz-Snyder, R., & Shprintzen, R. J. (2003). Thickness and histological and histochemical properties of the superior pharyngeal constrictor muscle in velocardiofacial syndrome. *Archives of Facial Plastic Surgery, 5*, 503–510.

2

Clefts of the Lip and Palate

INTRODUCTION

A cleft is an abnormal opening or fissure in a body part or organ. According to *Stedman's Medical Dictionary*, 25th edition, clefts of the lip and palate are congenital anomalies that result from "incomplete merging or fusion of embryologic processes normally uniting in the formation of the face" (Spraycar, 1995, p. 352). Embryologic merging of the upper lip occurs roughly between the 5th and 7th weeks of gestation, while fusion of the palatal shelves occurs roughly between the 8th and 10th weeks (Burdi, 2006; Burdi & Faist, 1967; Carlson, 1998). If these embryologic processes are interrupted or delayed, then a cleft may occur. Clefts may occur due to internal (e.g., genetic, intrauterine) and external (e.g., teratogenic) events. Clefts involving the oral structures are some of the most frequently occurring congenital defects. Clefts can involve the upper lip, upper gum ridge (alveolus), hard palate, and soft palate (velum) and can vary in severity. Clefts can involve only one side of the lip or palate (unilateral) or both sides (bilateral). Clefts can extend completely through the lip and palate or only partially through these structures. In general, unilateral clefts are less severe than bilateral clefts, and an incomplete cleft is less severe than a complete cleft.

The purpose of this chapter is to describe the nature of cleft lip and palate anomalies. The chapter begins with a description of the types of clefts that occur with a focus on embryologic classification. The following sections include normal embryology, formation of clefts, causes of clefts, and epidemiology of clefts relative to prevalence and recurrence. The chapter concludes with a brief overview of the implications of clefts relative to feeding, hearing, and speech development—issues that are of most concern to speech-language pathologists and that are covered in detail later in this book.

TYPES OF CLEFTS

Embryologic Classification

Clefts may be best described using the embryologic classification system of Kernahan and Stark (1958). They developed a system that, through various modifications, has become perhaps the most accepted for classifying clefts. Kernahan and Stark described the location of clefts relative to the *incisive foramen*, an anatomical landmark that was consistent with embryological development and demarcation of the *primary* and *secondary* palates. Accordingly, Kernahan and Stark proposed a three-group classification system that consisted of clefts of (a) the primary palate only, (b) the secondary palate only, and (c) both the primary and secondary palates. This system is consistent with the American Cleft Palate-Craniofacial Association's document, "Core Curriculum for Cleft Lip/Palate and Other Craniofacial Anomalies" (2007).

Kernahan and Stark (1958) considered clefts involving the lip and alveolar ridge as part of the *primary palate* that develops from the 5th to 7th week after conception (see Embryology later in this chapter). The primary palate consists of the central portion of the lip and the *premaxilla*, a wedge-shaped portion of the alveolar bone anterior to the *incisive foramen* (see Figure 1–6 in Chapter 1). The incisive foramen is an opening in the maxilla for the passage of nerves and blood vessels. It is anatomically marked by the incisive papilla. Embryologic merging (or fusion) of the primary palate begins at the incisive foramen and proceeds in an anterior direction, outward toward the lip along the incisive suture lines. A complete cleft of the primary palate, therefore, includes both the soft tissue and muscle of the lip, and the alveolar bone up to the incisive foramen. An incomplete cleft of the primary palate involves just the soft tissue and muscle of the lip. An incomplete cleft of the primary palate (i.e., cleft lip only) is considered less severe than a complete cleft of the primary palate due to the fact that alveolar bone developed normally.

Kernahan and Stark (1958) considered clefts involving the hard and soft palate as part of the *secondary palate* that develops from 8 to 10 weeks after conception. The secondary palate includes the bony palatal shelves and the velum. Embryologic fusion of these structures typically begins at the incisive foramen and proceeds in a posterior direction along the midline, backward to the uvula. Similar to clefts of the primary palate, clefts of the secondary palate can be complete or incomplete. A complete cleft of the secondary palate involves the soft and hard palate up to the incisive foramen. Often, this type of cleft is simply called a cleft palate or an isolated cleft palate. An incomplete cleft of the secondary palate means that the cleft did not extend to the incisive foramen, and part of the hard and, possibly, soft palate is intact. A cleft of only the soft palate would be an example of an incomplete cleft of the secondary palate. As described below, clefts of both the primary and secondary palates often occur together.

Isolated Clefts of the Primary Palate

Clefts that involve only the soft tissue and muscle of the lip are considered incomplete clefts of the primary palate (Figure 2–1A). These clefts are typically described as clefts of the lip. Clefts of the lip can be unilateral (right or left side) or bilateral (both sides). In rare cases, clefts of the lip can be microform (also called *forme fruste*). This is a defect in the underlying muscle (orbicularis oris) without overlying tissue separation.

Clefts that extend through both the lip and alveolus to the incisive foramen are considered complete clefts of the primary palate (Figure 2–1B). These clefts—also often described as clefts of the lip—can be unilateral or bilateral.

A complete cleft of the primary palate can have a considerable effect on nasal anatomy. Because the bone of the premax-

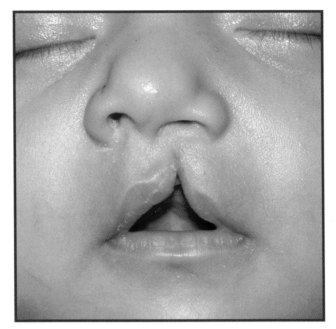

A

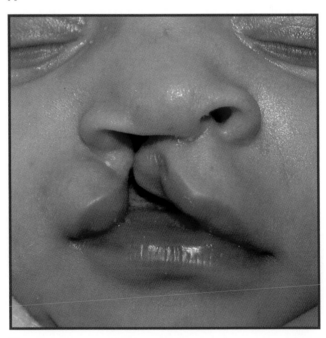

B

Figure 2–1. A. Left unilateral *incomplete* cleft of the primary palate (left cleft lip). Cleft does not fully extend into the floor of the nostril; alveolar ridge is minimally affected. **B.** Right unilateral *complete* cleft of the primary palate (right cleft lip and alveolus). Cleft extends completely through alveolar ridge. Note collapse of alar rim and nasal tip. (Courtesy of Joseph A. Napoli, MD, DDS, Plastic, Maxillofacial, and Craniofacial Surgery, Alfred I. duPont Hospital for Children, Wilmington, DE.)

illa forms the base (or floor) of the nose, alveolar clefts typically cause collapse of the alar cartilage and rim of the nose on the side of the cleft (see Figure 2–1B). Because the anatomy of the nose is complex, nasal deformities are a surgical challenge to correct. It is not uncommon for individuals with complete clefts of the primary palate to undergo one or more lip or nasal revisions following initial repair of the lip and nasal deformity.

Isolated Clefts of the Secondary Palate

A complete cleft of the secondary palate involves both the soft and hard palates. In such a case, the palatal structures are open completely from the uvula to the incisive foramen (Figure 2–2). Complete clefts of the secondary palate can also be unilateral or bilateral. This distinction pertains to whether both shelves of the hard palate are separated from the *vomer* bone (bilateral) or if one side of the hard palate is attached to the vomer (unilateral). As described in Chapter 1, the vomer is a pyramidal-shaped bone that helps form the nasal septum and separates the oral and nasal cavities. Bilateral clefts of the secondary palate are more severe than unilateral clefts in that a wider opening is usually present and more extensive surgery is required for the repair. Some surgeons will use tissue flaps taken from the covering of the vomer bone to repair wide bilateral clefts. Of interest, the teenager pictured in Figure 2–2 did not have palatal surgery and wore an obturator appliance to cover the cleft (see Chapter 11). Typical reasons for an infant not to have palatal surgery are financial and medical. As noted in the next chapter, isolated clefts of the secondary palate are associated with syndromes and other medical conditions (e.g., cardiac anomalies) more frequently than isolated clefts of the primary palate or clefts of both the primary and secondary palate. Palate surgery is often delayed, or not done, when an infant has life-threatening medical conditions.

A cleft of the secondary palate that does not extend completely to the incisive foramen is considered incomplete. An incomplete cleft may involve only

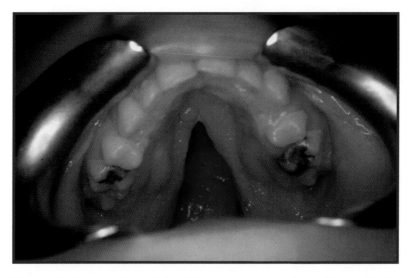

Figure 2–2. Complete cleft of the secondary palate. Cleft extends from the uvula through the soft and hard palate to the incisive foramen.

the uvula and soft palate (Figure 2–3) or extend into part of the hard palate. An incomplete cleft that involves only the uvula may be part of a submucous cleft (discussed in the next section). Clefts that involve the soft palate usually result in complete separation of the paired palatal muscles. As described in Chapter 1, the muscle that elevates and retracts the soft palate during speech and swallowing is levator veli palatini. When a cleft of the soft palate occurs, this muscle along with palatopharyngeus inserts onto the posterior border of the hard palate. This condition is referred to as the *cleft muscle of Veau*. Tensor veli palatini and palatoglossus also fail to insert at midline of the velum and become nonfunctional. As discussed in Chapter 5, one of the primary goals of palatal surgery is to restore the velar muscles into a functional unit to allow for normal speech, swallowing, and hearing.

Submucous Cleft Palate. A submucous cleft palate is an unusual type of cleft of the secondary palate. Essentially, it is a failure of the underlying velar muscles to attach at midline but without disruption of the overlying oral mucosa. Calnan (1954) described this condition as an "imperfect muscle union across the velum . . . so that speech is nasal in quality and may even be unintelligible" (p. 264). Submucous cleft palate is typically diagnosed based on a triad of anatomical anomalies or markers (Figure 2–4). First, the uvula is split or

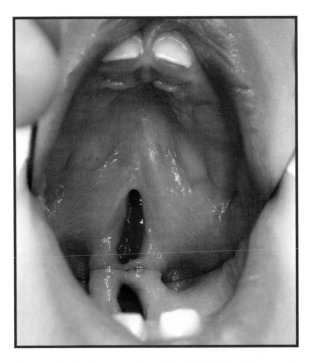

Figure 2–3. Incomplete cleft of the secondary palate. Cleft extends from the uvula through the soft palate; hard palate is intact. Note: Photo taken via mirror placed in mouth. Mirror pushes cleft uvula together. (Courtesy of Joseph A. Napoli, MD, DDS, Plastic, Maxillofacial, and Craniofacial Surgery, Alfred I. duPont Hospital for Children, Wilmington, DE.)

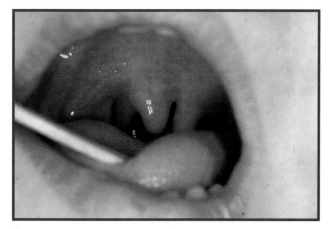

A

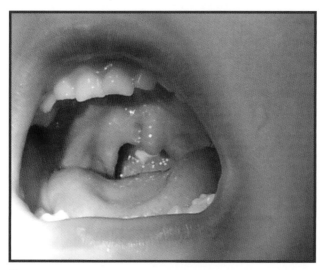

B

Figure 2–4. A. Bifid uvula as part of submucous cleft palate (SMCP). **B.** Asymmetric bifid uvula as part of SMCP. Uvula is held together by surface tension of tissue. Note large adenoid pad on posterior pharyngeal wall. **C.** Bifid uvula as part of SMCP. Soft palate appears V-shaped during phonation. Note large tonsils.

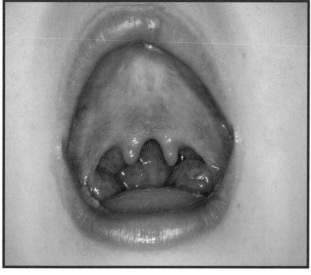

C

bifid. The bifidity may be quite obvious, affecting the entire uvula (Figure 2–4A), or subtle, involving only the tip or part of the uvula. At times, a bifid uvula may appear intact because it is held together by surface tension of the split tissues (Figure 2–4B). Second, the velum appears short, translucent, or V-shaped (Figure 2–4C). This appearance, also called a *zona pellucida*, is due to the insertion of the velar muscles into the posterior hard palate that leaves the midline of the velum hypoplastic. The V-shaped appearance may be most apparent during phonation of a vowel, as shown in Figure 2–4C. Third, the posterior border of the hard palate may have a bony deficiency. This defect is usually discernable only by digital palpation. Calnan noted that the bony deficiency "may vary from a slight notching to a large V-shaped bony defect" that could extend to the incisive foramen (p. 265).

A submucous cleft palate may be difficult to detect at birth. It may be missed if the underlying muscle defect is limited and the infant is not experiencing feeding difficulties. In some cases, a submucous cleft palate may not be detected until a child is 3 or even 4 years of age and experiencing delayed or hypernasal speech. At times, an *occult* submucous cleft palate may be diagnosed. This is characterized by the presence of speech symptoms such as hypernasality in the absence of any anatomical evidence of submucous cleft palate based on an oral examination (Croft, Shprintzen, Daniller, & Lewin, 1978; Kaplan, 1975). Usually, nasopharyngoscopy is needed to identify velar abnormality (see Chapter 9). Diagnosis of the occult defect is confirmed by the appearance of an abnormal sagittal groove in the nasal surface of the velum that is due to hypoplasticity or insertion of velar muscles onto the hard palate. Kaplan (1975),

however, made the point that "definitive" diagnosis of occult submucous cleft palate can only be achieved as part of surgical exploration of the muscles of the velum. Finally, a bifid uvula may be present without the occurrence of submucous cleft palate. Shprintzen, Schwartz, Daniller, and Hoch (1985) reported that at least two of 25 children with bifid uvula showed no other anatomical markers for submucous cleft palate. In such cases, the velar muscles developed normally with only the uvula failing to fuse in utero. Clinicians should be alerted that such a condition will not affect speech, and surgical intervention will not be needed. The individual may even be unaware of the structural difference.

Clefts of the Primary and Secondary Palate

Often, clefts occur that affect both the primary and secondary palates. As discussed later in the chapter, this type of cleft actually occurs more frequently than isolated clefts of the primary or secondary palate. Typically, these clefts are described using terms such as "left unilateral complete cleft lip and palate" (Figure 2–5A) or "bilateral complete cleft lip and palate" (Figure 2–5B–D). At times, a bilateral cleft may be complete on one side and incomplete on the other side (Figure 2–6). When a complete cleft lip and palate is bilateral, the *premaxilla* may protrude forward considerably (see Figure 2–5C). As noted previously, the premaxilla is a wedge-shaped segment of bone that contains the central and lateral incisor teeth. The middle portion of the lip tissue that remains attached to the premaxilla when a bilateral cleft occurs is called the *prolabium*. Surgical implications of a protruding premaxilla are discussed in Chapter 5.

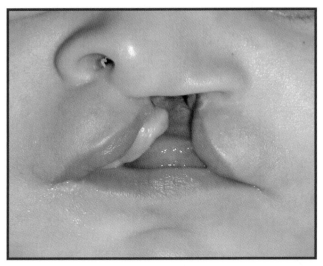

A

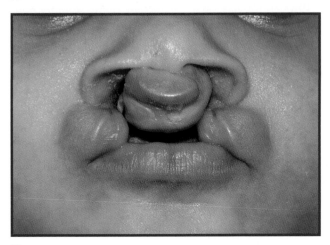

B

Figure 2–5. A. Complete unilateral cleft of the primary and secondary palate (left cleft lip and palate). **B.** Complete bilateral cleft of the primary and secondary palate (bilateral cleft lip and palate). Note protruding premaxilla and prolabium. *continues*

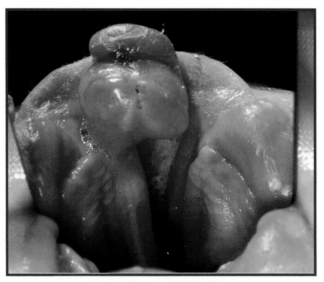

C

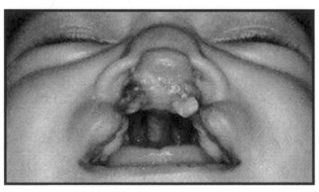

D

Figure 2–5. *continued* **C.** Intra-oral view of infant in B. Note that premaxilla is attached to the vomer bone but not to either palatal shelf. **D.** Complete bilateral cleft lip and palate. Note eruption of teeth from premaxilla. (A–C courtesy of Joseph A. Napoli, MD, DDS, Plastic, Maxillofacial, and Craniofacial Surgery, Alfred I. duPont Hospital for Children, Wilmington, DE.)

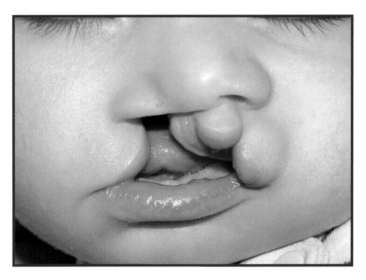

Figure 2–6. Bilateral cleft lip and palate. Cleft is complete on the right but incomplete on the left as the nostril base is intact. (Courtesy of Joseph A. Napoli, MD, DDS, Plastic, Maxillofacial, and Craniofacial Surgery, Alfred I. duPont Hospital for Children, Wilmington, DE.)

Other Classification Systems

Numerous systems have been devised to describe and classify the types of clefts that are clinically encountered. Several of these systems are briefly reviewed below. Although this is done primarily for historical perspective, we have, at times, encountered surgeons and other professionals who still use some of these classification systems to describe clefts.

As expressed by Kernahan and Stark (1958), the aim of all classification systems is the uniform and efficient communication of information among professionals to enhance both patient care and research. To achieve this aim, systems have been devised that range from relatively simple verbal descriptors of cleft type to elaborate visual displays that attempt to convey both cleft type and severity. Although a more comprehensive system may con-

vey greater information, it may come with a price of being overly complicated to use. Obviously, a classification system must be relatively easy to understand and use to become accepted.

One of the first attempts to establish a uniform classification system was described by Davis and Ritchie (1922). They proposed a three-group system to describe the location of clefts relative to the alveolar ridge as an anatomical landmark. Group I, called prealveolar, included clefts that were anterior to the alveolar ridge. Group II, called postalveolar, included clefts that were posterior to the alveolar ridge. Group III included clefts that involved the alveolar ridge. Veau (1931) described a four-group system (Figure 2–7): Group 1 consisted of clefts of the soft palate only; Group 2 consisted of clefts of both the soft and hard palates; Group 3 included unilateral clefts that involved

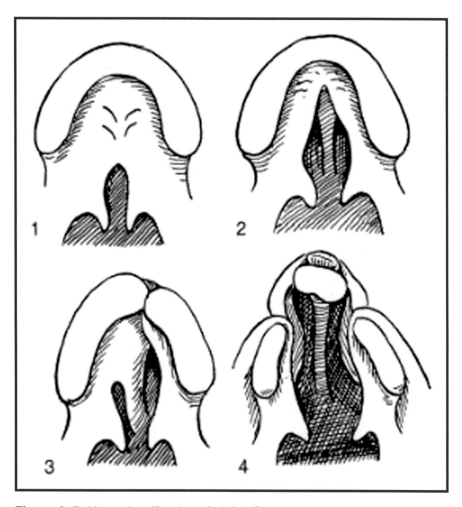

Figure 2–7. Veau classification of clefts: Group 1, soft palate; Group 2, soft and hard palate; Group 3, complete unilateral (right or left) lip and palate; and Group 4, complete bilateral lip and palate. (Punjabi, A., & Hardesty, R. A. [2006]. Classification and anatomy of cleft palate. In S. J. Mathes (Ed.), *Plastic surgery. Volume 4: Pediatric plastic surgery.* Philadelphia, PA: Saunders Elsevier. Reprinted with permission.)

the lip, alveolus, and palate; and Group 4 included bilateral clefts that involved the lip, alveolus, and palate.

Others have attempted to either refine the classification of Kernahan and Stark (1958) or develop new systems. Kernahan (1971) proposed a symbolic classification system that extended the earlier work of Kernahan and Stark (1958). In this system,

the figure Y is used to represent the possible locations of oral clefts using nine blocks (Figure 2–8). In this system, blocks 1 and 4 represent the lips, blocks 2 and 5 represent the alveolus, blocks 3 and 6 represent the hard palate from the alveolus to the incisive foramen (the circle in the figure), blocks 7 and 8 represents the hard palate, and block 9 represents the soft palate.

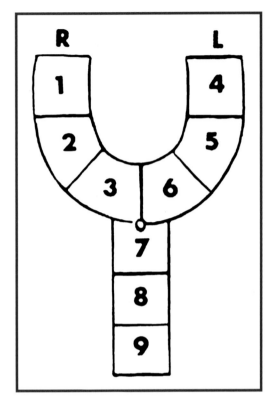

Figure 2–8. Kernahan's striped Y classification of clefts. Blocks 1 and 4, lips; Blocks 2 and 5, alveolus; Blocks 3 and 6, hard palate from alveolus to incisive foreman; Blocks 7 and 8, hard palate; and Block 9, soft palate. (Kernahan, D. A. [1971]. The striped Y—A symbolic classification for cleft lip and palate. *Plastic and Reconstructive Surgery, 47,* 469. Reprinted with permission.)

A concise description of a cleft can be conveyed to other professionals by shading or stippling the blocks affected by the cleft. In addition, the system promotes computer software documentation due to the numeric coding of the blocks.

Kriens (1990) proposed a similar symbolic classification system, LAHSHAL, using alphabetic characters. In this system, the extent of the cleft is specified by use of letters that represent the lips (L), alveolus (A), and hard (H) and soft (S) palates. Thus, LAHSHAL denotes a bilateral cleft of both the primary and secondary palates, and LAHS denotes a right unilateral cleft of both the primary and secondary palates (the side of the patient is opposite of the lettering). In our experience, we have not seen the LAHSHAL system used extensively.

EMBRYOLOGY OF THE PRIMARY AND SECONDARY PALATES

To facilitate an understanding of the types and occurrence of oral clefts, a basic knowledge of normal embryologic development is essential. The following material is summarized from an online tutorial developed at the University of North Carolina (UNC) at Chapel Hill, "Embryo Images: Normal and Abnormal Mammalian Development" (https://syllabus.med.unc.edu/courseware/embryo_images/).

Formation of the Primary Palate

At approximately the 2nd week of human gestation, the embryo has a flat, disc-shaped appearance and consists of two cell layers, the *epiblast* and the *hypoblast.* During a process called *gastrulation,* cells of the epiblast begin to invaginate or fold in at the caudal (tail) end of the embryo. This process leads to the formation of three distinct cell layers: the *ectoderm* (previously the epiblast), the *mesoderm* (formed from the epiblast), and the *endoderm* (previously the hypoblast). These three cell layers will continue to grow and eventually form all of the specialized cells and organs of the fetus. Ectodermal cells will develop into *neural* and *surface* ectoderm that will compose the central nervous system and outer covering of the body, respectively. Mesodermal cells will contribute to the formation of bone and connective tissue, and endodermal cells will contribute to the development of the digestive system.

The rapid folding and growth of the embryo change its appearance from a flat disc to a more human-like form by the end of the 4th week. At this time, the embryo has developed into a C-shaped form with its cranial and caudal ends tightly curved (Figure 2–9). The head and neck of the embryo at this stage comprise approximately half its length. Also at this stage, the developing forebrain, first and second pharyngeal arches, the inner ear, heart, and upper limb are clearly discernable. The forebrain and pharyngeal arches develop from *neural crest* cells that migrate from the dorsal (back) side of the embryo to the front. The first pharyngeal arch has both maxillary and mandibular prominences that will eventually develop into the upper and lower jaws. The second

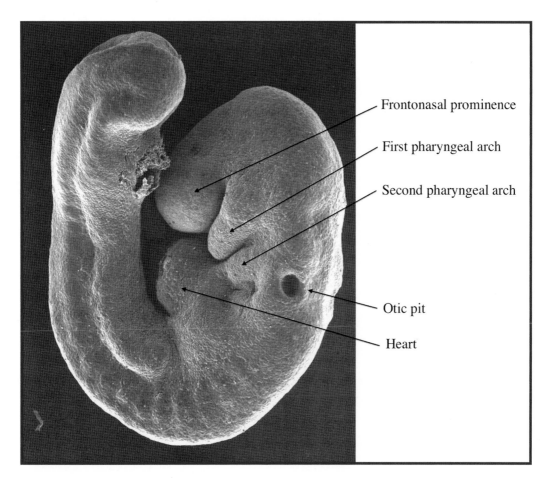

Frontonasal prominence

First pharyngeal arch

Second pharyngeal arch

Otic pit

Heart

Figure 2–9. Scanning electron micrograph of mouse embryo at Gestation Day 9 (human age approximately 27 days). (Courtesy of Kathleen K. Sulik, PhD, Department of Cell Biology and Physiology, University of North Carolina at Chapel Hill.)

pharyngeal arch will contribute to formation of the hyoid bone and ear.

Figure 2–10 shows development of the head of the embryo during the 5th week of gestation. Two nasal pits (indentions) are formed by migration of neural crest cells from the forebrain that develop *medial* and *lateral* tissue prominences. The nasal pits are lined with neural ectodermal cells called the *olfactory placodes.* This tissue will eventually form the olfactory nerve. Below the nasal pits is an opening that will develop into the mouth (*stomodeum*). During the 6th week of gestation, the upper lip is formed by the union of the medial and lateral nasal prominences with each other and with the *lateral maxillary prominence,* tissue that developed from the first pharyngeal arch. The medial nasal prominences continue to merge in the midline to complete formation of the upper lip, resulting in the *philtral ridges* (Figure 2–11).

Formation of the Secondary Palate

The secondary palate begins to form after the primary palate at approximately 8 weeks' gestation. Initially, the paired palatal shelves are in a floppy, vertical position with the developing tongue

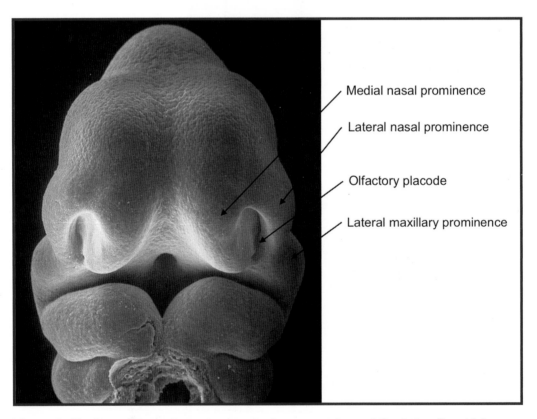

Medial nasal prominence

Lateral nasal prominence

Olfactory placode

Lateral maxillary prominence

Figure 2–10. Scanning electron micrograph of mouse embryo at Gestation Day 10 (human age approximately 5th week). (Courtesy of Kathleen K. Sulik, PhD, Department of Cell Biology and Physiology, University of North Carolina at Chapel Hill.)

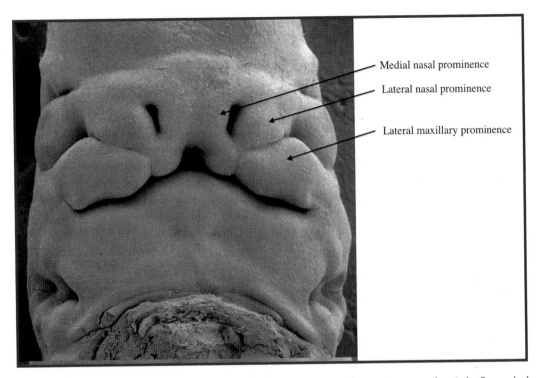

Figure 2–11. Scanning electron micrograph of human embryo at approximately 6 weeks' gestation. (Courtesy of Kathleen K. Sulik, PhD, Department of Cell Biology and Physiology, University of North Carolina at Chapel Hill.)

interposed between the shelves (Figure 2–12). The palatal shelves are part of the lateral maxillary prominences that develop from the first pharyngeal arch. During the 9th week, the shelves begin to elevate and assume a horizontal position above the tongue before fusing. As illustrated in Figure 2–12, however, the tongue presents an obstacle to palatal shelf elevation and fusion. Some embryologists have proposed that the tightly curled embryo needs to grow in order to allow extension of the neck and forward growth of the mandible, resulting in lowering of the tongue *prior* to palatal elevation (Diewert, 1974; Zeiler, Weinstein, & Gibson, 1964). Others, however, have suggested that mandibular growth and tongue low-

ering actually occur following palatal fusion and that palatal fusion itself triggers tongue lowering and forward growth of the mandible (Kjaer, Bach-Peterson, Graem, & Kjaer, 1993). It is also possible that mouth-opening reflexes are responsible for lowering the tongue prior to shelf elevation (Humphrey, 1969).

Regardless of the actual mechanism of tongue lowering, the palatal shelves elevate and begin to approximate each other in the midline (Figure 2–13). Fusion begins at the incisive foramen and continues in a posterior direction until completed at the uvula. Complete fusion of the secondary palate, including muscles and tissues of the soft palate, is usually complete by the 12th week of gestation. Burdi

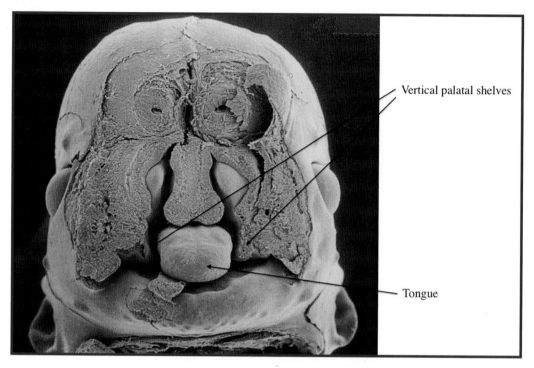

Figure 2–12. Scanning electron micrograph of mouse embryo at Gestation Day 14 (human age approximately 8 weeks). (Courtesy of Kathleen K. Sulik, PhD, Department of Cell Biology and Physiology, University of North Carolina at Chapel Hill.)

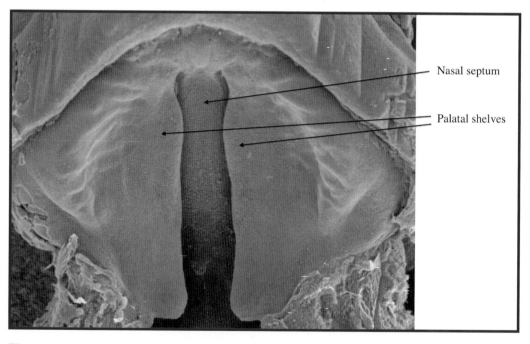

Figure 2–13. Scanning electron micrograph of human embryo at approximately 9 weeks' gestation. (Courtesy of Kathleen K. Sulik, PhD, Department of Cell Biology and Physiology, University of North Carolina at Chapel Hill.)

and Silvey (1969) have shown that formation of the secondary palate is delayed by approximately 1 week in female embryos. This longer window needed for development may contribute to the higher rate of clefts of the secondary palate in females as compared to males, at least in Caucasians (see below), due to a greater chance of environmental factors that can disrupt palatal fusion. Finally, it should be noted that in the UNC online embryo images, palatal fusion is illustrated as beginning in the middle of the hard palate and proceeding in both directions simultaneously. This pattern, however, is more typical of the mouse embryo. Bush and Jiang (2012), for example, have noted the occurrence of anterior but not posterior clefts of the secondary palate in mice following specific gene manipulations. Although this is an unusual type of cleft in humans, both authors have seen this pattern clinically.

HOW CLEFTS FORM

Based on the foregoing review of embryological development, it should be apparent that the occurrence of a cleft reflects the breakdown in the formation of specific oral-facial structures at specific times and locations. A complete left unilateral cleft of the primary palate, for example, will occur approximately during the 5th to 7th weeks of gestation due to an interruption of growth or fusion of the lateral maxillary prominence to the lateral and medial nasal prominences on the left side of the embryo. Typically, the earlier the interruption occurs, the more severe is the cleft. Likewise, a complete cleft of the secondary palate will occur approximately during the 8th to 10th weeks of gestation due to an interruption of growth or fusion of the palatal shelves in the midline from the incisive foramen to the uvula. Why such disruptions or malformations in embryological development occur is discussed in the next section.

CAUSES OF CLEFTS

A cleft arises from a failure in growth or fusion of the normal craniofacial developmental process (Leslie & Marazita, 2013). Cleft lip or palate (CL/P) can occur as an isolated defect or as a feature of a syndrome (see Chapter 3). Isolated or nonsyndromic CL/P refers to a cleft that is not associated with a major defect or multiple defects. Although an additional single minor anomaly may be identified, it is one that commonly occurs in the general population (e.g., club foot, also referred as talipes equinovarus) (Christensen, 1999), is causally unrelated to the cleft (Shprintzen, Siegel-Sadewitz, Amato, & Goldberg, 1985), and has minimal medical consequences (Saal, 2008). In their population-based study of oral clefts, Vallino-Napoli, Riley, and Halliday (2006) reported that two thirds of the clefts recorded were nonsyndromic conditions. With respect to cleft type, Jugessur, Farlie, and Kilpatrick (2009) reported that 70% of CL/P cases and 50% of all cleft palate only cases were nonsyndromic.

The primary cause or etiology of nonsyndromic CL/P is the interaction of genetic and environmental risk factors (Figure 2–14). More recently, there has been growing support for environmental risk factors (e.g., maternal smoking) and teratogens (e.g., maternal alcohol use) as causative factors in the development of a cleft (Leslie & Marazita, 2013).

Syndromic cleft refers to a cleft that is associated with two or more minor anomalies (multiple system defect) or

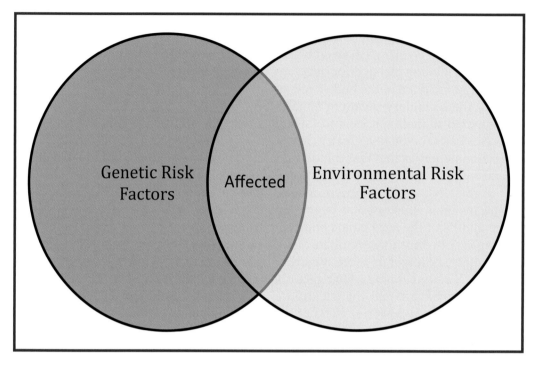

Figure 2–14. The interaction between genetic and environment risk factors causing cleft lip/palate.

syndromes. The cleft in this case is but one feature of several associated features that co-occur with the syndrome or disorder. The risk of recurrence for syndromic clefts is for the syndrome and not for the cleft. Approximately one third of infants with CL/P have other congenital anomalies (Vallino-Napoli et al., 2006). As of this writing, there are more than 400 recognizable syndromes known to have either a cleft lip or palate as a primary feature (http://www.ncbi.nlm.nih.gov/omim) of which about half are due to Mendelian inheritance (Marazita & Mooney, 2004). As reported by Leslie and Marazita (2013), 75% have a known genetic cause involving a single gene mutation, chromosome abnormality, or teratogen. These are discussed in Chapter 3.

EPIDEMIOLOGY OF CLEFTS

Prevalence

Cleft lip with or without cleft palate (CL±CP) is one of the most frequently occurring birth defects in the United States. Determination of prevalence rates, however, is difficult due to multiple factors that may affect estimates including sex, race or ethnicity, socioeconomic level, and method of ascertainment (e.g., reviewing birth records versus live examination of patients). Also, it has been suggested that estimates may be artificially low due to the difficulty of detecting submucous cleft palate (Peterson-Falzone, Hardin-Jones, & Karnell, 2010).

Murray (2002) reported an overall rate of cleft occurrence of 1-in-500 to 1-in-1000 live births worldwide, not taking race, sex, or cleft type into consideration. Marazita and Mooney (2004) reported rates of 1-in-500 to 1-in-2000 depending on the specific population. Parker et al. (2010) surveyed population-based birth data covering 21 major birth defects from 24 states in the United States during the years 2004 to 2006. They reported that CL±CP was the second most frequent birth defect with an estimated annual occurrence of 1-in-940 live births, adjusted for maternal race and age. The most frequently occurring birth defect was Trisomy 21 (Down syndrome) with an adjusted occurrence of 1-in-737 live births. This study also reported that the prevalence of CL±CP showed considerable variability across states, presumably reflecting differences in case ascertainment methods and environmental factors.

Prevalence of CL±CP also varies widely as a function of type of cleft, race or ethnicity, and sex. In general, cleft lip and palate occur approximately twice as often as either cleft lip or cleft palate only (Millard & McNeill, 1965). Unilateral clefts tend to occur more frequently than bilateral clefts (Jensen, Kreiborg, Dahl, & Fogh-Andersen, 1988; Shaw, Croen, & Curry, 1991), and unilateral clefts occur more frequently on the left than the right (Fraser & Calnan, 1961; Jensen et al., 1988). Relative to race, American Indians and Asians have the highest rates of clefts, followed by Caucasians, followed by individuals of sub-Saharan African descent (Murray, 2002; Vanderas, 1987). Vanderas (1987), for example, reported a rate as high as in 1-in-267 live births among American Indians. Clefts also vary according to sex and race. CL±CP occurs more frequently in Caucasian males than in females (Donahue, 1965). Cleft palate only, however, occurs more frequently in Caucasian

females than in males (Calzolari et al., 1988). Altemus (1966) reported that both CL±CP and cleft palate only occur more often in males versus females of African descent, and Emanuel, Huang, Gutman, Yu, and Lin (1972) reported the converse in Chinese individuals.

Meskin, Gorlin, and Isaacson (1964) provided estimates of the occurrence of bifid (or cleft) uvula in the absence of overt cleft palate. These investigators studied two samples of individuals. The first sample was 1,864 dental patients, and the second sample was 7,837 entering college students. Meskin et al. reported an overall occurrence rate of bifid uvula as 1.44%. Of interest, more males than females were affected. Meskin et al. explained this apparent reversal of sex bias relative to clefts of the secondary palate as possibly due to severity. That is, Meskin et al. noted that some studies showed less of a sex difference when clefts of the secondary palate affected only the soft palate (e.g., Knox & Braithwaite, 1963). Stewart, Ott, and Lagace (1972) screened 10,836 school-age children in Colorado. They reported 100 of the children had isolated bifid uvula (less than 1%) and nine had submucous cleft palate (1 in 1,200).

Risk of Recurrence

In general, nonsyndromic clefts tend to recur in a family based on several factors, including (a) the number of affected individuals in the family, (b) how closely related the individuals are, and (c) the severity of clefts of related individuals. Recurrence rates can be determined empirically or theoretically. Table 2–1 shows theoretical recurrence rates for CL±CP adapted from Tenconi, Clementi, and Turolla (1988). The first entry in the table

Table 2–1. Theoretical Recurrence Risk (%) for Cleft Lip With or Without Cleft Palate

Other Relatives	Neither Parent Affected	One Parent Affected	Both Parents Affected
None affected	0.08*	2.1	26.2
One sibling affected	2.4	7.6	29.0
One sibling affected, one not affected	2.3	7.1	28.1
Two siblings affected	7.7	14.0	31.3
One sibling affected, five not affected	1.9	5.5	24.5

Note. *0.08% = 0.008 per 100, 2.1% = 0.021 per 100, 7.6% = 0.076 per 100, and so on.

Source: Adapted from Tenconi, R., Clementi, M., & Turolla, L. (1988). Theoretical recurrence risks for cleft lip derived from a population of consecutive newborns. *Journal of Medical Genetics, 25*, 243–246. With permission.

shows the risk (0.08%) for having a child with CL±CP when neither parent nor other family members are affected. As shown in the third column of the table, risk is significantly increased as both the number of affected relatives and degree of relationship are increased. The recurrence risk increases to 26.2%, for example, when both parents are affected. It should be emphasized that maternal cigarette smoking can double this already high risk as nicotine is a fetal teratogen.

IMPLICATIONS OF CLEFTS FOR FEEDING, SPEECH, AND HEARING

Clefts of the Primary Palate

Prior to surgery, clefts of the lip only typically do not affect feeding in the infant. If necessary, the mother is usually able to manually assist the infant in obtaining a good lip seal at the nipple for either bottle or breastfeeding (see Chapter 4). Complete clefts of the primary palate (i.e., lip and alveolus), however, may affect feeding to some extent by limiting the infant's ability to seal or compress the nipple. These problems are more likely to occur in bilateral complete clefts. Although most clinicians believe that children with cleft lip only rarely have speech problems, this may not be entirely accurate. Vallino, Zuker, and Napoli (2008) studied various parameters of speech, language, hearing, and dentition in 95 three-year-old children with cleft lip, some with a cleft extending into the alveolus. Their findings showed that 13% had articulation errors that were not considered age appropriate, and 18% had a language disorder. These rates are higher than in the general population but lower than rates for children with cleft lip and palate. If a cleft of the lip and alveolus is severe (i.e., wide), then speech may be affected secondary to later dental or occlusal anomalies (see Chapter 8). Finally, eustachian tube function and hearing are typically not affected when clefts of the primary palate occur. The frequency of early ear infections in children with clefts of the primary palate is about the same as in the general population (Paradise, Bluestone, & Felder, 1969). Vallino et al. (2008), however, reported slightly higher rates of both middle ear effusion and mild conductive hearing loss in children with cleft lip only (see Chapter 6).

Clefts of the Secondary Palate

Complete clefts of the secondary palate typically have substantial adverse effects on feeding, hearing, and babbling prior to surgery. The normal suck, swallow, and breathing cycle of the infant may be disrupted due to an open palate and the inability to generate either positive or negative sucking pressures. As described in Chapter 4, parents typically must use special nipples and bottles to facilitate feeding. Likewise, adequate oral air pressure usually cannot be generated to produce stop consonants until the palate is repaired. As described in Chapter 7, children with complete clefts of the secondary palate typically experience delayed babbling, especially stop consonants, prior to palate repair (Chapman, Hardin-Jones, Schulte, & Halter, 2001). Even following palate surgery, speech is often delayed well into the second year of life (Chapman, 2008). In our experience, it is not uncommon for parents to report that a child is still not attempting words with stop consonants 4 to 6 months following palate repair. Although it is possible that these children simply require some period of time to learn to use new palatal structures, there may be other factors at play. One possible contributing factor is the almost universal conductive hearing loss in infants with unrepaired cleft palate

(Paradise et al., 1969). Although definitive research is lacking, at least one study has suggested a relationship between early hearing status and linguistic development in children with repaired cleft palate. Broen, Devers, Doyle, Prouty, and Moller (1998) obtained hearing thresholds on children with cleft palate at 3-month intervals from 9 to 30 months of age. They also obtained standardized measures of language development at 30 months of age. Broen et al. reported that the children with clefts experienced poorer hearing at 9, 12, and 15 months of age and reduced language scores at 30 months of age compared to control children without clefts. Of interest, when the investigators reanalyzed the language data using hearing level as a covariate, the differences between groups were eliminated, suggesting that early hearing difficulty may have contributed to later linguistic performance.

Older children with repaired clefts of both the primary and secondary palates are often susceptible to articulation problems even when velopharyngeal function is adequate. This may occur due to dental and occlusal hazards that are present during acquisition of the phonetic inventory. Sibilant and tongue-tip alveolar stop-plosives are especially misarticulated in school-age children. There is evidence that the presence of maxillary arch anomalies may contribute to articulation difficulties in children with repaired cleft lip and palate (see Chapter 8).

Submucous Cleft Palate

Submucous cleft palate may or may not affect early feeding, hearing, and babbling depending on the extent of muscle function. Relative to speech, McWilliams (1991) examined the records of 130 patients at the University of Pittsburgh Cleft Palate Center (Pittsburgh, Pennsylvania) for the presence of "frank" submucous cleft palate. This was defined as the presence of the triad of anatomical anomalies in most cases. The age of diagnosis varied from 6 days to 20 years. McWilliams reported that 44% of the patients exhibited normal speech and did not require surgical intervention. She advised that "a submucous cleft should be repaired in infancy only when feeding problems or unremitting ear disease is observed" (p. 247). It is our opinion, however, that the decision for surgery should be based primarily on speech as both feeding and ear disease can be effectively managed by other means. Finally, because it may be difficult to detect submucous cleft palate in the newborn, health care personnel should be suspicious of any otherwise healthy newborn that has difficulty with either breastfeeding or bottle-feeding. In such cases, a thorough oral examination should be done to rule out the presence of submucous cleft palate.

CHAPTER SUMMARY

Oral clefts can best be described using an embryological classification based on the incisive foramen. Clefts of the primary palate involve structures that are anterior to the incisive foramen—the alveolus and upper lip. Embryological formation of the primary palate begins at 6 to 7 weeks' gestation and involves growth and fusion of the lateral maxillary prominence, lateral nasal prominence, and medial nasal prominence, structures that evolve from the first pharyngeal arch. Fusion of the primary palate begins at the incisive foramen and continues to the upper lip along the incisive sutures. Clefts of the second-

ary palate involve structures that are posterior to the incisive foramen—the hard palate, soft palate, and uvula. Embryological formation of the secondary palate begins after the primary palate at 8 to 9 weeks' gestation and involves the elevation and fusion at midline of the two vertical palatal shelves. Fusion begins at the incisive foramen and continues in a posterior direction to the uvula. Some clefts of the secondary palate are submucous in that palatal fusion does not occur but the defect is covered by oral mucosa. Either genetic or environmental factors can disrupt embryological development and cause clefts. Genetic factors can include mutant genes and chromosomal abnormalities. Environmental factors can include teratogens such as maternal smoking and alcohol use. Most clefts are likely caused by a combination of genetic and environment factors. The prevalence of clefts worldwide varies according to factors including cleft type, sex, and race, with a general estimate of approximately 1-in-500 to 1-in-1000 live births. The recurrence of a cleft within a family also varies according to factors such as severity of the cleft, number of affected relatives, and closeness of affected relatives. Oral clefts, especially clefts of the secondary palate, can significantly impact early feeding, hearing, and babbling of an infant. Clefts of both the primary and secondary palates can significantly impact facial aesthetics, nasal function, and speech and resonance of the older child and even adult.

REFERENCES

Altemus, L. A. (1966). The incidence of cleft lip and palate among North American negroes. *Cleft Palate Journal, 3,* 357–361.

American Cleft Palate-Craniofacial Association. (2007). *Core curriculum for cleft lip/palate and other craniofacial anomalies*. Retrieved from http://acpa-cpf.org/core_curriculum/

Broen, P. A., Devers, M. C., Doyle, S. S., Prouty, J. M., & Moller, K. T. (1998). Acquisition of linguistic and cognitive skills by children with cleft palate. *Journal of Speech, Language, and Hearing Research, 41*(3), 676–687.

Burdi, A. R. (2006). Developmental biology and morphogenesis of the face, lip and palate. In S. Berkowitz (Ed.), *Cleft lip and palate* (2nd ed., pp. 3–12) New York, NY: Springer.

Burdi, A. R., & Faist, K. (1967). Morphogenesis of the palate in normal human embryos with special emphasis on the mechanisms involved. *American Journal of Anatomy, 120*, 149–160.

Burdi, A. R., & Silvey, R. G. (1969). Sexual differences in closure of the human palatal shelves. *Cleft Palate Journal, 6*, 1–7.

Bush, J. O., & Jiang, R. (2012). Palatogenesis: Morphogenetic and molecular mechanisms of secondary palate development. *Development, 139*(2), 231–243.

Calnan, J. (1954). Submucous cleft palate. *British Journal of Plastic Surgery, 7*, 264–282.

Calzolari, E., Cavazzuti, G. B., Cocchi, G., Contrino, C., Magnani, C., Moretti, M., . . . Volpato, S. (1988). Epidemiological and genetic study of 200 cases of oral cleft in the Emilia Romagna region of northern Italy. *Teratology, 38*(6), 559–564.

Carlson, B. M. (1998). *Human embryology and developmental biology* (2nd ed.). St. Louis, MO: Mosby.

Chapman, K. L. (2008). The acquisition of speech and language in children with cleft palate: Interactions and influences. In K. T. Moller & L. E. Glaze (Eds.), *Cleft palate: Interdisciplinary issues and treatment—For clinicians by clinicians* (pp. 243–291). Austin, TX: Pro-Ed.

Chapman, K. L., Hardin-Jones, M., Schulte, J., & Halter, K. A. (2001). Vocal development of 9-month-old babies with cleft palate. *Journal of Speech, Language, and Hearing Research, 44*(6), 1268–1283.

Christensen, K. (1999). The 20th century Danish facial cleft population-epidemiological and genetic-epidemiological studies. *Cleft Palate-Craniofacial Journal, 36*(2), 96–104.

Croft, C. B., Shprintzen, R. J., Daniller, A., & Lewin, M. L. (1978). The occult submucous cleft palate and the musculus uvulae. *Cleft Palate Journal, 15*, 150–154.

Davis, J. R., & Ritchie, H. P. (1922). Classification of congenital clefts of the lip and palate. *Journal of the American Medical Association, 79*, 1323.

Diewert, V. (1974). A cephalometric study of orofacial structures during secondary palate closure in the rat. *Archives of Oral Biology, 19*, 303–315.

Donahue, R. F. (1965). Birth variables and the incidence of cleft palate: Part 1. *Cleft Palate Journal, 2*, 282–290.

Emanuel, I., Huang, S. W., Gutman, L. T., Yu, F. C., & Lin, C. C. (1972). The incidence of congenital malformations in a Chinese population: The Taipei collaborative study. *Teratology, 5*(2), 159–169.

Fraser, F. C., & Calnan, J. (1961). Cleft lip and palate: Seasonal incidence, birth weight, birth rank, sex, site, associated malformations, and parental age. A statistical surgery. *Archives of Diseases of Children, 36*, 420–423.

Humphrey, T. (1969). The relationship between human fetal mouth opening reflexes and closure of the palate. *American Journal of Anatomy, 125*, 317–344.

Jensen, B. L., Kreiborg, S., Dahl, E., & Fogh-Andersen, P. (1988). Cleft lip and palate in Denmark, 1976–1981: Epidemiology, variability, and early somatic development. *Cleft Palate Journal, 25*, 258–269.

Jugessur, A., Farlie, P. G., & Kilpatrick, N. (2009). The genetics of isolated orofacial clefts: Ffrom genotypes to subphenotypes. *Oral Diseases, 15*, 437–453.

Kaplan, E. (1975). The occult submucous cleft palate. *Cleft Palate Journal, 12*, 356–368.

Kernahan, D. A. (1971). The striped Y—A symbolic classification for cleft lips and palates. *Plastic and Reconstructive Surgery, 47*, 469.

Kernahan, D. A., & Stark, R. B. (1958). A new classification for cleft lip and palate. *Plastic and Reconstructive Surgery, 22*, 435.

Kjaer, I., Bach-Petersen, S., Graem, N., & Kjaer, T. (1993). Changes in human palatine bone location and tongue position during the prenatal palatal closure. *Journal of Craniofacial Genetics and Developmental Biology, 13,* 18–23.

Knox, G., & Braithwaite, F. (1963). Cleft lips and palates in Northumberland and Durham. *Archives of Disease in Childhood, 38*(197), 66.

Kriens, O. (1990). Documentation of cleft lip, alveolus, and palate. In J. Bardach & H. L. Morris (Eds.), *Multidisciplinary management of cleft lip and palate.* Philadelphia, PA: W.B. Saunders.

Leslie, E. J., & Marazita, M. L. (2013). Genetics of cleft lip and cleft palate. *American Journal of Medical Genetics Part C (Seminars in Medical Genetics), 163C,* 246–258.

Marazita, M. L., & Mooney, M. P. (2004). Current concepts in the embryology and genetics of cleft lip and cleft palate. *Clinics in Plastic Surgery, 31*(2), 125–140.

McWilliams, B. J. (1991). Submucous clefts of the palate: How likely are they to be symptomatic? *Cleft Palate-Craniofacial Journal, 28*(3), 247–251.

Meskin, L. H., Gorlin, R. J., & Isaacson, R. J. (1964). Abnormal morphology of the soft palate: I. The prevalence of cleft uvula. *Cleft Palate Journal, 1,* 342–346.

Millard, D. R., & McNeill, K. A. (1965). The incidence of cleft lip and palate in Jamaica. *Cleft Palate Journal, 2,* 384–388.

Murray, J. C. (2002). Gene/environment causes of cleft lip and/or palate. *Clinical Genetics, 61*(4), 248–256.

Paradise, J. L., Bluestone, C. D., & Felder, H. (1969). The universality of otitis media in 50 infants with cleft palate. *Pediatrics, 44*(1), 35–42.

Parker, S. E., Mai, C. T., Canfield, M. A., Rickard, R., Wang, Y., Meyer, R. E., . . . Correa, A. (2010). Updated national birth prevalence estimates for selected birth defects in the United States, 2004–2006. *Birth Defects Research Part A: Clinical and Molecular Teratology, 88*(12), 1008–1016.

Peterson-Falzone, S. J., Hardin-Jones, M. A., & Karnell, M. P. (2010). *Cleft palate speech* (4th ed.). St. Louis, MO: Mosby.

Punjabi, A., & Hardesty, R. A. (2006). Classification and anatomy of cleft palate. In S. J. Mathes (Ed.), *Plastic surgery. Volume 4: Pediatric plastic surgery* (pp. 55–68). Philadelphia, PA: Saunders Elsevier.

Saal, H. M. (2008). The genetics evaluation and common craniofacial syndromes. In A. W. Kummer (Ed.), *Cleft palate and craniofacial anomalies: Effects on speech and resonance* (pp. 86–118). Clifton Park, NY: Delmar Cengage Learning.

Shaw, G. M., Croen, L. A., & Curry, C. J. (1991). Isolated oral cleft malformations: Associations with maternal and infant characteristics in a California population. *Teratology, 43,* 225–228.

Shaw, G. M., Wasserman, C. R., O'Malley, C. D., Nelson, V., & Jackson, R. J. (1999). Maternal pesticide exposure from multiple sources and selected congenital anomalies. *Epidemiology, 10*(1), 60–66.

Shprintzen, R. J., Schwartz, R. H., Daniller, A., & Hoch, L. (1985). Morphologic significance of bifid uvula. *Pediatrics, 75*(3), 553–561.

Shprintzen, R. J., Siegel-Sadewitz, V. L., Amato, J., & Goldberg, R. B. (1985). Anomalies associated with cleft lip, cleft palate, or both. *American Journal of Medical Genetics, 20*(4), 585–595.

Spraycar, M. (Ed.). (1995). *Stedman's medical dictionary* (26th ed.). Baltimore, MD: Williams and Wilkins.

Stewart, J. M., Ott, J. E., & Lagace, R. (1972). Submucous cleft palate: Prevalence in a school population. *Cleft Palate Journal, 9,* 246–250.

Tenconi, R., Clementi, M., & Turolla, L. (1988). Theoretical recurrence risks for cleft lip derived from a population of consecutive newborns. *Journal of Medical Genetics, 25*(4), 243–246.

Vallino, L. D., Zuker, R., and Napoli, J. A. (2008). A study of speech, language, hearing, and dentition in children with cleft lip only. *Cleft Palate Craniofacial Journal, 45*(5), 485–494.

Vallino-Napoli, L. D., Riley, M. M., & Halliday, J. L. (2006). An epidemiologic study of orofacial clefts with other birth defects in Victoria, Australia. *Cleft Palate Craniofacial Journal, 43,* 571–576.

Vanderas, A. P. (1987). Incidence of cleft lip, cleft palate, and cleft lip and palate among races: A review. *Cleft Palate Journal, 24*(3), 216–225.

Veau, V. (1931). *Division palatine.* Paris, France: Masson.

Zeiler, K., Weinstein, S., & Gibson, S. (1964). A study of the morphology and the time of closure of the palate in the albino rat. *Archives of Oral Biology, 9,* 545–554.

3

Syndromes and Associated Anomalies

INTRODUCTION

Speech and language impairment is a common feature among a number of syndromes. There are many factors associated with these conditions that predispose individuals to speech and language impairment, including, but not limited to, structural anomalies, hearing loss, cognitive impairment, delayed development, and psychosocial circumstances. Gene mutations play a prominent role in the etiology of many disorders, and in others, environmental factors may also contribute to the cause. Certain families of gene mutations may cause a group of craniofacial anomalies with similar and overlapping features (Trainor & Richtsmeier, 2015). The clinician, who understands the nature of a specific anomaly and of the impact of the associated structural and functional problems, is in an optimal position to offer best care in terms of assessment and management (Siegel-Sadewitz & Shprintzen, 1982; Sparks, 1984).

In this chapter an overview of genetics is provided, and the terminology used to categorize and identify congenital anomalies is presented. We describe a select group of craniofacial anomalies that have a unique pathological basis for communication impairment. The defects are classified based on three different presumed pathogenetic commonalities: (a) conditions in which cleft lip and palate is a predominant feature, (b) branchial arch anomalies, and (c) craniosynostosis. The conditions within each category have similar features and functional problems and may have like speech, language, and hearing problems.

BASIC GENETICS: DNA, GENES, AND CHROMOSOMES

Genetics is the study of genes and heredity. A genome is an organism's complete set of genetic or hereditary instructions. The Human Genome Project, completed in 2003 was an extraordinary research effort to sequence and map all of the genes of the human being (All about the Human Genome Project [HGP], n.d.). Understanding this "genetic blueprint" has enabled scientists and clinicians to understand the genetic factors in a number of disorders.

The hereditary unit of all organisms is DNA (deoxyribonucleic acid), a double-stranded molecule that resembles a twisted ladder (double helix) (Figure 3–1).

The sides (or backbone) of this DNA "ladder" are made up of sugar and phosphate. There are four nucleic bases—adenine (A), guanine (G), cytosine (C), and thymine (T)—that must be properly matched in a specific way: A always binds with T, and C always binds with G. This is referred to as complementary base pairing. This pairing between base pairs forms the "rung" of the DNA ladder. The sequence of these bases along the sides of the ladder serves as instructions in assembling protein and RNA messages and in essence is the genetic code. The precision of this DNA sequence is so important that one change in the DNA can alter a gene causing a genetic defect.

Genes are the basic physical units of inheritance and the mechanism by which traits are passed from one generation to

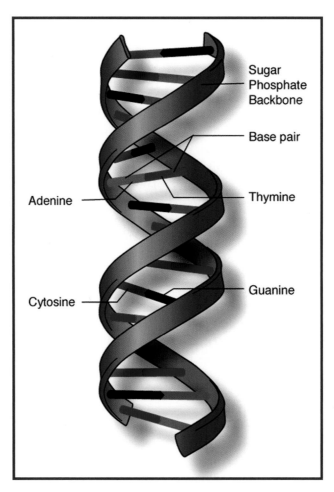

Figure 3–1. Double-helix model of DNA. National Institutes of Health, National Human Genome Research Institute, *Talking glossary of genetic terms*. Retrieved from http://www.genome.gov/glossary/)

the next. Every person has two copies of a gene, one from each parent. Humans have between 20,000 and 25,000 genes.

Genes are small segments of DNA that control specific traits (Figure 3–2). They are a special sequence of nucleotides designed to carry instructions for making a particular protein essential to the growth and development of the body's cells, tissues, and organs. For example, one gene called *FGFR3* provides instruction for a protein called fibroblast growth factor receptor 3, which plays an important role in embryo development and cell growth and division. Genes are distributed on chromosomes and arranged in a specific sequence and location or locus of the chromosome (Figure 3–2).

Alleles refer to variations of a gene located on specific locations on the chromosome (Nussbaum, McInnes, & Willard, 2004). There are two alleles at each gene location, one inherited from each parent. A *genotype* is a person's genetic makeup and refers to the pair of alleles at a given location. *Phenotype* is the constellation of observable traits or characteristics produced by the genotype plus environmental influences (e.g., hair color).

A person is said to be homozygous for a trait if he or she has two copies of the same allele for a gene (e.g., AA or aa) and heterozygous if there are two different alleles of a gene (e.g., Aa) (Nussbaum et al., 2004) (Figure 3–3). Alleles can be dominant or recessive. A dominant allele will

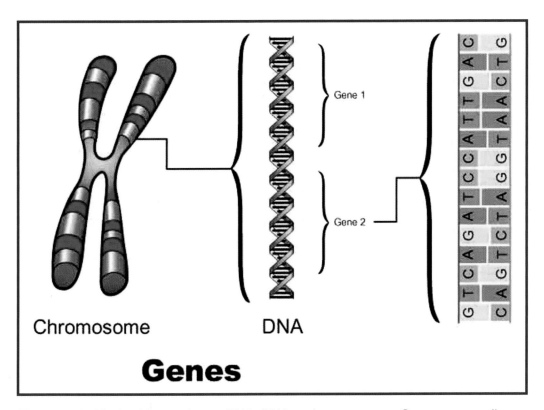

Figure 3–2. Nucleotides make up DNA. DNA makes up genes. Genes are small segments of chromosomes. (Plant and Soil Sciences eLibrary [http://passel.unl.edu], hosted at the University of Nebraska Institute of Agriculture and Natural Resources. Reprinted with permission.)

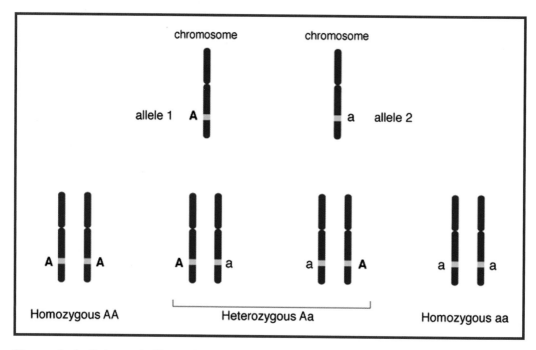

Figure 3–3. Schematic illustration of chromosomes showing alleles. Homozygotes have identical alleles (AA or aa). Heterozygotes have two different alleles (Bb or bB). The dominant alleles are capitalized and recessive alleles are lower case. (National Institutes of Health, National Human Genome Research Institute, *Talking glossary of genetic terms*. Retrieved from http://www.genome.gov/glossary/)

show its effect in a person who has one copy of the allele passed from one parent (i.e., heterozygous). A recessive allele will show its effect in a person who has two copies of the allele, one from each parent (i.e., homozygous). Those who have both a dominant and recessive allele are considered carriers for the recessive allele. The importance of these terms will be clearer when we later discuss gene mutations and single-gene disorders.

Chromosomes consist of very long strands of DNA and contain hundreds and thousands of genes (Figure 3–4).

Each chromosome has a constriction called a centromere that joins the two identical halves (chromatids) of the chromosomes. The centromere of the chromosome also divides the chromosome into two arms, a long arm (q) and short arm (p). The normal human has 46 chromosomes consisting of 23 homologous pairs, one half of each pair comes from the mother and the other half comes from the father. The 23 pairs of chromosomes include 22 autosome pairs (numbered 1 through 22 according to size), and one pair are sex chromosomes, termed X and Y (XX = female, XY = male).

When a chromosome is stained and viewed through a microscope, cytogenetic regions that are depicted as light and dark bands can be seen on the two arms of the chromosome and labeled according to their locations. The bands are numbered consecutively away from the centromere on both the long and short arms (Bickmore, 2001). Chromosomes are classified accord-

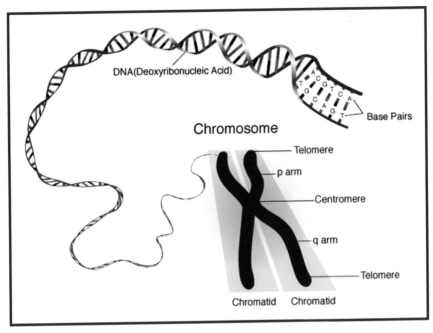

DNA(Deoxyribonucleic Acid)

Base Pairs

Chromosome

Telomere

p arm

Centromere

q arm

Telomere

Chromatid   Chromatid

Figure 3–4. Chromosome structure. Note that the chromosome contains long strands of DNA. (National Institutes of Health, National Human Genome Research Institute, *Talking glossary of genetic terms*. Retrieved from http://www.genome.gov/glossary/)

ing to their length and the location of their centromere and subsequently matched and paired based on their corresponding patterns. A pictorial representation of the pattern of chromosomes commonly is referred to as a karyotype (Figure 3–5).

There is a conventional way to describe the location of a gene on a particular chromosome that is helpful in understanding a genetic disorder. The first number or letter used presents the chromosome. (Recall that numbers 1 through 22 are autosomes, and letters X and Y are sex chromosomes.) The arm of the chromosome is then identified (q representing the long arm and p the short arm). The position of the gene, identified by the pattern of light and dark bands on the stained chromosome, is generally represented by two numbers representing a region and a

band, and sometimes followed by a decimal point and a number representing a sub-band. For example, when describing the gene location for velocardiofacial syndrome, it is written as 22q11.2 deletion, meaning that the gene is located on the long arm of chromosome 22 in region 1, band 1, sub-band 2.

MUTATIONS

Although most variations in our genetic code are inconsequential, there are some variations that result in a faulty gene or mutation that is directly responsible for causing a defect (Nussbaum et al., 2004). A mutation is any change in the nucleotide sequence of DNA that alters an individual gene resulting in extra gene material (insertion) or loss of genetic material (deletion)

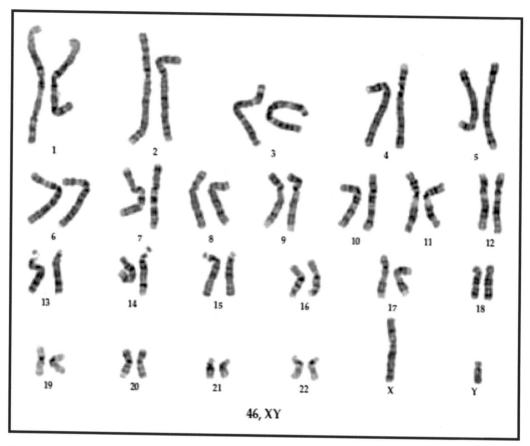

46, XY

Figure 3–5. Karyotype of a normal male (46, XY). (Used with permission of Mayo Foundation for Medical Education and Research. All rights reserved.)

or a chromosome structure or number (Nussbaum et al., 2004) (Figure 3–6).

In other words, mutations change the correct code of DNA that results in a defective protein structure. A specific gene mutation can have a phenotypic effect and clinical consequences. For example, a mutation in the *FGFR3* gene can cause premature closure of the bones of the skull or craniosynostosis resulting in an anomaly with distinct craniofacial features that include abnormal skull shape, underdevelopment of the midface, and wide-set eyes (detailed later in the chapter).

Many mutations happen spontaneously and are new or de novo, meaning that the mutation occurred for the first time in a family. On the other hand, a mutation can also be transmitted and thus hereditable.

There are three categories of genetic disorders: single-gene disorders, chromosome disorders, and multifactorial disorders (Nussbaum et al., 2004).

SINGLE-GENE DISORDERS

A single-gene disorder (Mendelian disorder) is determined by a mutation at a single gene locus on an autosome or sex (X) chromosome, and whether it is either dom-

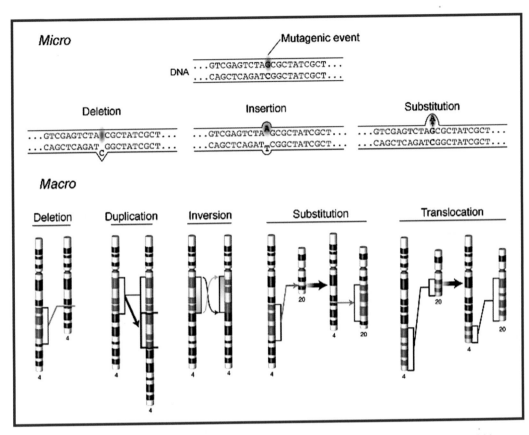

Figure 3–6. The effects of gene mutations. (National Institutes of Health, National Human Genome Research Institute, *Talking glossary of genetic terms*. Retrieved from http://www .genome.gov/glossary/)

inant or recessive. A single-gene disorder typically follows a predictable pattern of inheritance and recurrence risk. There are three basic patterns of inheritance: autosomal dominant, autosomal recessive, and sex-linked inheritance. As described later in the chapter, many of the craniofacial conditions are the result of a single-gene defect.

In order to understand the occurrence of a trait, geneticists will construct a pedigree. A pedigree is a pictorial representation of the genetic history of a family through several generations. It is used to discern the inheritance pattern of a trait or disorder that is consistent with one of the three basic modes of Mendelian inheritance (dominant, recessive, or X-linked). Pedigree symbols are used to identify family members and their relationships (Figure 3–7).

In the next section, we describe the modes of Mendelian inheritance and show the pedigrees used to depict them.

Autosomal Dominant Inheritance

Typically, in an autosomal dominant disorder the child inherits an abnormal gene on one of two autosomes (numbered chromosomes) from one parent who is

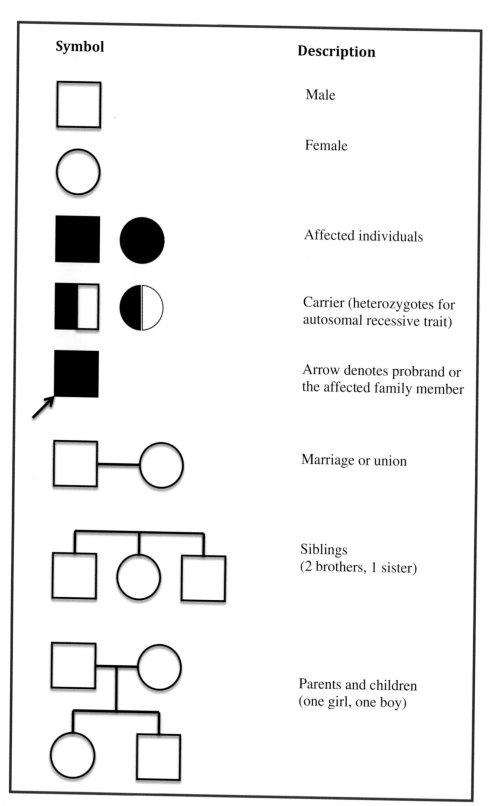

Symbol	Description
□	Male
○	Female
■ ●	Affected individuals
◨ ◐	Carrier (heterozygotes for autosomal recessive trait)
■ (with arrow)	Arrow denotes probrand or the affected family member
□—○	Marriage or union
□ ○ □	Siblings (2 brothers, 1 sister)
□—○ with ○ □	Parents and children (one girl, one boy)

Figure 3–7. Principle pedigree symbols.

affected and a copy of the normal gene from the other parent who is not affected. Effectively, the abnormal gene on one autosome overrides the effect of the corresponding normal gene on the other autosome. Because the abnormal gene can be inherited from an affected parent, there is a 50% chance that with each pregnancy the abnormal gene causing the defect will be passed to the offspring who would then be affected. An autosomal dominant disorder may occur as result of a new gene mutation, in which case the disorder may occur for the first time in a family but from this point forward the trait follows the autosomal dominant inheritance pattern. Table 3–1 summarizes the principles of autosomal dominant inheritance, and this is illustrated in the pedigree shown in Figure 3–8.

Autosomal Recessive Inheritance

In an autosomal recessive disorder, the affected child will have received two copies of the gene mutation: one copy from each parent. Each parent is a gene carrier but neither has the disorder. If both parents are carriers, they have with each pregnancy a 25% chance of having an affected child, a 25% chance of having an unaffected child, and a 50% chance of having an infant who is unaffected but who is a carrier. Sometimes, it is only when a child is diagnosed with an autosomal recessive condition that the parents become aware that they are carriers. The principles of autosomal recessive inheritance are summarized in Table 3–2, and this is illustrated in the pedigree shown in Figure 3–9.

Sex-Linked Inheritance

A sex-linked (X-linked) disorder results from a gene mutation located on the X chromosome. Standard practice has been to classify X-linked disorders as X-linked dominant or recessive. Based on the general rules of X-linked inheritance, in an X-linked dominant disorder the daughters of affected males always inherit the disorder, and an affected female can transmit the trait to both sexes; in an X-linked recessive inheritance, carrier females transmit the trait to their sons who are almost exclusively affected. However, X-linked disorders do not always follow

Table 3–1. Principles of Autosomal Dominant Inheritance

1. Any child of an affected person has a 50% chance of inheriting the trait.

2. Males and females are equally likely to be affected.

3. Except for new mutations, every affected person has an affected parent.

4. Unaffected siblings of an affected person do not transmit the trait to their offspring.

5. The clinical manifestation ranges from very mild to very severe (variable expressivity).

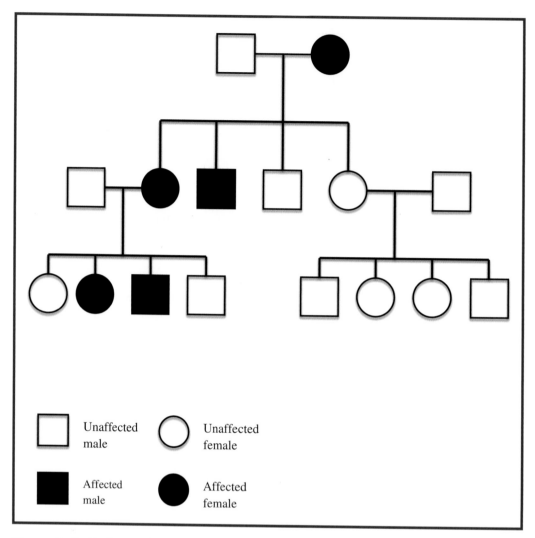

Figure 3–8. Pedigree showing autosomal dominant inheritance.

Table 3–2. Principles of Autosomal Recessive Inheritance

1. The parents of an affected child are unaffected carriers of the condition.

2. The child born to two carrier parents has a one in four chance of being affected, two in four chance of being a carrier, and one in four chance of being unaffected.

3. All children of two affected parents will have the trait.

4. Males and females are equally likely to be affected.

5. The risk of recurrence is higher if both parents have one or more ancestors in common (consanguinity).

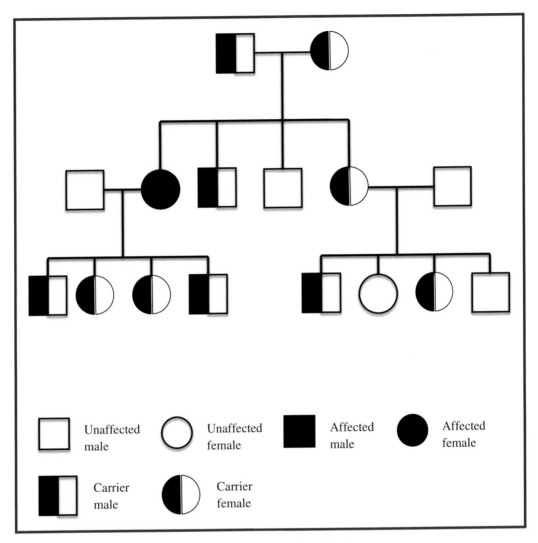

Figure 3–9. Pedigree showing autosomal recessive inheritance.

this rule, and penetrance and expressivity can be variable (defined later). The research by Dobyns et al., 2004) showed that the rules differentiating X-linked dominant and X-linked recessive inheritance have failed to explain the variability of X-linked disorders, or why many female carriers with an X-linked recessive disorder can have abnormal phenotypes. As a result, Dobyns et al. (2004) suggest that clinicians discontinue the terms *X-linked dominant* and *X-linked recessive* in favor of describing such disorders simply as *X-linked inheritance*. Table 3–3 summarizes the revised principles of X-linked inheritance (Dobyns et al., 2004), and this is illustrated in the pedigree shown in Figure 3–10.

Table 3–3. Revised Principles of X-Linked Inheritance

1. In hemizygous males	No male-to-male transmission can occur.
	Sons never inherit the trait.
	Daughters of affected males are carriers or affected.
	Affected males are related through heterozygous females.
2. In heterozygous females	Penetrance is higher and expressivity is more severe in hemizygous males and heterozygous females.
	When female penetrance is low, males are typically affected.
	When female penetrance is higher, more females than males are affected.

Source: Summarized from Dobyns et al. (2004) (p. 141).

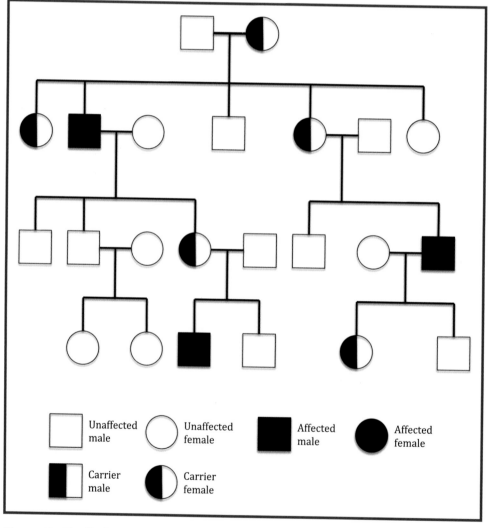

Figure 3–10. Pedigree showing X-linked inheritance.

Penetrance and Expressivity

Individuals having a certain genotype can show variability in phenotype. The two terms used to describe this phenotypic variability are *penetrance* and *expressivity*. Penetrance refers to the percentage of individuals who have the genetic mutation and actually exhibit any of the clinical features of the disorder. Penetrance can be complete or incomplete. Complete penetrance (100%) means that everyone who has the gene shows the clinical trait. Incomplete penetrance means only some people with a gene for a specific disorder will exhibit the trait, and others will not. For example, 80% penetrance means that about 80% of the people with the gene will show the characteristics of the disorder.

Expressivity refers to the range of clinical features that a person with the disorder can present. Variable expressivity refers to the variation in the number, type, and severity of clinical features that can occur between individuals with the same condition. For example, the features of Treacher Collins syndrome can vary widely; people may have features that are so mild that they may be missed or overlooked, while others may have features that are more severe and pronounced. The concepts of expressivity and penetrance are illustrated in Figure 3–11.

CHROMOSOME DISORDERS

Chromosome abnormalities can be caused by changes in structure or number. The structure of a chromosome can be changed in several ways. A portion of the chromosome can be deleted (a deletion) resulting

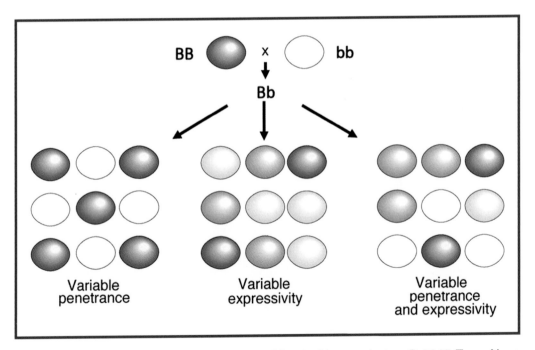

Figure 3–11. Penetrance and expressivity. (Used with permission © 2015 Terra Nova Genomics, Steven M. Carr.)

in missing genetic material or duplicated resulting in extra genetic material (a duplication). An example of a syndrome resulting from a deletion is 22q11.2 (described later in the chapter); an example of a syndrome resulting from duplication is Fragile X. In Fragile X syndrome, multiple repeats of the fragile X mental retardation 1 (*FMR1*) gene occur that leads to cognitive impairment of various degrees. A translocation is a rearrangement of the chromosome and occurs when one part of the chromosome is transferred to another chromosome. There are two types of translocation: balanced and unbalanced. In a balanced translocation, the genetic material is rearranged but does not result in extra or deleted material. A person with a balanced translocation is phenotypically normal but at risk for transmitting an unbalanced chromosome makeup to an offspring. In an unbalanced translocation, the exchange of genetic material from one chromosome to another is uneven resulting in a deletion or duplication. An unbalanced translocation causes congenital abnormalities and developmental delay. Inversion translocation occurs when one part of the chromosome has broken off and reattached upside down. A ring chromosome occurs when a part of the chromosome has broken off and reattached in the shape of a ring. Types of structural chromosome abnormalities are shown in Figure 3–12.

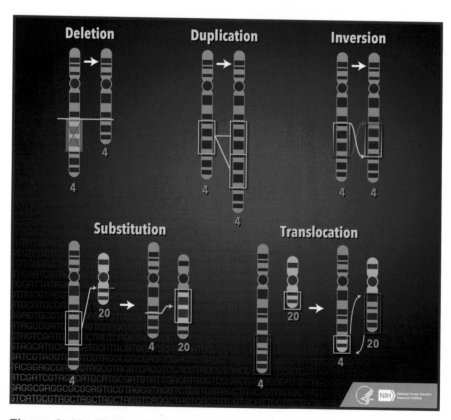

Figure 3–12. Structural chromosome abnormalities. (Note: Ring chromosome is not shown.) (National Human Genome Research Institute. Retrieved from https://www.genome.gov/11508982. Courtesy of Darryl Leja, NHGRI, NIH, and Ernesto Del Aguila III, NHGRI, NIH.)

Numerical chromosomal abnormalities are caused by abnormal cell division during meiosis resulting in a total that is not 46. Thus, a person may have an extra chromosome in addition to the normal pair (trisomy), or a missing chromosome (monosomy) in which one chromosome of a given pair is absent or missing. For example, in Trisomy 21 there are three copies of chromosome 21 resulting in a total of 47 chromosomes rather than 46, whereas in monosomy X (Turner syndrome or 45X), the person has one X chromosome rather than the usual pair of XX resulting in a total of 45 chromosomes. Polyploidy refers to a duplication of the 23 pairs of chromosomes.

MULTIFACTORIAL DISORDERS

Multifactorial inheritance has been explained using the Threshold Model (Fraser, 1976). The premise is that a person has a genetic predisposition toward a given disorder, and when combined with environmental influences, the disorder presents itself. Figure 3–13 illustrates the threshold model depicting this interaction.

Liability refers to all the genetic and environmental factors that contribute to the development of a multifactorial disorder. As shown in the figure, the liability of a person generally follows a normal distribution in the general population. A person having a genetic liability above a certain threshold will have the disorder, if exposed to certain environmental conditions. Nonsyndromic cleft lip and/or palate is the most common congenital defect associated with multifactorial inheritance.

In contrast to single-gene patterns of inheritance, multifactorial inheritance does not follow any recognizable inheritance pattern. The recurrence risk for multifactorial inheritance ranges from as low as 2% to as high as 10% depending on the traits and characteristics of the disorder (Smith, 1971). The recurrence risk increases as more family members are affected by a given disorder (see Chapter 2). Table 3–4 summarizes the major characteristics of multifactorial inheritance, and this is illustrated in the pedigree shown in Figure 3–14.

TERATOGENS

Unlike a genetic mutation, a teratogen is an agent (i.e., drugs, infection, environmental chemicals) that interferes with the

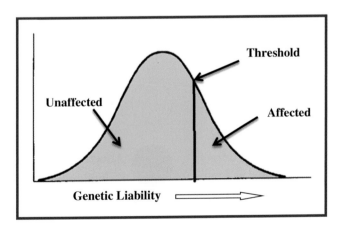

Figure 3–13. Threshold liability curve.

Table 3–4. Principles of Multifactorial Inheritance

1. The recurrence risk of the trait increases if more than one family member is affected.

2. The recurrence risk of the trait is higher in first-degree relatives (i.e., siblings, parents) than in more distant relatives.

3. The more severe the defect, the higher is the recurrence risk.

4. Consanguinity slightly increases the risk for an affected child.

5. The risk of recurrence within a family decreases as the degree of relationship becomes more remote.

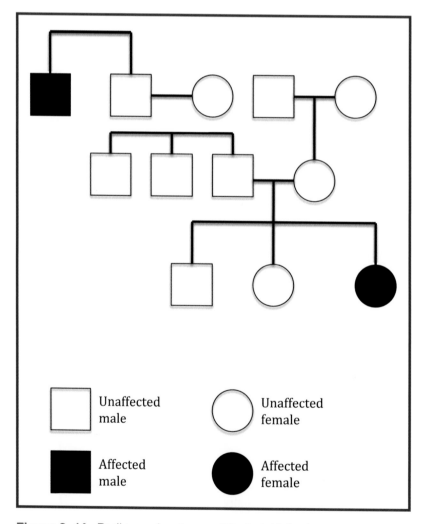

Figure 3–14. Pedigree showing multifactorial inheritance.

development of the fetus. It is not genetic. The risk for a child having a birth defect caused by a teratogen depends on the time of exposure, duration and strength of the teratogen, and genetic susceptibility of the fetus (Gilbert-Barness, 2010). The fundamental difference between birth defects caused by teratogens and genetic mutagens is that the teratogen acts directly on the developing embryo, whereas mutagens cause hereditable alterations in the genetic material (Nussbaum et al., 2004). Thus, the recurrence risk in a disorder caused by a teratogen is low if the teratogen is avoided in a future pregnancy.

There are many different teratogens that cause birth defects, in which a cleft may be associated. They include, alcohol, maternal infections, drugs and chemicals, radiation, and maternal metabolic factors. Alcohol is a common teratogen causing intrauterine growth retardation and abnormal facies including cleft palate, maxillary hypoplasia, and smooth philtrum. These individuals also have cognitive and learning challenges. Fetal alcohol spectrum disorder is a completely preventable disorder if the woman does not drink alcohol during her pregnancy.

Maternal infections that pass through the placenta and directly into the fetal bloodstream can threaten the development of the fetus. The effects of rubella and cytomegalovirus are well known. High doses of radiation can cause gene mutations resulting in abnormalities in the developing embryo (e.g., microcephaly).

GENETIC TESTING

Genetic testing consists of methods to detect heritable conditions. Cytogenetics is the branch of science that studies the number and structure of chromosomes and their relationship to a disease or disease process (Pergament, 2008). Cytogenetic techniques are valuable and widely used in the diagnosis of genetic disorders. Referral for cytogenetic testing is dependent on a thorough genetic evaluation that includes a comprehensive family history, pregnancy and birth history, and developmental and physical examination (Zaslav, Marino, Jurgens, & Mercado, 2013). In this section, we describe three techniques most often used to identify genetic disorders. They are Giesma banding (G banding), fluorescence in situ hybridization (FISH), and microarray comparative genomic hybridization (aCGH).

Giesma banding (G banding) is the most common method used to produce a karyotype for chromosome analysis (see Figure 3–5). A Giesma stain is used to produce light and dark bands that result in a pattern that is unique to each chromosome. G banding is useful in detecting numerical and structural chromosome abnormalities. The limitation to G banding is the inability to detect small deletions or microdeletions. Thus, *in conjunction* with chromosomal analyses, advanced techniques such as fluorescence in situ hybridization (FISH) and microarray comparative genomic hybridization (aCGH) are used to map specific genes or portions of genes.

FISH is a technique used to study specific regions of a chromosome. It is an approach for detecting microdeletions of a specific gene on a given chromosome that cannot be detected by standard chromosome analysis such as G banding. FISH uses a fluorescent DNA probe specific to a chromosome, chromosome region, or gene that can be used to diagnose a chromosome abnormality (Nussbaum et al., 2004). A probe is a single strand of DNA that is intended to bind to a complementary DNA strand on a portion of the chromosome the clinician is looking for. When the probe binds to a chromosome, the fluorescent tag allows the clinician to identify it. If there is a small deletion in the region of the complementary probe, the probe will not bind to its complementary sequence. An example of a FISH assay for 22q11.2 deletion syndrome is shown in Figure 3–15.

The limitations of FISH are that it does not screen for all chromosome changes and that the FISH probes are specific to one particular deletion or duplication within one band of a chromosome so that it can only find what it is looking for (National Human Genome Research Institute, 2015).

Wherein FISH there is a single target and known chromosome region, aCGH targets the entire genome for abnormalities caused by deletions and duplications of pieces of DNA (Oostlander, Meijer, & Ylstra, 2004). Using tens of thousands of sequences of DNA or probes, this technique compares the DNA of a patient with a reference or control DNA in order to detect differences (Theisen, 2008). aCGH also uses single-strand DNA obtained from a control sample stained with one color (e.g., red) and a single DNA strand from the patient stained with another color (e.g., green). The probe and control DNA are mixed together and placed on a chip (grid on a glass slide) so that the base pairs will bind with their matching probes. This chip is then scanned in a machine called a *microarray* to produce a fluorescence ratio of the patient DNA to control DNA binding signals determined

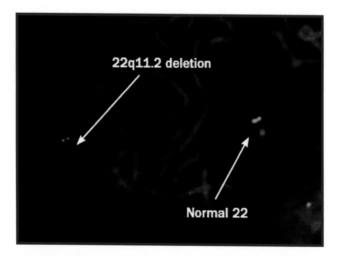

Figure 3–15. Positive fluorescence in situ hybridization (FISH) assay for 22q11.2 deletion syndrome. Two green control probes are present, indicating chromosome 22. The single red signal can be seen on the normal chromosome 22. The red signal is missing on the chromosome 22 with the deletion. (Used with permission of Mayo Foundation for Medical Education and Research. All rights reserved.)

at positions along the genome (Theisen, 2008; Rare Chromosome, 2015). Whether the patient has the correct amount of DNA or too much or too little is based on the ratio provided. The aCGH results for a patient with 22q11.2 deletion are presented in Figure 3–16.

CLASSIFYING CONGENITAL BIRTH DEFECTS

In normal development, a tissue, structure, or organ is genetically programmed to be the appropriate size and shape. This orderly process is referred to as *morphogenesis*.

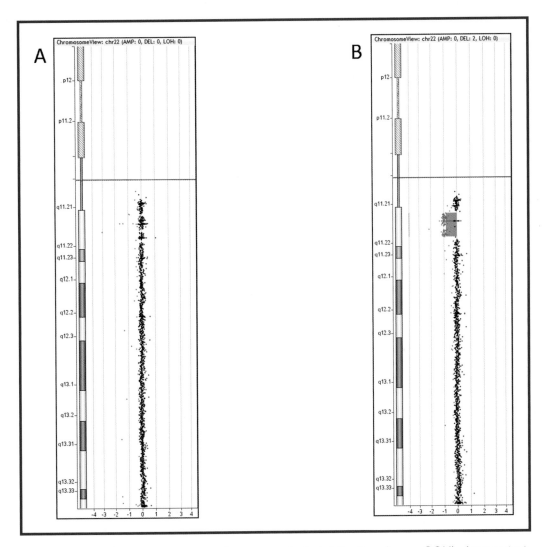

Figure 3–16. Oligoarray comparative genomic hybridization (array CGH) demonstrating the 22q11.21 microdeletion. **A.** A normal chromosome 22. **B.** A chromosome 22 with the 22q11.21 microdeletion between LCR22-A and D (red shaded area) that causes the DiGeorge/velocardiofacial syndrome. (Array CGH courtesy of Fady M. Mikhail, MD, PhD, FACMG, Department of Genetics, University of Alabama, Birmingham.)

Yet, as we know this does not always happen, and there is an interruption in the developmental process causing malformed features referred to as *dysmorphogenesis*. This interruption can occur early during the first trimester in which case the structure may never have had the chance to develop normally, or as late as the third trimester when the structure started to develop normally but the development was disrupted, and from that point forward normal development could not be completed (Davies & Evans, 2003; Spranger, et al., 1982). There are four categories of morphological abnormalities: malformation, deformation, disruption, and dysplasia.

A *malformation* represents a morphological defect of an organ or region due to an intrinsically abnormal developmental problem with the formation, growth, or differentiation of an organ or structure (Jones, 2006; Spranger et al., 1982). A common example of a malformation would be cleft palate. A *deformation* is an abnormal shape caused by an extrinsic mechanical force acting on an originally normally formed structure (Davies & Evans, 2003; Spranger et al., 1982). An example of a deformation is clubfoot. A *disruption* is the destructive breakdown of a normally developing tissue (Spranger et al., 1982). The most common example of a disruption is amniotic band constriction in which thin bands of tissue tear away from inside the amniotic sac (amnion) and attach to parts of the baby's body, cutting off the blood supply to the developing structure and preventing further growth. *Dysplasia* is a structural anomaly resulting from a breakdown in the organization of tissues from which normal structures are formed (Jones, 2006; Spranger et al., 1982). An example of a dysplasia would be Stickler syndrome (described later in the chapter).

Some congenital birth defects occur in recognizable patterns that may be pathogenically or causally related, occur together based on a statistical basis, or occur by chance alone (Spranger et al., 1982). Patterns of anomalies are categorized as syndromes, sequences, and associations.

A *syndrome* is a recognizable pattern of multiple anomalies that occur together and are thought to be pathogenetically related and have a known or suspected cause (Spranger et al., 1982). Individuals with a syndrome will look alike even though they are unrelated (e.g., Trisomy 21, 22q11.2 deletion syndrome, Treacher Collins syndrome). A *sequence* is a pattern of multiple anomalies occurring as a result of a single known or presumed prior anomaly or mechanical factor causing a cascade of secondary anomalies (Springer et al., 1982). Pierre Robin sequence is a familiar example. An *association* is a nonrandom occurrence of a pattern of multiple congenital anomalies in two or more individuals, which are not known to be a syndrome or a sequence, and although not *pathogenetically* or causally related anomalies, they occur more frequently together than would be expected by chance alone (Davies & Evans, 2003; Spranger et al., 1985). Examples of an association are VATER and CHARGE associations.

MALFORMATIONS OF THE CRANIOFACIAL COMPLEX

In this section we describe malformations based on pathogenetic commonalities: those in which a cleft is a predominant feature, branchial arch anomalies, and craniosynostosis. The list is by no means exhaustive. To be sure, these and the many other craniofacial conditions are complex. For each category we have selected disorders often seen by the cleft palate-craniofacial team. Their clinical features and communication characteristics are presented. Tables 3–5 through 3–7 highlight structural anomalies common to each category and the impact on speech and hearing.

Conditions Commonly Associated With Cleft Palate

We present here four craniofacial conditions in which a cleft or palatal anomaly is frequently associated. They are Van der Woude syndrome, Pierre Robin sequence, Stickler syndrome, and 22q11.2 deletion syndrome.

Table 3–5. Structural Abnormalities Associated With Malformations in Which Cleft Palate Is Predominant and the Impact on Speech and Hearing

Structural Abnormality	Functional Impact	Impairment
Mandibular hypoplasia	Airway obstruction	Breathing
Cleft palate, noncleft palatal dysfunction	Resonance	Hypernasality
Class II +/– open bite, various dental anomalies	Articulation	Distortions on sibilants and affricates
Eustachian tube dysfunction	Hearing	Mild to moderate conductive hearing loss

Table 3–6. Structural Abnormalities Associated With Branchial Arch Anomalies and the Impact on Speech and Hearing

Structural Abnormality	Functional Impact	Impairment
Mandibular hypoplasia	Airway obstruction	Breathing
Class II +/– anterior open bite malocclusion	Articulation	Distortions on sibilants and affricates. Depending on the severity of the open bite, may observe reverse placement on tip alveolar consonants and lingualabial productions of bilabial consonants
External and middle ear anomalies	Hearing	Mild to moderate conductive hearing loss
Abnormal supralaryngeal vocal tract	Voice quality	Muffled, cul-de-sac
Cleft palate, noncleft palatal dysfunction	Resonance	Hypernasality

Table 3–7. Structural Abnormalities Associated With Craniosynostosis and the Impact on Speech and Hearing

Structural Abnormality	Functional Impact	Impairment
Midface hypoplasia	Resonance	Hyponasality
	Airway obstruction	Breathing
Class III +/– anterior open bite malocclusion	Articulation	Distortions on sibilants and affricates. Reverse placement on tip alveolar consonants and lingualabial productions of bilabial consonants
Outer and middle ear anomalies	Hearing	Mild to moderate conductive hearing loss
Eustachian tube dysfunction	Otitis media with effusion	Conductive hearing loss
Cleft palate (more common in Apert syndrome)	Resonance	Hypernasality

Van der Woude Syndrome

Clinical Features. Van der Woude syndrome (VWS) (Van der Woude, 1954) is the most common syndromic form of clefting (Schutte, Sander, Malik, & Murray, 1996), occurring in approximately 2% of individuals having a cleft (Burdick, Bixler, & Puckett, 1985; Rintala & Ranta, 1980; Schinzel & Klauser, 1986). It is an autosomal dominant disorder with variable expressivity and high penetrance (Cêrvenka, Gorlin, & Anderson, 1967). The estimated prevalence of VWS varies from 1:40,000 to 1:100,000 live births (Burdick, 1986; Cêrvenka et al., 1967; Gordon, Davies, & Friedberg, 1969; Janku et al., 1980; Rintala & Ranta, 1981; Van der Woude, 1954) with no reported sex difference. The cause of VWS has been mapped to mutations in the gene encoding IRF6 (interferon regulatory factor 6), on the long arm of chromosome 1 (Kondo et al., 2002). IRF6 is a protein responsible for the formation and development of tissue in the skull and face.

Orofacial Features. The salient features of VWS are lower lip pits and cleft lip with or without cleft palate (Figure 3–17).

Submucous cleft palate, bifid uvula, and incomplete unilateral and bilateral cleft lip have also been documented (Shprintzen, Goldberg, & Sidoti, 1980), but they occur with less frequency. The lip pits are usually circular and located symmetrically and bilaterally on the upper border of the lower lip.

Other oral features associated with VWS include hypodontia (Rintala & Ranta, 1981; Schinzel & Klauser, 1986; Schneider, 1973), missing upper teeth (Ranta & Rintala, 1983), ankyloglossia, and oral synechiae between the upper

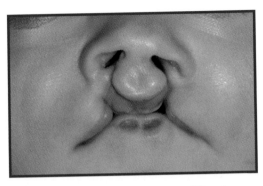

Figure 3–17. Infant with Van der Woude syndrome showing lower lip pits and bilateral cleft lip and palate. (Photo courtesy of Joseph A. Napoli, MD, DDS, Plastic, Maxillofacial, and Craniofacial Surgery, Alfred I. duPont Hospital for Children, Wilmington, DE.)

and lower gum pads (Shaw & Simpson, 1980).

Developmental Features. Cognitive and developmental challenges are not typically associated with VWS.

Ear Anomalies and Hearing. The structures of the ears in VWS are normal. The middle ear disease associated with cleft palate may cause a mild transient conductive hearing loss.

Speech and Language. Individuals with VWS do not typically present with distinguishing speech, language, hearing, or cognitive features (Peterson-Falzone, Hardin-Jones, & Karnell, 2010). In the absence of any cognitive delay or other problems that have an impact on communication development, it is reasonable to suggest that the concerns about communication would be similar to those involving the effect of a cleft including VPI and conductive hearing loss (Peterson-Falzone et al., 2010).

Pierre Robin Sequence

Clinical Features. In 1923, Pierre Robin (Robin, 1923) described a series of infants who presented with a triad of symptoms characterized by micrognathia (small jaw),[1] glossoptosis (posterior displacement of the tongue), and airway obstruction (Figure 3–18).

Since then, the presence of a cleft palate has broadened this definition (Tan, Kilpatrick, & Farlie, 2013) to one that many clinicians have come to identify with Pierre Robin sequence (PRS). To be sure, a cleft need not be present in order for a definitive diagnosis of PRS to be made. PRS is a feature that has been

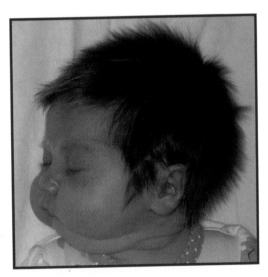

Figure 3–18. An infant with Pierre Robin sequence and severe micrognathia.

---

[1]The terms *micrognathia* and *retrognathia* are often confused. Micrognathia refers to a small mandible, whereas retrognathia refers to an abnormal posteriorly positioned mandible. The terms are not synonymous.

associated with more than 40 syndromes (Cohen, 1999; Evans, Sie, Hopper, Glass, Hing, & Cunningham, 2013), including Stickler, Treacher Collins, and 22q11.2 deletion syndromes.

PRS is a sequence (not a syndrome) in which a single primary anomaly causes a cascade of other anomalies. As well described by Tan et al. (2013), the primary defect is micrognathia in which the small oral volume leaves little space for the tongue to move downward and forward during embryonic development, preventing elevation of the palatal shelves and failure of the palate to fuse, resulting in a cleft palate.

The estimated prevalence of PRS varies from 1:8,500 to 1:14,000 live births with equal distribution among males and females (Evans et al., 2013; Printzlau & Andersen, 2004; Tan et al., 2013). This variation in prevalence may be attributed to the variability in diagnostic criteria used among clinicians to label PRS in a newborn (Evans et al., 2013; Tan et al., 2013). In the absence of any co-occurring birth defects or syndrome, the risk of recurrence is very low as PRS is not an inheritable condition.

Oral Features. The mandible is micrognathic. Whether the mandibular growth "catches up" over time has been controversial. Perhaps it can be said that the growth likely correlates with the etiology of the condition or underlying syndrome (Bromberg, Pasternak, Walden, & Rubin, 1961; Evans et al., 2013; Shprintzen, 1988). Cleft palate, when present, is typically wide and U-shaped (Figure 3–19) with fewer infants presenting with a V-shaped cleft (LeBlanc & Golding-Kushner, 1992; Marques, Barbieri, & Bettiol, 1998; Rintala, Ranta, & Stegars, 1984; Shprintzen, 1988).

Combined with the small jaw, glossoptosis can give rise to airway obstruction and feeding problems (Figure 3–20).

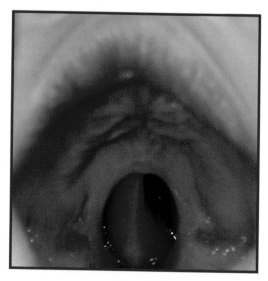

Figure 3–19. U-shaped cleft palate in Pierre Robin sequence. (Photo courtesy of Joseph A. Napoli, MD, DDS, Plastic, Maxillofacial, and Craniofacial Surgery, Alfred I. duPont Hospital for Children, Wilmington, DE.)

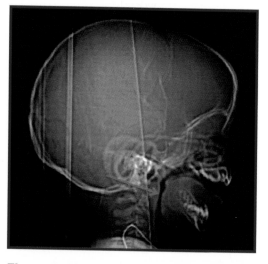

Figure 3–20. Lateral x-ray showing airway in infant with Pierre Robin sequence. Note base of tongue as potential site of airway obstruction.

Although not all infants with PRS experience airway obstruction, for those who do the focus of treatment is on maintaining an airway for breathing and preventing complications such as hypoxia, respiratory failure, and death (Evans et al., 2011). Strategies for maintaining the airway can be nonsurgical or surgical depending on the nature and seriousness of airway obstruction (see Chapter 5).

Feeding difficulties may lead to poor nutrition requiring nasogastric or orogastric tube management (Evans, Rahbar, Rogers, Mulliken, & Volk, 2006; Peterson-Falzone et al., 2010).

Developmental Features. Cognition in PRS is considered to be similar to that of children with isolated cleft palate (Peterson-Falzone et al., 2010). This has been our experience as well. It is, of course, important to be aware that a child with PRS may also experience speech and language disorders as a result of general developmental delay, prolonged hospitalization, environmental deprivation, and other psychosocial factors (Peterson-Falzone, 1981).

Ear Anomalies and Hearing. In PRS, the structures of the ears are normal. Middle ear fluid with effusion associated with cleft palate is common, causing a conductive hearing loss.

Speech and Language. The factors associated with PRS that can cause communication impairment are velopharyngeal inadequacy (VPI), malocclusion, and conductive hearing loss.

VPI or unrepaired cleft palate results in hypernasal resonance and other associated speech problems. If the mandible is underdeveloped enough to cause a Class II malocclusion, articulation may be affected. Dentally related articulation disorders are discussed in Chapter 8.

Glossopexy and tracheostomy, procedures used to treat airway obstruction, can interfere with early speech development. LeBlanc and Golding-Kushner (1992) suggested that glossopexy or tongue-lip adhesion (described in Chapter 5) cause delayed babbling and initiation of first words but that the delays seem to be temporary. The only long-term effect reported was a tendency for the tongue-tip sounds to be created with the tongue blade, resulting in a production that was judged to be visually aberrant but perceptually normal.

Long-term tracheostomy can impede articulation development. With the cannula in place, the tongue is maintained in a retracted position and its movement restricted. As a consequence, children can development maladaptive speech sound productions such as backing to velar and /h/ or stop replacement for fricatives and affricatives (Kamen & Watson, 1991).

Language skills are generally consistent with those found in children with cleft palate.

Stickler Syndrome (Hereditary Arthro-Ophthalmology)

Clinical Features. Stickler syndrome (SS) is among the most common of connective tissue disorders associated with a cleft, and also the most common syndrome associated with PRS (Cohen, 1979). Individuals with Stickler syndrome have a distinctive face and ocular, auditory, and musculoskeletal abnormalities (Stickler & Pugh, 1967) (Figure 3–21).

Inheritance is autosomal dominant with complete penetrance and variable expressivity (Stickler et al., 1965). The estimated prevalence of Stickler syndrome

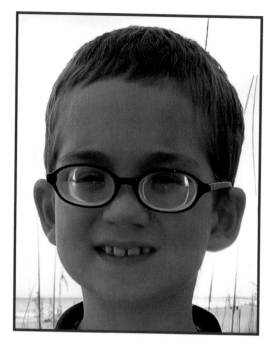

Figure 3–21. Facial features of a 7-year-old child with Stickler syndrome.

ranges from 1:7,500 to 1:9,000 newborns (Robin, Moran, Warman, and Ala-Kokko, 2011).

There are three types of Stickler syndrome classified according to the specific gene mutation. Approximately 70% to 75% of cases are SS Type I caused by a mutation in the *COL2A1*gene on chromosome 12q11.3 (Ahmad et al., 1990; Knowlton, et al., 1989; Rose et al., 2005; Snead & Yates, 1999). SS Types II and III are caused by mutations in the *COL 11A1* gene on chromosome 11 and *COL 11A2* gene on chromosome 6p21, respectively, and are more rare. Ocular abnormalities are associated with Types I and II.

Ocular and Musculoskeletal Features. The primary vision problem in SS is severe bilateral myopia or nearsightedness that is often present before the age of 10 years (Snead & Yates, 1999; Stickler, Hughes,

& Houchin, 2001). It is quite common to see a young child with SS wearing glasses with heavy lenses. A number of other eye problems such as retinal degeneration and retinal detachment have been reported (Seery, Pruett, Liberfarb, & Cohen, 1990; Stickler et al., 1965). The significant nature of the ocular problems underscores the need for early diagnosis and long-term follow-up.

Joint problems tend to develop early in individuals with SS and signs of osteoarthritis often begin to manifest in the teenage years. Because of the joint problems, physical activities tend to be restricted. Other reported problems include mitral valve prolapse (Liberfarb & Goldblatt, 1986), and dental anomalies such as natal teeth, maleruption and enamel hypoplasia (Herrmann, France, Spranger, Opitz, & Wiffler, 1975).

Orofacial Features. Flattened midface, malar hypoplasia, micrognathia, hypoplastic and wide nasal bridge, anteverted nares, and prominent appearing eyes are characteristic features in SS (Figure 3–21). Similar to those with PRS, the micrognathia and glossoptosis may be severe enough to cause airway and feeding problems (Peterson-Falzone et al., 2010).

Cleft palate and submucous cleft palate are present in about 20% of the cases with SS (Gorlin, Cohen, & Hennekam, 2001). Bifid uvula, short palate, and palatal immobility may also be present (Gorlin et al., 2001; Weingeist et al., 1982).

Ear Anomalies and Hearing. Hearing loss is prevalent in SS. The type and degree of the impairment are often age dependent (Acke, Dhooge, Malfait, & Leenheer, 2012; Stickler et al., 2001; Szymko-Bennett, et al., 2001). Whereas conductive hearing loss is common in young children, a sloping high frequency sensorineural hearing loss is more prevalent in older children and adults (Acke et al., 2012; Nowak, 1998; Szmko-Bennett et al., 2001). Both types of hearing loss can co-occur resulting in a mixed hearing loss.

Developmental Features. In most cases, intelligence is normal in persons with SS, but they may face educational challenges as a consequence of their vision and hearing problems (Snead & Yates, 1999).

Speech and Language. The factors contributing to speech and language problems in SS are similar to those reported for PRS. They include VPI, malocclusion, and hearing loss (refer to section on Pierre Robin sequence).

Differential Diagnosis. Because infants with SS often present with symptoms associated with PRS, the diagnosis may be delayed (Stickler et al., 2001). Hermann et al. (1975) reported that as many as 50% of individuals with PRS will, after further examination have SS. Thus, in a child who presents symptoms suggestive of PRS, it is routine practice for the geneticist to order an ophthalmologic examination and cytogenetic testing to rule out or confirm a diagnosis of SS.

22q11.2 Deletion Syndrome (Velocardiofacial Syndrome, DiGeorge Syndrome, Shprintzen Syndrome)

Clinical Features. The 22q11.2 deletion syndrome is a genetic disorder with an estimated prevalence of 1:4,000 to 1:6,000 live births, making it a relatively common disorder in the general population (Botto et al., 2003; DuMontcel, Mendizabal, Aymé, Lévy, & Philip, 1996) (Figure 3–22).

It is caused by a small gene deletion located at a specific region (11.2) on the long arm (q) of chromosome 22. Inheritance is autosomal dominant with variable expressivity.

Although the loss of a gene at this locus is responsible for a number of characteristic phenotypic features, there is considerable variation ranging from mild to severe (Digilio, Marino, Caploino, & Dallapiccola, 2005; McDonald-McGinn et al., 1999). Several disorders that were once considered separate entities are now considered variants of the same genetic deletion on chromosome 22q11.2 (Solot et al., 2000.). They include velocardiofacial syndrome, DiGeorge syndrome, Shprintzen syndrome, conotruncal anomaly face syndrome, and Cayler cardiofacial syndrome.

The most common features of 22q11.2 deletion syndrome are facial anomalies, cardiac defects, cleft palate or velopharyngeal dysfunction, immune deficiencies and hypocalcemia, learning challenges, and communication impairment (Goldmuntz, et al., 1999; Shprintzen et al., 1978). There are over 180 listed features associated with 22q11.2 deletion syndrome (Shprintzen, 2000, 2008), and it is possible that the spectrum of anomalies could continue to widen.

Because not all infants exhibit the classic symptoms of 22q11.2 deletion syndrome, it may not be identified immediately at birth (Saal, 2008). For some, the presenting symptoms may be hypernasal speech or delays in speech and language development for which the initial contact is the speech-language pathologist (Gorlin & Baylis, 2009). For others, the initial contact may be the cardiologist (McDonald-McGinn et al., 1997). Because of the high prevalence of cardiac defects associated with this disorder, neonates

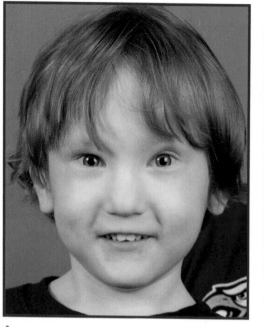 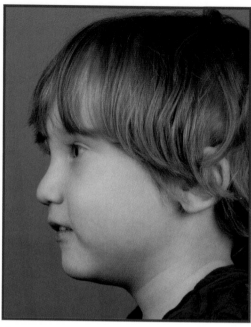

A   B

Figure 3–22. Frontal (**A**) and profile (**B**) views of a 4-year-old child with 22q11.2 deletion syndrome.

and infants with heart problems are commonly referred for cytogenetic testing to rule out or confirm a diagnosis of 22q11.2 deletion syndrome.

Cardiac Defects and Other Features. Congenital heart defects are present in approximately 75% of those with 22q11.2 deletion syndrome (McDonald-McGinn et al., 1999; Marino et al., 2001). The most common cardiac malformations are conotruncal defects including ventricular septal defect and tetralogy of Fallot (Goldmuntz et al., 1998; Marino, Digilio, Toscano, Giannotti, & Dallapiccola, 1999; Marino et al., 2001; Young, Shprintzen, & Goldberg, 1980). Medial displacement of the internal carotid artery, a vascular anomaly, is present in a number of individuals (D'Antonio & Marsh, 1987; Finkelstein

et al., 1993; MacKenzie-Stepner et al., 1987; Ross, Witzel, Armstrong, & Thomson, 1996). Obvious pulsations of the artery along the posterior pharyngeal wall have been observed during endoscopic examination. Knowledge of the placement of the carotid artery is important in order to circumvent carotid arterial injury during pharyngeal flap surgery to correct VPI.

Other features of 22q11.2 deletion syndrome are hypocalcemia or low calcium (Ryan et al., 1997) and immune deficiency disorder caused by low T cells, which are important for fighting off infection (Gennery, 2012; Smith, Driscoll, Emanuel, McDonald-McGinn, Zackai & Sullivan, 1998; Sullivan, McDonald-McGinn, & Zackai, 2002; Zemble et al., 2010). Children with severe immunodeficiency frequently miss school may require home schooling. Rib anomalies and hand (e.g., clinodactyly or curvature of fifth finger) and feet anomalies (e.g., toe syndactyly or webbing) have also been reported (Ming et al., 1997).

Orofacial Features. The distinctive orofacial features of 22q11.2 deletion syndrome are long face with vertical maxillary excess, micrognathia, small mouth with everted upper lip, thin upper lip, and long philtrum, bulbous nose, and hypoplastic nares (see Figure 3–22).

Palatal anomalies can include overt cleft palate, submucous cleft palate, and occult submucous cleft palate. Cleft lip only and cleft lip and palate are rare (Gorlin et al., 2001).

Palate dysfunction in the absence of a cleft occurs with a relatively high frequency. Noncleft conditions include pharyngeal hypotonia, hypoplasia or agenesis of the musculus uvula, and platybasia (flattening of the skull base) that can cause increased distance between the velum and the posterior pharyngeal wall to such an extent that VP closure cannot be attained during speech (Arvystas & Shprintzen, 1984; Havkin, Tatum, & Shprintzen, 2000; Ruotolo et al., 2006; Williams, Shprintzen & Rakoff, 1987). Other conditions causing palatal dysfunction include a congenital short velum, reduced lateral pharyngeal wall movement, small adenoid size that increases the VP space, and abnormalities of the pharyngeal muscles (Arvystas & Shprintzen, 1984; Finkelstein et al., 1993).

Ear Anomalies and Hearing. The ears are typically low set, and there may be abnormal folding of the pinna (see Figure 3–22). Stenotic external auditory canals and ossicular anomalies have been reported (Black, Spanier, & Kohut, 1975).

Up to 90% of the children with 22q11.2 deletion have chronic otitis media causing conductive hearing loss (Digilio et al., 1999; Reyes, LeBlanc, & Bassila, 1999). Cases of sensorineural and mixed hearing loss have also been documented (Digilio et al., 1999; Reyes et al., 1999; Solot et al., 2000). Hearing loss can compound the communication deficits in a population that is known to exhibit speech and language delays.

Developmental Features. Early delays in development, hypotonia and delayed motor development, and speech and language delays, all of which can vary in severity, are common findings in individuals with 22q11.2 deletion syndrome (Gerdes et al., 1999; Goldberg et al., 1983; McDonald-McGinn et al., 1997; Moss et al., 1999; Shprintzen et al., 1981; Solot et al., 2000; Solet et al., 2001; Swillen et al., 1997). Cognitive and learning challenges can range from mild to severe. The rate of learning disabilities in this population is estimated at 99% to 100% (Goldberg, Motzkin, Marion, Scambler & Shprintzen, 1993; Shprintzen et al., 1981). Attention deficit with hyperactivity disorder, attention deficit disorder, emotional instability and anxiety have been reported (Goldberg et al., 1993). Some children may exhibit impulsivity and others may be withdrawn and shy (Golding-Kushner, Weller, & Shprintzen, 1985; Swillen et al., 1997; Swillen, et al., 1999). These individuals are also at risk for developing psychiatric and mental health conditions such as schizophrenia, bipolar disorder, and depression (Baker & Skuse, 2005; Murphy, Jones, & Owen, 1999; Shprintzen, Goldberg, Golding-Kushner, & Marion, 1992).

Speech and Language. Speech and language impairment is a hallmark feature of 22q11.2

deletion syndrome. Peterson-Falzone et al. (2010) stated that "Virtually every publication on speech and language development in children with VCFS speaks of delayed acquisition of first words, delayed appearance of first sentences, delayed acquisition of phonologic knowledge, and problems in the ability to produce and coordinate the speech movements required to articulate sounds clearly" (p. 77). Some have suggested that children with 22q11.2 deletion syndrome may in fact, have a distinct communication profile (D'Antonio, Scherer, Miller, Kalbfleisch, & Bartley, 2001; Scherer, D'Antonio, & Rodgers, 2001; Solot et al., 2001). The factors associated with 22q11.2 deletion syndrome that can contribute to speech and language problems include general articulatory/phonologic delay, VPI, oromotor impairment, hearing loss, and developmental and cognitive delays.

Resonance. Hypernasality is exceedingly prevalent in 22q11.2 syndrome often ranging in degree from moderate to severe. Although a cleft palate or submucous cleft palate may be responsible for VPI, it is important to understand that many of these individuals have hypernasal speech caused by VP dysfunction in the *absence* of a cleft.

Articulation. Young children with 22q11.2 deletion syndrome often show a delay in phonologic development and a greater number of developmental errors (D'Antonio et al. 2001; Persson, Lohmander, Jönsson, Óskarsdottir, & Söderpalm, 2003; Solot et al., 2000, 2001). In their prospective study, Persson et al. (2003) showed that children with 22q11.2 deletion syndrome did not reach 90% correct place and manner of articulation until around

the age of 6 years. D'Antonio et al. (2001) compared the speech characteristics of children with 22q11.2 deletion syndrome to those who had some phenotypic characteristics of the disorder but were not affected. Children ranged in age from 3 to 10 years. They found that younger children with 22q11.2 deletion presented with greater speech impairment than older children with or without the disorder. Specifically, they reported severe speech production impairment in children 3 to 7 years and mild speech impairment in those ages 7 to 10 years. The young children often exhibited smaller consonant inventories, a greater number of developmental errors, a greater severity of articulation disorders, and a higher frequency of glottal stop use, a finding reported by others (Persson et al., 2003; Rommel et al., 1999; Solot et al., 2001).

Oromotor speech disorders including apraxia and dysarthria have been reported (Baylis, Munson & Moller, 2008; D'Antonio et al., 2001; Gerdes et al., 1999; Kummer, Lee, Stutz, Maroney & Brandt, 2007; Solot et al., 2000, 2001). The low facial tone often seen in these children contributes to drooling, open mouth posture at rest, and dysarthic speech (Solot et al., 2000).

Intelligibility. Studies show a relatively high rate of reduced intelligibility at various ages in 22q11.2 deletion syndrome (Persson et al., 2003). Rommel et al. (1999) reported that only 34% of their study group could be well understood during early childhood by their parent. However, the age of these children were not specified. Solot et al. (2000) found an equal distribution among speech intelligibility ratings of mild, moderate, and severe difficulty with intelligibility in a group of 31 children older than 5 years of age. Persson et al. (2003) studied the speech intelligibility of 65 individuals with 22q11.2 deletion syndrome ranging in age from 3 to 33 years and found that only 17% of the children between 5 and 10 years were judged to be intelligible all or most of the time and that the intelligibility of those 10 years and older was lower than expected. Although several of the adolescents and adults could be understood easily, there were others who experienced extreme difficulties in being understood. Intelligibility of speech may be affected by articulation, phonological, and oromotor impairment as well as resonance and errors related to hearing loss.

Language. Language impairment is common in children with 22q11.2 deletion syndrome (Goorhuis-Brouwer, Dikkers, Robinson, & Kerstjens-Frederikse, 2003; Scherer et al., 1999, 2001; Solot et al., 2000, 2001). It is evident in early childhood and may continue to be present well into adolescence and adulthood. The degree of language impairment may vary from mild to severe.

Scherer et al. (1999) compared speech and language development in four children with 22q11.2 deletion aged 6 to 30 months with three other groups: typically developing, cleft lip and palate, and cleft palate only. They observed that children with 22q11.2 deletion syndrome exhibited expressive-receptive language skills that were impaired from the onset of language and that the delay widened through 30 months of age. They also reported a severely restricted vocabulary use, delayed speech and expressive language development beyond a level predicted by their other developmental or receptive language performance, and severe limita-

tions in speech sound inventories and early vocabulary development that far exceeded those shown by the children with cleft lip and palate and cleft palate. They concluded that young children with 22q11.2 deletion syndrome emerge from a critical speech and language-learning period with severe limitations in their communication abilities. In a following study, Scherer et al. (2001) compared communication between children with 22q11.2 deletion and Trisomy 21. Their findings showed that children with Trisomy 21 demonstrated a flat communication profile across all language measures with delays relative to their chronological age, whereas children with 22q11.2 deletion exhibited a vocabulary, pattern of sound types, and reduced babbling length below cognitive and other language ages. Solot et al. (2000, 2001) also reported language delays with or without cognitive delays in children with 22q11.2 deletion ranging from infancy to early adolescence. Preschool children showed universal delay in language acquisition milestones and expressive language skills that were lower than receptive language skills. Language impairment persisted in the school-age group. In contrast, Glaser, Mumme, Blasey, Morris, Daboun, Antonarakis, Reiss, and Eliez (2002) compared the language skills of 25 children with and without 22q11.2 deletion, matched for IQ, and described a lower receptive than expressive language skills when compared to their unaffected counterparts.

Persson, Niklasson, Óskarsdottir, Johansson, Jönsson, and Söderpalm (2006) reported difficulties with language use in school-aged children, specifically in the ability to convey relevant information in a retelling task. Utterances were marked by low grammatical complexity and short sentences. D'Antonio et al. (2001) observed that as children with 22q11.2 deletion get older, speech development improves but expressive and receptive language skills continue to be delayed. Thus, language impairment can be a long-term challenge in these individuals.

As shown, speech and language impairment in individuals with 22q11.2 deletion syndrome is a pervasive and complex problem. Speech sound development and expressive and receptive language skills are delayed in young children. Specific language impairment and higher-level language/social-pragmatic difficulties are present in older children (Solot et al., 2000; Swillen, Devriendt, Ghesquiere, & Fryns, 2001).

Branchial Arch Anomalies

During embryologic development, abnormal morphogenesis of the branchial arches (also called pharyngeal arches) gives rise to defects of the face and ears (see Chapters 1 and 2). Malformations involving the first branchial arch affect the eyes, ears, palate, and mandible, and those involving the second branchial arch affect pinna and ossicular development and facial symmetry.

Two craniofacial conditions involving the branchial arches will be described: oculo-auriculo-vertebral spectrum (OAVS) and Treacher Collins syndrome (TCS).

Oculo-Auriculo-Vertebral Spectrum (OAVS) (Hemifacial Microsomia and Goldenhar Syndrome)

Clinical Features. Oculo-auriculo-vertebal spectrum (OAVS) is a complex cra-niofacial anomaly that typically affects the external ear, middle ear, mandible, temporomandibular joint, and facial muscles (Figueroa & Pruzansky, 1982; Poswillo, 1973). It is a heterogenous condition with a wide range of phenotypic expression from mild to severe (Cohen, Rollnick, & Kaye, 1989) (Figures 3–23 through 3–25).

Among the many names given to this constellation of malformations, perhaps the two most familiar to clinicians are hemifacial microsomia (HFM) and Goldenhar syndrome. Hemifacial microsomia has been described as an asymmetrical condition affecting primarily aural, oral, and mandibular development (Cohen et al., 1989; Gorlin et al., 2001). Typically, involvement is limited to one side, and although it may occur bilaterally, one side may be more severely affected than the other. Goldenhar syndrome is considered a variant of HFM that includes additional features, epibulbar dermoids, and vertebral anomalies (Cohen et al., 1989; Gorlin et al., 2001).

Over time, so much overlap between the two conditions had been reported that no clear distinction could be made between them, and both are considered part of the OAVS spectrum (Gorlin et al., 2001).

The majority of cases of OAVS occur sporadically but some familial instances have been observed (Gorlin et al., 2001). The estimated prevalence ranges from 1:3,000 to 1:5,600, with a male preponderance (Grabb, 1965; Jones, 2006; Rollnick, Kaye, Nagatoshi, Hauck, & Martin, 1987).

Ocular, Vertebral, and Other Anomalies. Ocular defects include epibulbar dermoids (small benign tumor on surface of the

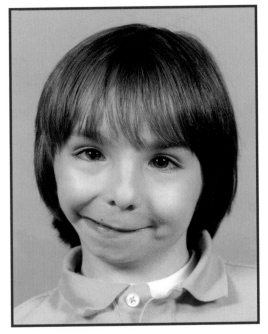

A

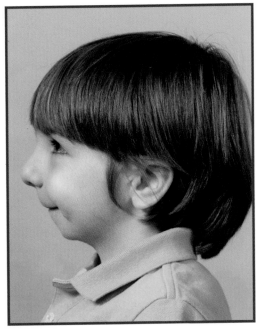

B

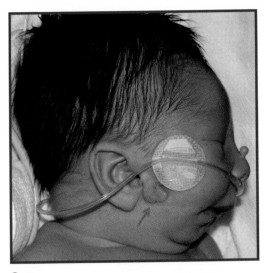

C

Figure 3–23. Frontal (**A**) and profile (**B**) views of a 6-year-old boy with oculo-auriculo-vertebral spectrum (OAVS) with unilateral involvement. The mandible is hypoplastic on the right side. **C.** Preauricular tag (*arrow*) in an infant with OAVS. Note the deviated retruded mandible and nasal appendage. (Photo courtesy of Joseph A. Napoli, MD, DDS, Plastic, Maxillofacial, and Craniofacial Surgery, Alfred I. duPont Hospital for Children, Wilmington, DE).

eye), coloboma (notch) of the upper lid, microphthalmia (abnormally small eyeball), and anophthalmia (absent eye). Vertebral anomalies may occur in up to 60% of those who are given the diagnosis of Goldenhar syndrome (Figueroa & Friede, 1985) and include the presence of fused ribs, hemivertebrae, and scoliosis (Anderson & David, 2005; Cohen et al., 1989) (Figure 3–26). Renal, cardiac, and cerebral anomalies occur occasionally (Cohen et al. 1989; Digilio et al., 2008).

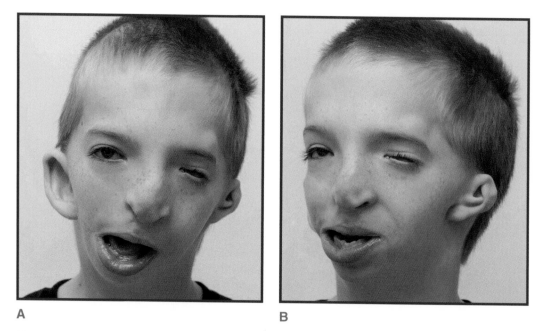

Figure 3–24. Frontal (**A**) and three-quarter-turn (**B**) views of a 13-year-old boy with oculo-auriculo-vertebral spectrum (OAVS) affecting the face bilaterally. He has a cleft lip and palate, left ear microtia, and left anophthalmia.

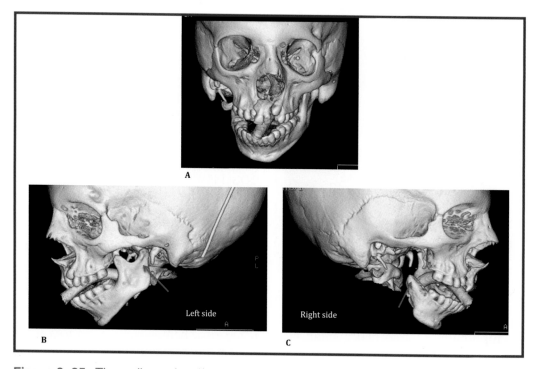

Figure 3–25. Three-dimensional computerized tomography (3D CT) of the boy shown in Figure 3–24. The frontal view (**A**) shows mandibular deviation to the right side and cleft lip and palate. The left lateral view (**B**) is the normal side. Note presence of condylar process (*arrow*). The right lateral view (**C**) is the affected side. Note absence of condylar process (*arrow*).

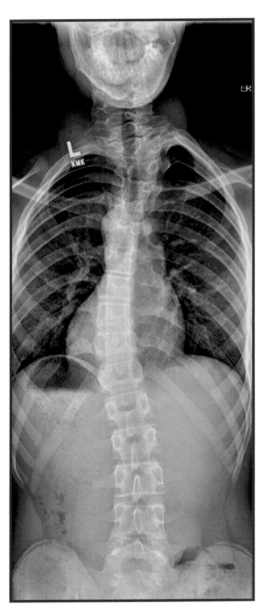

Figure 3–26. X-ray showing scoliosis in a 19-year-old with oculo-auriculo-vertebral spectrum.

Orofacial Features. A prominent feature of OAVS is mandibular asymmetry in which the chin is deviated to the affected side. Involvement typically occurs unilaterally with the right side more commonly affected (Rollnick et al., 1987). When involvement occurs bilaterally, one side is usually more affected than the other, but it may be symmetrical as well (Converse, Wood-Smith, McCarthy, Coccaro, & Becker, 1974; Farkas, Ross, & James, 1977; Ross, 1975). The mandibular ramus does not form in approximately one third of the cases with OAVS, and some individuals have a lateral facial cleft or macrostomia (McCarthy, 2007).

The estimated prevalence of cleft lip with or without cleft palate is 7%, with cleft palate occurring more frequently at a rate of about 15% (Rollnick et al., 1987). Submucous cleft palate is an occasional finding (Belenchia & McCardle, 1985; D'Antonio, Rice, & Fink, 1998). Some individuals with OAVS exhibit VPI in the absence of a cleft related to palatal and pharyngeal asymmetry. In these cases, the VPI is caused by lack of palatal elevation on the affected side and limited or absent lateral pharyngeal wall motion also on that side (Luce, McGibbon, & Hoopes, 1977; Shprintzen, Croft, Berkman, & Rakoff, 1980). The palate can be observed to elevate asymmetrically toward the unaffected side during the production of "ah."

D'Antonio et al. (1998) described pharyngeal and laryngeal anomalies in a cohort of 23 patients with OASV, including small, underdeveloped larynx with foreshortened vocal folds; omega-shaped epiglottis; narrow airway dimension; small, curled, anteriorly directed epiglottis; and asymmetrical movement of the arytenoids or larynx at rest or during phonation.

The tongue and palatal muscles can be hypoplastic or paralyzed (Cohen et al., 1989). With unilateral involvement, the tongue when protruded will deviate to the affected side (Figure 3–27).

Involvement of the cranial nerves, particularly the facial nerve, can cause

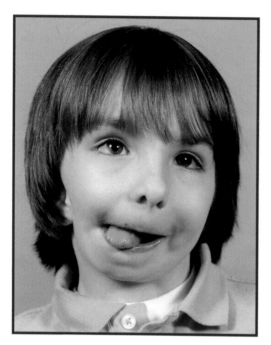

Figure 3–27. Child with oculo-auriculo-vertebral spectrum shown in Figure 3–23. The tongue is shown to deviate to the right or affected side when protruded.

facial asymmetry, drooping of the corner of the mouth, and inability to hold the lips tightly together (Carvalho, Song, Vargervik, & Lalwani, 1999; Rabhar et al., 2001). During smiling or crying, the corner of the mouth may be drawn or pulled to the unaffected side.

Ear Anomalies and Hearing. Preauricular tags and ear pits appearing in the front of the pinna are common, and may be unilateral or bilateral (Figure 3–23C). The pinna can be malformed in a variety of ways, ranging from a slightly misshaped form to small (microtia) to complete absence (anotia) (Figure 3–24) (Bergstrom & Baker, 1981; Phelps, Lloyd, & Poswillo, 1983; Rollnick et al., 1987; Skarżyński, Porowski, & Rodskarbi-Fayette, 2009).

In almost all individuals with unilateral mandibular hypoplasia, the microtic ear is on the same side (ipsilateral) to the mandibular hypoplasia (Rollnick et al., 1987). There is a tendency for a more severely affected ear to be associated with a more severely involved mandible (Figueroa & Pruzansky, 1982).

The external auditory canal can be stenotic or atretic. The middle ear may be hypoplastic or atretic and the ossicles malformed or fused (Rahbar et al., 2001). Abnormalities of the cochlear are rare (Phelps et al., 1983; Rabhar et al., 2002). Outer, middle, and inner ear malformations can co-occur.

The outer and middle ear malformations cause a permanent conductive hearing loss that can range from mild to moderately severe. The inner ear anomalies cause a sensorineural hearing loss, the prevalence of which is said to be higher than once previously thought (Bassila & Goldberg, 1989; Carvalho et al., 1999; Phelps et al., 1983; Rahbar et al., 2001). A mixed hearing loss is possible.

Developmental Features. Intelligence is normal in most with OAVS; however, cognitive and developmental challenges have been observed (Jones, 2006).

Speech and Language. Factors associated with OAVS that can contribute to speech problems include VPI caused by a cleft palate or palatal and pharyngeal asymmetry; malocclusion caused by the mandibular defect; cranial nerve anomalies affecting oromtor function; and hearing loss.

There are few studies of speech and language in this population. Van Lierde, Van Cauwenberge, Stevens, and Dhooge (2004) studied speech and language skills in four children with OAVS (Goldenhar syndrome) aged 4.5 to 10.5 years and found a variety of articulation errors among the participants. Articulation errors were often secondary to malocclusion most commonly characterized by dentalization and interdentalization of sibilants and tip-alveolar consonants. Phonological processing errors included initial and final consonant deletion, cluster reduction, and deletion of unstressed syllable.

Language impairment was documented in three of the four children, including problems with receptive morphology, sentence expression, and comprehension. Belenchia and McCardle (1985) reported on a child with OAVS who presented with delayed language abilities at 12 months of age, but after intervention, these skills were judged to be age appropriate. If severe enough, hearing loss can have an adverse effect on speech and language learning.

Given the small number of subjects in which language was studied, it is difficult to make generalizations. Suffice it to say, children with OAVS are at risk for speech and language problems, the extent to which it occurs warrants further study with a larger population.

Treacher Collins Syndrome (Mandibulofacial Dysostosis)

Clinical Features. Treacher Collins syndrome (TCS) is a craniofacial disorder that is characterized by malar hypoplasia, downward slanting palpebral fissures, ocular coloboma, micrognathia, and ear deformities (Figure 3–28).

In some individuals, malar hypoplasia can be severe enough to be characterized by an actual clefting or absence of the cheekbones. The degree to which the phenotypic features of TCS are expressed ranges from mild to severe. The severity of expression of TCS in the affected parent is not well correlated with the severity of expression in subsequent generations.

TCS is caused by a mutation in the *TCOF1* gene on chromosome 5q32-q33.1. Inheritance is autosomal dominant with variable expressivity. The estimated birth prevalence is approximately 1:50,000 births (Trainor, Dixon, & Dixon, 2009).

Orofacial Features. The mandible is hypoplastic and malformed, characterized by a small vertical ramus, varying degrees of condylar hypoplasia, prominent antegonial notch, and downward curvature of the lower border of the mandible. These features may result in limited mandibular opening and dental crowding. Limited mandibular opening may impair access to the oral cavity for hygiene and treatment (i.e., cleft palate repair, pharyngoplasty, prosthetic speech appliance) (Peterson-Falzone & Figueroa, 1986). The deformity of the mandible and maxilla can result in a Class II malocclusion and anterior open bite that can worsen with age (Figure 3–29).

Cleft palate is present in approximately 30% to 35%, and cleft lip only is rare. Approximately 30% to 40% have other types of velopharyngeal problems including submucous cleft palate, short palate, noncleft palatal dysfunction due to poor muscle function, or oromotor difficulty (Peterson-Falzone & Pruzansky, 1976; Vallino-Napoli, 2002).

Peterson-Falzone and Figueroa (1986) have described the pharyngeal space in TCS as crowded (Figure 3–30). The oropharyngeal lumen is narrow, and the pharyngeal musculature is hypoplastic (Peterson-Falzone & Pruzansky, 1976; Shprintzen, Croft, Berkman, & Rakoff,

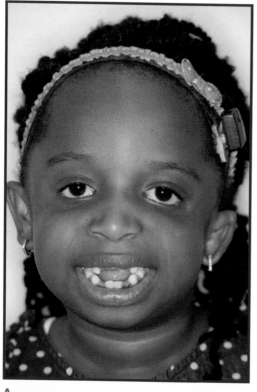

A

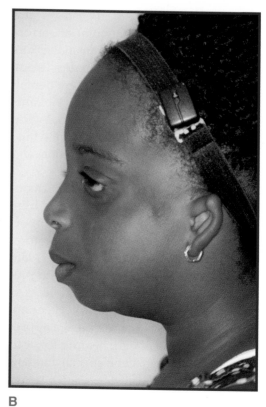

B

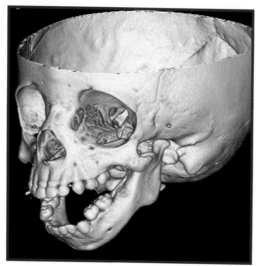

C

Figure 3–28. Frontal (**A**) and profile (**B**) views of a 7-year-old with Treacher Collins syndrome. In **A**, note the downward slant of palpebral fissures, hypoplastic zygomatic arches, and open bite malocclusion. In **B**, note the mandibular hypoplasia and microtia. The three-dimensional CT reconstruction shows missing zygomatic arch and open bite malocclusion (**C**).

1979). If severe, the retrognathia can decrease the pharyngeal diameter. The cranial base in TCS is acute, and as this angulation progresses over time the posterior pharyngeal wall moves forward, which further reduces the pharyngeal

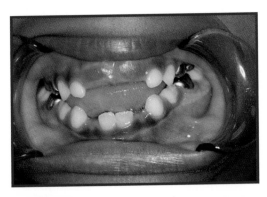

Figure 3–29. Close-up of open-bite maloc-clusion of the child shown in Figure 3–28. Note the tendency for lingual protrusion created by the gap between the upper and lower teeth.

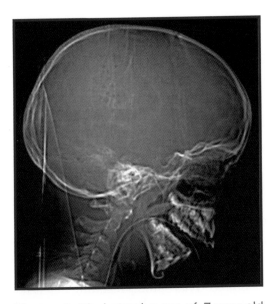

Figure 3–30. Lateral x-ray of 7-year-old child with Treacher Collins syndrome. Note the angle of the mandible, open-bite maloc-clusion, and obliterated airway.

space (Figueroa, 1991; Kreiborg & Dahl, 1993). Posterior choanal atresia, a condi-tion in which the back of the nasal airway (choanae) is blocked, has been reported (Perkins, Sie, Mitzcuk, & Richardson, 1997).

Individuals with TCS are prone to upper airway obstruction occurring at the level of the oropharynx or nasopharynx (see Figure 3–30), and it may be severe enough to require mandibular distraction or tracheostomy (see Chapter 5).

Ear Anomalies and Hearing. Ear abnormali-ties are prominent features of TCS. Defor-mities of the pinna and middle ear are bilateral and usually but not always sym-metrical. The pinna deformities range from minor to severe microtia (see Figure 3–28).

The external auditory canal is typi-cally stenotic or atretic. The middle ear cavity can be hypoplastic and ankylosed or absent ossicles (Hutchinson, Caldarelli, & Valvassori, 1977; Phelps et al., 1981; Pron, Galloway, Armstrong, & Posnick, 1993). The mastoid bone may be poorly pneumatized (Hutchinson et al., 1977; Jahrsdoefer and Jacobson, 1995). Inner ear structures are generally normal in TCS (Pron et al., 1993).

The outer and middle ear anoma-lies cause conductive hearing loss rang-ing from moderate to moderately severe degree with a configuration that is either flat or reverse sloping (Pron et al., 1993). Sensorineural and mixed hearing loss can and does occur in TCS but to a lesser extent (Phelps, Poswillo, & Lloyd, 1981; Pron et al., 1993; Sando, Suehiro, & Wood, 1983).

Developmental Features. Intelligence is usu-ally normal in TCS (Gorlin et al., 2001). Overall development is comparable to that of the general population.

Speech and Language. Factors associ-ated with TCS that can contribute to speech problems are VPI, malocclusion, a crowded oral space, supralaryngeal abnormalities, and hearing loss. The combined effects of the structural and functional abnormalities in those with TCS can compromise intelligibility (Åsten, Akre, & Persson, 2014).

Resonance and Phonation. It is often a challenge to describe resonance in patients with TCS. Certainly, VPI can cause hypernasal speech. However, the crowding of the nasopharyngeal and oropharyngeal airway can alter the perception of "true" hypernasality, making it difficult to judge (Peterson-Falzone, 1981; Vallino, Peterson-Falzone, & Napoli, 2006). The aberrant shape of the supralaryngeal vocal tract can also modify resonance so that some describe it as "muffled" or cul de sac (Peterson-Falzone, 1981; Vallino et al., 2006). Choanal atresia can cause hyponasal speech (Åsten et al., 2014).

Articulation. Vallino-Napoli (2002) reviewed the articulation of 30 patients with TCS ranging from 1.6 to 21 years of age. Findings showed that all patients had articulation errors related to the Class II open bite malocclusion. Phonemes most frequently affected were sibilants, lingual alveolar stops, and bilabial stops. Errors on sibilants were characterized by interdentalizations or lateralizations, a finding also reported by Åsten et al. (2014). Lingual alveolar stops were often interdentalized, and bilabial stops produced labiodentally. Other errors were related to VPI or nondevelopmental phonological process such as an /h/ substitution for fricatives and affricates. Some errors were attributed to the presence of the cannula of the tracheostomy tube. The relatively small size of the oral cavity or pharyngeal hypoplasia in combination with a retracted tongue position can be a contributory factor in the production of pha-

ryngeal stops, fricative, and affricates (Vallino-Napoli, 2002). Many of these findings have also been reported by Åsten et al. (2014).

Language. The literature provides limited data regarding language skills in TCS. Hearing loss can contribute to language impairment, but the effect can be minimized if a child is fit with hearing aids, which can be as early as 3 months of age. If present, developmental delay and intellectual disabilities can cause delays in language development.

Craniosynostosis

Craniosynostosis is a condition in which two or more cranial sutures close prematurely, preventing the skull from growing normally, resulting in a misshaped head. The shape of the head depends on which of the four sutures are fused: sagittal, coronal, metopic, or lambdoidal (Figure 3–31). Two of the more common types of skull deformities associated with craniosynostosis are bicoronal synostosis (brachycephaly) (Figure 3–32) and sagittal synostosis (scaphocephaly) (Figure 3–33). Bicoronal synostosis is caused by premature fusion of both coronal sutures resulting in a head that is spherically shaped. Sagittal synostosis is caused by premature fusion of the sagittal sutures creating a long and narrow head shape.

Craniosynostosis can occur in isolation or as part of a syndrome. When occurring as an isolated condition, the head is misshapen with little to no consequence to the facial skeleton and appearance (Thompson & Britto, 2004). The cause is unknown, and the risk of recurrence is low.

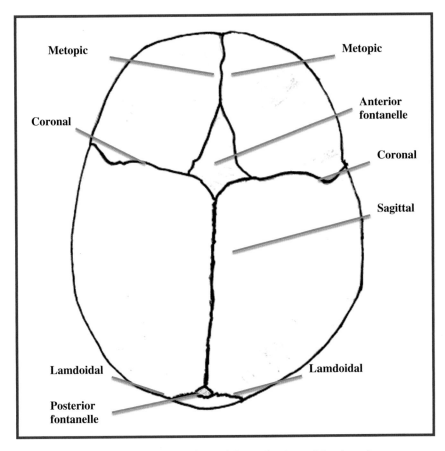

Figure 3–31. Cranial sutures viewed from the top of the head.

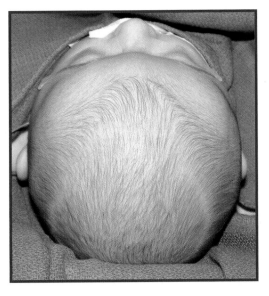

Figure 3–32. Bilateral coronal synostosis (brachycephaly). The head is spherically shaped. (Photo courtesy of Joseph A. Napoli, MD, DDS, Plastic, Maxillofacial, and Craniofacial Surgery, Alfred I. duPont Hospital for Children, Wilmington, DE).

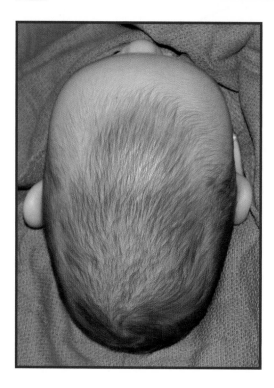

Figure 3–33. Sagittal synostosis (scapho-cephaly). The shape of the head is elongated. (Photo courtesy of Joseph A. Napoli, MD, DDS, Plastic, Maxillofacial, and Craniofacial Surgery, Alfred I. duPont Hospital for Children, Wilmington, DE).

Syndromic craniosynostosis is caused by a mutation in the *FGFR* gene. The role of this gene is to provide instruction to the FGFR protein for bone growth during embryologic development. A mutation on this gene alters the protein, causing premature fusion of the bones of the skull, hands, and feet. The features associated with *FGFR* mutations are hypertelorism, midface hypoplasia, small beaked nose, and prognathism. Syndromic craniosynostosis follows an autosomal dominant pattern of inheritance. Although there are as many as 60 conditions that have craniosynostosis as a feature, we focus on the phenotypic and communication features of three: Apert syndrome, Crouzon syndrome, and Pfeiffer syndrome.

Apert Syndrome (Acrocephalosyndactyly)

Clinical Features. Apert syndrome is characterized by craniosynostosis, midface retrusion, hypertelorism, and hand and feet abnormalities (Figure 3–34). The estimated birth prevalence of Apert syndrome is 15.5 per 1,000,000,000 births (Cohen et al., 1992).

The most commonly involved sutures are the coronal sutures in which early fusion results in a skull that is short in the anteroposterior dimension and elongated vertically (see Figure 3–32). The characteristic facial features are a protuberant frontal region and flat occiput, depressed nasal bridge, beak-like nose, midface hypoplasia, and trapezoidal mouth shape, particularly in the neonatal period (Kreiborg & Cohen, 1992). Patients also exhibit hypertelorism, strabismus, and downward slanting palpebral fissures. The orbits are shallow, causing the eyes to bulge anteriorly or to bulge anteriorly with respect to the orbit, conditions respectively referred to as ocular exophthalmos or proptosis.

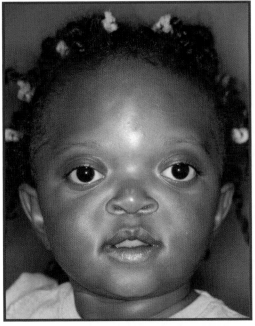 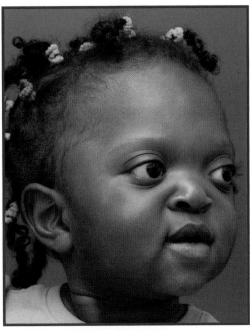

A   B

Figure 3–34. Frontal (**A**) and three-quarter-turn (**B**) views of a toddler with Apert syndrome.

Syndactyly (webbing or bony fusion) of the hands and feet is the most distinguishing feature of Apert syndrome, setting it apart from other craniosynostosis syndromes. It usually occurs symmetrically and with varying severity (Figures 3–35 and 3–36). Figure 3–37 shows X-rays of skeletal abnormalities associated with syndactyly of the hands and feet.

Orofacial Features. The maxilla is hypoplastic and retruded, and the mandible, relative to the maxilla, looks prognathic (referred to as relative prognathism). The deformity of the maxilla and the relationship to the mandible cause a Class III malocclusion and anterior open bite and posterior crossbite.

The upper dental arch is severely constricted, and there is dental crowding. There is also crowding in the mandible but to a lesser degree (Kreiborg & Cohen, 1992). Dental anomalies include delayed eruption of the primary and secondary teeth, ectopic eruption, and shovel-shaped incisors (Kreiborg & Cohen, 1992) with minor anomalies including supernumerary teeth, impacted teeth, missing teeth, and crossbite.

Abnormalities of the palate are common among individuals with Apert syndrome. Reported rates of overt cleft of the soft palate vary between 30% to 40% of the cases and bifid uvula in approximately 34% (Gorlin et al., 2001; Kreiborg & Cohen, 1992) (Figure 3–38). The palate is often highly arched and narrow, with a deep narrow groove, giving it a byzantine or V-shaped appearance. There are lateral swellings on both sides of the palatine process caused by progressive accumulation of soft tissue attributed to excess acid mucopolysaccharide content (Figure

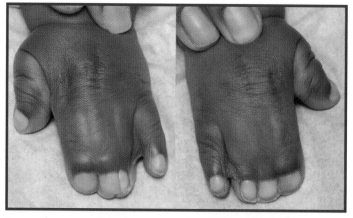

A

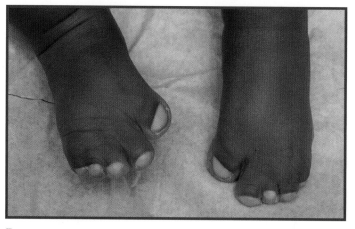

B

Figure 3–35. Syndactyly of the hands (**A**) and feet (**B**) in a toddler with Apert syndrome.

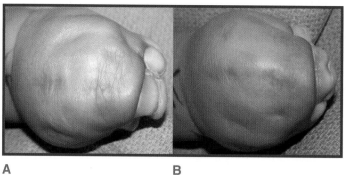

A   B

Figure 3–36. Syndactyly of the hands (**A**) and feet (**B**) that is more severe than that shown in Figure 3–35. (Photo courtesy of Joseph A. Napoli, MD, DDS, Plastic, Maxillofacial, and Craniofacial Surgery, Alfred I. duPont Hospital for Children, Wilmington, DE).

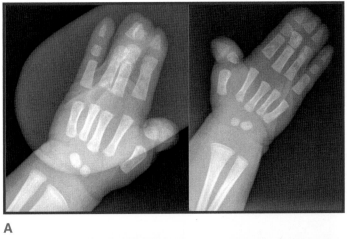

A

B

Figure 3–37. X-rays of skeletal abnormalities of hands (**A**) and feet (**B**) of the toddler with Apert syndrome shown in Figure 3–35.

3–38) (Solomon, Medenica, Pruzansky, & Kreiborg, 1973; Peterson & Pruzansky, 1974). Submucous cleft palate and short palate occur with less frequency.

The pharynx is shallow and reduced in height and depth. The midface hypopla-sia and shallow oropharynx cause an open-mouth posture at rest, anterior tongue car-riage, and obligatory mouth breathing. The soft palate is often abnormally long and thick, and the height and width of the posterior choanae are reduced (Peterson

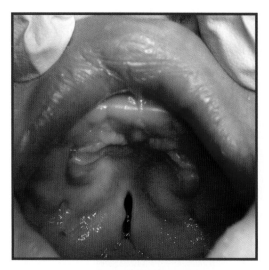

Figure 3–38. Cleft palate in Apert syndrome. Note the lateral swellings on both sides of the palatine process. (Photo courtesy of Joseph A. Napoli, MD, DDS, Plastic, Maxillofacial, and Craniofacial Surgery, Alfred I. duPont Hospital for Children, Wilmington, DE).

& Pruzansky, 1974). These conditions can be severe enough to cause breathing problems requiring physical management (see Chapters 5 and 13).

Tracheal anomalies including a solid cartilaginous tube, tracheal sleeve anomaly, and distal tracheal stenosis have been reported (Cohen & Kreibog, 1990, 1992b). Some individuals will have choanal atresia (Perkins et al., 1997).

Ear Anomalies and Hearing. Almost all individuals with Apert syndrome have low-set ears (Farkas, 1978). The pinnae may be macrotic, microtic, or posteriorly rotated (Bergstrom, Hemenway, & Sando, 1972; Farkas, 1978), and the external auditory canal can be constricted or stenotic (Lindsay, Black, & Donnelly, 1975; Phillips & Miyamoto, 1986). Middle ear anomalies include ossicular chain and stapes fixation (Phillips & Myamoto, 1986). Otitis media

with effusion (OME) is prevalent, caused by a crowded nasopharyngeal space that inhibits normal eustachian tube function (Gould & Caldarelli, 1982; Selder, 1973) (see Chapter 6). The outer and middle ear anomalies cause mild to moderate conductive hearing loss. The presence of OME can exacerbate an already existing loss caused by the structural ear anomalies. Inner ear anomalies causing a sensorineural hearing loss and mixed loss are rare.

Developmental Features. Intellectual disabilities are common; however, normal intelligence has been reported in a few cases (Cohen & Krieborg, 1990). Reports of IQ have consistently shown low scores (average: low 60 to low 70) and learning disabilities (Da Costa et al., 2006; Lefebvre, Travis, Arndt, & Munro, 1986; Patton, Goodship, Hayward, & Landsdown, 1988; Renier et al., 1996). These studies had a number of limitations including subject ascertainment, assessment scale used, and report of full scale IQ that combined performance and verbal scales. In their study of cognition in 10 children with Apert syndrome aged 4;1 to 5;11 years, Shipster, Hearst, Dockrell, Kilby, and Hayward (2002) did in fact, study performance IQ separately from verbal IQ and found that performance IQ fell within the average range (from 88 to 107). Further, IQ scores were considerably higher than reported in previous studies. In their review of this study, Da Costa et al. (2005) commented that the children were young, and it is unclear as to whether they will make developmental gains over time. This remains to be seen.

Problems with attention control and concentration span and parent report of hyperactivity have been documented (Sarimski, 1998; Shipster et al., 2002).

Speech and Language. There are only a few studies of the communication skills in Apert syndrome. Factors associated with Apert syndrome that can cause speech problems include midface hypoplasia and shallow nasopharynx, malocclusion, hearing loss, oromotor dysfunction, and developmental and cognitive impairment. Multiple hospitalizations, surgery, and recovery periods can interrupt opportunities to develop communication skills (e.g., limited play opportunities, regular school attendance) (Elfenbein, Waziri, & Morris, 1981; Shipster, 2004).

Resonance and Phonation. Hyponasal speech is a characteristic feature in Apert syndrome (Peterson-Falzone & Vallino, 1993; Shipster et al., 2002). Some causes of hyponasality include midface hypoplasia; reduced pharyngeal height, width, and depth; long, thick palate (Peterson & Pruzansky, 1974); and choanal stenosis or atresia.

Voice abnormalities including breathiness, reduced loudness, inappropriate high pitch, diplophonia, and "wet" voice have been reported (Shipster et al., 2002).

Articulation. Articulation errors are secondary to Class III malocclusion characterized by blade productions of alveolar consonants and interdentalizations of sibilants (Peterson-Falzone & Vallino, 1993; Shipster et al., 2002). Where the lips cannot approximate, the bilabial stops are produced labiodentally. In the patients they reviewed, Peterson-Falzone & Vallino (1993) also reported errors on /r/ and /l/.

Delayed phonological development is common. Immature phonological processing patterns characterized by stopping of fricatives and affricates, velar fronting, final consonant deletion, voicing for voiceless consonants, and palatoalveolar sounds have been reported (Peterson-Falzone & Vallino, 1993; Shipster et al., 2002).

Some infants with Apert syndrome and unrepaired cleft palate are able to produce bilabial and tip-alveolar stop consonants correctly. The significant midface retrusion seems to effectively obliterate the nasopharyngeal airway to an extent that is sufficient enough to maintain intraoral pressure.

Oromotor Skills. Shipster et al. (2002) reported persistent drooling in 4- and 5-year-olds with Apert syndrome, an age when in most typically developing children it should have subsided (Shipster et al., 2002). Dysarthria has also been documented (Shipster, 2004).

Language. Elfenbein et al. (1981) reported on the language skills of 6 children with craniofacial anomalies, of which 4, ranging in age from 7;0 to 13;0 years, had Apert syndrome. Three children had a receptive and expressive language impairment. In their discussion of this study, Shipster et al. (2002) pointed out that it is unclear whether these difficulties were commensurate with cognitive function or a function of a specific language impairment.

In a later study of 10 children with Apert syndrome (4;1 to 5;11 years), Shipster et al. (2002) reported that 8 children exhibited expressive language difficulties ranging from moderate to severe. Of these, 4 also exhibited severe receptive language impairment. They also found a significant difference between nonverbal composite scores on cognitive testing and receptive language for five children and expressive language for 4 children. Based on these results, Shipster et al. suggested that some children with Apert syndrome may have specific difficulties with language development that are not fully attributed to a general cognitive deficit. This is an area that warrants further study.

Crouzon Syndrome (Craniofacial Dysostosis)

Clinical Features. Crouzon syndrome is characterized by craniosynostosis, mid face hypoplasia, shallow eye orbits, ocular proptosis, and hypertelorism (Figure 3–39).

It is caused by premature closure of the coronal, sagittal, and lambdoidal sutures resulting in a skull shape called brachycephaly (Figure 3–32). Unlike Apert syndrome, individuals with Crouzon syndrome do not have syndactyly, but they do share many of the same structural and functional features as those seen in Apert syndrome.

The estimated birth prevalence of Crouzon syndrome is about 16.5 per million births (Cohen & Kreiborg, 1992a).

Orofacial Anomalies. The maxilla is hypoplastic and retruded, and the mandible, relative to the maxilla, looks prognathic (relative prognathism). The deformity of the maxilla and the relationship to the mandible results in a Class III mal-

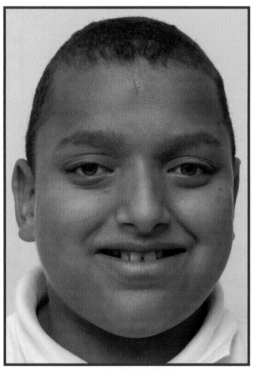
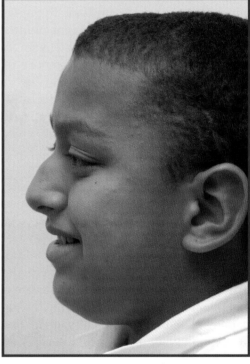

A   B

Figure 3–39. Frontal (**A**) and profile (**B**) views of a 10-year-old with Crouzon syndrome. He has mild proptosis and Class III malocclusion.

occlusion and anterior open bite and posterior crossbite (Kreiborg & Cohen, 1992).

The palate can be high and narrow and cleft of the secondary palate occasionally occurs (Gorlin et al., 2001). As with Apert syndrome, there may be lateral soft tissue swellings of the upper arch mucosa (Peterson & Pruzansky, 1974).

Ear Anomalies and Hearing. Abnormalities of the outer and middle ear structures are common, including external auditory canal atresia or stenosis (Orvidas, Fabray, Diacova, & McDonald, 1999) and ossicular fixation (Cremers, 1981). Middle ear effusion is often present. The presence of fluid behind the eardrum can compound an already existing permanent mild to moderate conductive hearing loss caused by the structural ear anomalies.

Developmental Features. Intelligence is usually within the normal range (Da Costa et al., 2006; Krieborg, 1981; Proudman, Clark, Moore, Abbot, & David, 1995; Noetzel, Marsh, Palkes, & Gado, 1985); few cases of borderline intellect have been reported (Noetzel et al., 1985). Although the prevalence of developmental delay in Crouzon syndrome is low, the diagnosis of craniosynostosis puts these children at-risk for delays and learning challenges. Routine monitoring is justified.

Resonance. Similar to Apert syndrome, hyponasal resonance in Crouzon syndrome is a characteristic feature, caused by midface hypoplasia and crowded nasopharynx that can become more severe with age (Peterson-Falzone, 1981;

Peterson-Falzone, Pruzansky, Parris, & Laffer, 1981).

Articulation. Articulation errors are often secondary to the Class III open-bite malocclusion and abnormal tongue posture (Peterson-Falzone & Vallino, 1993). Phonological impairment in school-age children with Crouzon has been reported (Shipster, 2004).

Language. Shipster (2004) reported that language impairment is more common in children with Crouzon syndrome who are severely affected than mildly affected. Hearing loss, developmental delay, and psychological factors can have an adverse affect on language (Peterson-Falzone, 1981).

Pfeiffer Syndrome

Clinical Features. The phenotypic features of Pfeiffer syndrome are craniosynostosis, midface hypoplasia, synostosis of the elbow, ocular hypertelorism, and small nose with low nasal bridge (Figure 3–40). Limb anomalies including broad, short thumbs and big toes are also characteristic features. The misshapen head in Pfeiffer syndrome is caused by premature closure of the coronal and lambdoidal sutures, and occasionally the sagittal sutures. As a result, there is frontal bossing of the forehead, midface hypoplasia, hypertelorism (widely spaced eyes), and exophthalmos.

The birth prevalence of Pfeiffer syndrome is estimated to be about 1 in 100,000 (Vogels & Fryns, 2006).

There are three subtypes of this disorder based solely on clinical features and severity (Cohen, 1993; Cohen & MacLean, 2000). Type 1 Pfeiffer is considered "classic Pfeiffer" with the aforementioned charac-

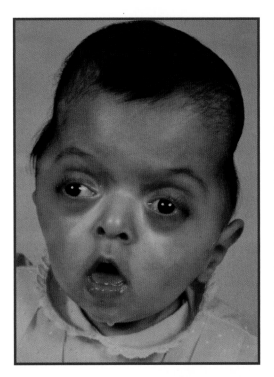

Figure 3–40. Toddler with Pfeiffer syndrome showing mild ocular hypertelorism, low nasal bridge, and maxillary hypoplasia. ("Audiologic and otologic characteristics of Pfeiffer syndrome" by L. D. Vallino-Napoli, 1996, *Cleft Palate-Craniofacial Journal*, *33*, 328. Copyright 1996 by American Cleft Palate Craniofacial Association. Reprinted with permission.)

teristics. Types 2 and 3 are more complex and have a poor prognosis (Cohen, 1993).

Orofacial Features. The midface hypoplasia usually leads to a Class III malocclusion. The maxillary dental arch is severely constricted and V-shaped. Dental anomalies include crowded teeth, supernumerary teeth, delayed dentition, ectopic eruption, missing teeth, and crossbite (Thompson & Britto, 2004).

The palate is often high-arched and narrow. Cleft palate is rare (Stoler et al., 2009). The soft palate is abnormally long

and thick. The pharynx is shallow and reduced in height and depth, and the height and width of the posterior choanae are often reduced. Together, these features can narrow the dimensions of the nasopharyngeal airway and cause upper airway obstruction and sleep apnea (Peteson-Falzone et al., 2001). The shallow oropharynx and anterior tongue carriage can cause obligatory mouth breathing.

Ear Anomalies and Hearing. A number of structural outer and middle ear anomalies have been reported including atresia or stenosis of the bony and cartilaginous portions of the external auditory canal and hypoplasia of the middle ear cavity, enlarged middle ear cavity (Vallino-Napoli, 1996) and ossicular fixation (Cremers, 1981). Middle ear effusion is often present and can further compound the mild to moderate conductive hearing loss caused by the external and middle ear anomalies (Vallino-Napoli, 1996). Inner ear abnormalities are rare (Desai, Rosen, Mulliken, Gopen, Meara, & Rogers, 2010).

Developmental Features. In the absence of cognitive and developmental delays, intelligence in Type 1 Pfeiffer syndrome is usually normal (Cohen & MacLean, 2000). To be sure, craniosynostosis is a risk factor for delays and learning challenges.

Speech and Language. There are few studies of communication skills in individuals with Pfeiffer syndrome. Factors associated with Pfeiffer syndrome contributing to speech impairment are similar to those in Apert and Crouzon syndromes. These include malocclusion, shallow or crowded nasopharynx, and hearing loss.

Hyponasal resonance is caused by the midface hypoplasia and crowded nasopharynx (Peterson-Falzone, 1981). Articulation errors are often secondary to the Class III open-bite malocclusion and abnormal tongue posture. Shipster (2004) reported phonological delay in some children with Pfeiffer syndrome.

Expressive language delay can be mild in Pfeiffer Type 1 and significant in Pfeiffer Types 2 or 3. Certainly, receptive language delay can be manifested in young preschool children, but it appears to be less impaired than expressive language (Shipster, 2004). Language skills can be adversely affected by hearing loss, developmental delay, and psychosocial factors (Peterson-Falzone, 1981).

CHAPTER SUMMARY

Genes play a prominent role in many craniofacial disorders. Traits may be heritable and passed from one generation to the next, or caused by new mutations to the DNA or gene. Some disorders occur as a result of multiple factors. Still, there are disorders for which the etiology is yet unknown. A craniofacial anomaly effects growth of the skull and face that, in turn, has an impact on articulation, resonance, and hearing. Best care for the individual with a craniofacial anomaly not only includes an understanding of the relationship between the structural defect and function, but of cognitive growth and development and individual differences. With this knowledge, the clinician can appropriately assess, diagnose, and successfully manage the communication problems in the unique population.

REFERENCES

Acke, F. R. E., Dhooge, I. J. M., Malfait, F., & Leenheer, E. M. R. (2012). *Orphanet Journal of Rare Diseases, 84.* Retrieved from http://www.ojrd.com/content/7/1/84/additional.

Ahmad, N. N., McDonald-McGinn, D. M., Zackai, E. H., Knowlton, R. G., LaRossa, D., DiMascio, J., & Prockop, D. J. (1993). A second mutation in the type II procollagen gene (COL2A1) causing Stickler syndrome (arthro-ophthalmopathy) is also a premature termination codon. *American Journal of Human Genetics, 52,* 39–45.

All About the Human Genome Project (HGP). (n.d.). Retrieved October 30, 2015, from http://www.genome.gov/10001772

Anderson, P. J., & David, D. J. (2005). Spinal anomalies in Goldenhar syndrome. *Cleft Palate-Craniofacial Journal, 42*(5), 477–480.

Arvystas, M., & Shprintzen, R. J. (1984). Craniofacial morphology in the velocardiofacial syndrome. *Journal of Craniofacial Genetics and Developmental Biology, 4,* 39–45.

Åsten, P., Akre, H., & Persson, C. (2014). Associations between speech features and phenotypic severity in Treacher Collins syndrome. *BMC Medical Genetics, 15,* 47. Retrieved from http//www.biomedcentral.com/1471-2350/15/47

Baker, K. D., & Skuse, D. H. (2005). Adolescents and young adults with 22q11 deletion syndrome: Psychopathology in an at-risk group. *British Journal of Psychiatry, 186,* 115–120.

Bassila, M. K., & Goldberg, R. (1989). The association of facial palsy and/or sensorineural hearing loss in patients with hemifacial microsomia. *Cleft Palate Journal, 26,* 287–291.

Baylis, A. L., Munson, B., & Moller, K. T. (2008). Factor affecting articulation skills with velocardiofacial syndrome and 193 children with cleft palate or velopharyngeal dysfunction. *Cleft Palate-Craniofacial Journal, 45,* 193–207.

Belenchia, P., & McCardle, P. (1985). Goldenhar's syndrome: A case study. *Journal of Communication Disorders, 18,* 383–392.

Bergstrom, L., & Baker, B. B. (1981). Syndromes associated with congenital facial paralysis. *Otolaryngology-Head and Neck Surgery, 89,* 336–342.

Bergstrom, L., Hemenway, W., & Sando, I. (1972). Pathological changes in congenital deafness. *Laryngoscope, 82*, 1777–1792.

Bickmore, W. A. (2001). *Karyotype analysis and chromosome banding* . eLS. doi:10.1038/npg .els.0001160

Black, F. O., Spanier, S. S., & Kohut, R. I. (1975). Aural abnormalities in partial DiGeorge syndrome. *Archives of Otolaryngology, 101*, 129–134.

Botto, L. D., May, K., Fernhoff, P. M., Correa, A., Coleman, K., Rasmussen, S. A., . . . Campbell, R. M. (2003). A population-based study of the 22q11.2 deletion: Phenotype, incidence, and contribution to major birth defects in the population. *Pediatrics, 112*(1 Pt 1), 101–107.

Bromberg, B. E., Pasternak, R., Walden, R. H., & Rubin, L. R. (1961). Evaluation of micrognathia with emphasis on late development of the mandible. *Plastic and Reconstructive Surgery, 28*, 537–548.

Burdick, A. B. (1986). Genetic epidemiology and control of genetic expression in Van der Woude syndrome. *Journal of Craniofacial Genetics and Developmental Biology Supplement, 2*, 99–105.

Burdick, A. B., Bixler, D., & Puckett, C. L. (1985). Genetic analysis in families with Van der Woude syndrome. *Journal of Craniofacial Genetics and Developmental Biology, 5*(2), 181–208.

Carvalho, G. J., Song, C. S., Vargervik, L., & Lalwani, A. K. (1999). Auditory and facial nerve dysfunction in patients with hemifacial microsomia. *Archives of Otolaryngology-Head and Neck Surgery, 125*, 209–212.

Čěrvenka, J., Gorlin, R. J., & Anderson, V. E. (1967). The syndrome of pits of the lower lip and cleft lip and/or palate. Genetic considerations. *American Journal of Human Genetics, 19*(3 Pt 2), 416–432.

Cohen, M. M., Jr. (1979). Syndromology's message for craniofacial biology. *Journal of Maxillofacial Surgery, 7*(2), 89–109.

Cohen, M. M., Jr. (1993). Pfeiffer syndrome update, clinical subtypes, and guidelines for differential diagnosis. *American Journal of Medial Genetics, 45*, 300–307.

Cohen, M. M., Jr. (1999). Robin sequence and complexes: Causal heterogeneity and pathogenetic/phenotypic variability. *American Journal of Medical Genetics, 84*(4), 311–315.

Cohen, M. M., Jr., & Kreiborg, S. (1990). The central nervous system in the Apert syndrome. *American Journal of Medical Genetics, 35*, 36–45.

Cohen, M. M., Jr., & Krieborg, S. (1992a). Birth prevalence studies of the Crouzon syndrome: Comparison of direct and indirect methods. *Clinical Genetics, 41*, 12–15.

Cohen, M. M., Jr., & Krieborg, S. (1992b). Upper and lower airway compromise in the Apert syndrome. *American Journal of Medical Genetics, 44*, 90–93.

Cohen, M. M., Jr., Kreiborg, S., Lammer, E. J., Cordero, J. F., Mastroiacovo, P., Erickson, J. D., . . . Martinex-Frias, M. I. (1992). Birth prevalence study of the Apert syndrome. *American Journal of Medical Genetics, 42*, 655–659.

Cohen, M. M., Jr., & MacClean, R. E. (Eds). (2000). *Craniosynosostosis: Diagnosis, evaluation, and management* (2nd ed.). New York, NY: Oxford University Press.

Cohen, M. M., Jr., Rollnick, B. R., & Kaye, C. I. (1989). Oculoauriculovertebral spectrum: An updated critique. *Cleft Palate Journal, 26*(4), 276–286.

Converse, J. M., Wood-Smith, J. G., McCarthy, J. G., Coccaro, P. J., & Becker, M. H. (1974). Bilateral facial microsomia. *Plastic and Reconstructive Surgery, 54*, 413–423.

Cremers, C. W. (1981). Hearing loss in Pfeiffer' syndrome. *International Journal of Pediatric Otolaryngology, 3*(4), 343–353.

D'Antonio, L. D., & Marsh, J. L. (1987). Abnormal carotid arteries in the velocardiofacial syndrome. *Plastic and Reconstructive Surgery, 80*, 471–472.

D'Antonio, L. L., Rice, R. D., & Fink, S. C. (1998). Evaluation of pharyngeal and laryngeal structure and function in patients with oculo-auriculo-vertebral spectrum. *Cleft Palate-Craniofacial Journal, 35*, 333–341.

D'Antonio, L. L., Scherer, N. J., Miller, L. L., Kalbfleisch, J. H., & Bartley, J. A. (2001).

Analysis of speech characteristics in children with velocardiofacial syndrome (VCFS) and children with phenotypic overlap without VCFS. *Cleft Palate-Craniofacial Journal, 38,* 455–467.

DaCosta, A. C., Savarirayan, R., Wrennall, J. A., Walters, I., Gardiner, N., Tucker, A., Anderson, V., & Meara, J. G. (2005). Neuropsychological diversity in Apert syndrome: A comparison of cognitive function. *Annals of Plastic Surgery, 54,* 450–455.

Da Costa, A. C., Walters, I., Savarirayan, R., Anderson, V. A., Wrennall, J. A., & Meara, J. G. (2006). Intellectual outcomes in children and adolescents with syndromic and nonsyndromic craniosynostosis. *Plastic Reconstructive Surgery, 118,* 175–181.

Davies, D. P., & Evans, D. J. R. (2003). Clinical dysmorphology: Understanding congenital abnormalities. *Clinical Pediatrics, 13,* 288–297.

Desai, U., Rosen, H., Mulliken, J. B., Gopen, Q., Meara, J. G., & Rogers, G. F. (2010). Audiologic findings in Pfeiffer syndrome. *Journal of Craniofacial Surgery, 21,* 1411–1418.

Digilio, M. C., Calzolari, F., Capolino, R., Toscano, A., Sarkozy, A., de Zorzi, A., . . . Marino, B. (2008). Congenital heart defects in patients with oculo-auriculo-vertebral spectrum (Goldenhar syndrome). *American Journal of Medical Genetics, 146A,* 1815–1819.

Digilio, M. C., Marino, B., Caploino, R., & Dallapiccola, B. (2005). Clinical manifestations of deletion 22q11.2 syndrome (DiGeorge/velo-cardio-facial syndrome). *Images in Paediatric Cardiology, 7,* 23–24.

Digilio, M. C., Pacifico, C., Tieri, L., Marino, B., Giannotti, A., & Dallapiccola, B. (1999). Audiological findings in patients with microdeletion 22q11 (DiGeorge/velocardiofacial syndrome). *British Journal of Audiology, 33,* 329–334.

Dobyns, W. B., Filauro, A., Tomson, B. N., Chan, A. S., Ho, A. W., . . . Ober, C. (2004). Inheritance of most X-linked traits is not dominant or recessive, just X-linked. *American Journal of Medical Genetics, 129A,* 136–143.

DuMontcel, S. T., Mendizabal, H., Aymé, S., Lévy, A., & Philip, N. (1996). Prevalence of 22q11 microdeletion. *Journal of American Genetics, 33,* 719.

Elfenbein, J. L., Waziri, M., & Morris, H. L. (1981). Verbal communication skills of children with craniofacial anomalies. *Cleft Palate Journal, 18,* 59–64.

Evans, A. K., Rahbar, R., Rogers, G. F., Mulliken, J. B., & Volk, M. S. (2006). Robin sequence: A retrospective review of 115 patients. *International Journal of Pediatric Otorhinolaryngology, 70,* 973–980.

Evans, K. N., Sie, K. C., Hopper, R. A., Glass, R. P., Hing, A. V., & Cunningham, M. L. (2011). Robin sequence: From diagnosis to development of an effective management plan. *Pediatrics, 127,* 936–948.

Farkas, L. G. (1978). Ear morphology in Treacher Collins', Apert's and Crouzon's syndromes. *Archives of Otorhinolaryngology, 220,* 153–157.

Farkas, L. G., Ross, R. B., & James, J. (1977). Anthropometry of the face in lateral facial dysplasia: The bilateral form. *Cleft Palate Journal, 14,* 41–51.

Figueroa, A. A., & Friede, H. (1985). Craniovertebral malformations in hemifacial microsomia. *Journal of Craniofacial Genetics and Developmental Biology Supplement, 1,* 67–78.

Figueroa, A. A., & Pruzansky, S. (1982). The external ear, mandible, and other components of hemifacial microsomia. *Journal of Maxillofacial Surgery, 10,* 200–211.

Finkelstein, Y., Zohar, Y., Machmani, A., Talmi, Y. P., Lerner, M. A., Hauben, D. J., & Frydman, M. (1993). The otolaryngologist and the patient with velocardiofacial syndrome. *Archives of Otolaryngology-Head and Neck Surgery, 119,* 563–569.

Fraser, F. C. (1976). The multifactorial/threshold concept—Uses and misuses. *Teratology, 14,* 267–280.

Gennery, C. (2012). Immunological aspects of 22q11.2 deletion syndrome. *Cellular and Molecular Life Sciences, 69,* 17–27. doi:10.1007/s00018-011-0842-z

Gerdes, M., Solot, C., Wang, P. P., Moss, E., LaRoss, D., Randall, P., . . . Zackai, E. H. (1999). Cognitive and behavioral profile of preschool children with chromosome 22q11.2 deletion. *American Journal of Medical Genetics, 85,* 127–133.

Gilbert-Barness, E. (2010). Review: Teratogenic causes of malformations. *Annals of Clinical & Laboratory Sciences, 40,* 99–113.

Glaser, B., Mumme, D. L., Blasey, C., Morris, M. A., Daboun, S. P., Antonarakis, S., . . . Eliez, S. (2002). Language skills in children with velocardiofacial syndrome (deletion 22q11.2). *Journal of Pediatrics, 140,* 753–758.

Goldberg, R., Motzkin, B., Marion, R., Scambler, P. J., & Shprintzen, R. J. (1993). Velocardio-facial syndrome: A review of 120 patients. *American Journal of Medical Genetics, 45,* 313–319.

Golding-Kushner, K. J., Weller, G., & Shprintzen, R. (1985). Velo-cardio-facial syndrome: Language and psychological profiles. *Journal of Craniofacial Genetics and Developmental Biology, 5,* 259–266.

Goldmuntz, E., Clark, B. J., Mitchell, L. E., Jawad, A. F., Cuneo, B. F., Reed, L., . . . Driscoll, D. A. (1998). Frequency of 22q11 deletions in patients with conotruncal defects. *Journal of the American College of Cardiology, 32,* 492–498.

Goorhuis-Brouwer, S. M., Dikkers, F. G., Robinson, R. H., & Kerstjens-Frederikse, W. S. (2003). Specific language impairment in children with velocardiofacial syndrome: Four cases. *Cleft Palate-Craniofacial Journal, 40,* 190–195.

Gordon, H., Davies, D., & Friedberg, S. (1969). Congenital pits of the lower lip with cleft lip and palate. *South African Medical Journal, 43,* 1275–1279.

Gorlin, R. J., & Baylis, A. (2009). Embryologic and genetic aspects of clefting and selected craniofacial anomalies. In K. T. Moller & L. E. Glaze (Ed.), *Cleft lip and palate: Interdisciplinary issues and treatment* (2nd ed., pp. 103–169.). Austin, TX: Pro-Ed.

Gorlin, R. J., Cohen, M. M., Jr., & Hennekam, R. C. M. (2001). *Syndromes of the head and neck* (4th ed.). New York, NY: Oxford University Press.

Gould, H. J., & Caldarelli, D. D. (1982). Hearing and otopathology in Apert syndrome. *Archives of Otolaryngology, 108,* 347–349.

Grabb, W. C. (1965). The first and second branchial arch syndrome. *Plastic and Reconstructive Surgery, 36,* 485–508.

Havkin, N., Tatum III, S. A., & Shprintzen, R. J. (2000). Velopharyngeal insufficiency and articulation impairment in velo-cardiofacial syndrome: The influence of adenoids on phonemic development. *International Journal of Pediatric Otolarynogology, 54,* 103–110.

Herrmann, J., France, T. D., Spranger, J. W., Opitz, J. M., & Wiffler, C. (1975). The Stickler syndrome (hereditary arthroophthalmopathy). *Birth Defects Original Article Series, 11*(2), 76–103.

Hutchinson, J., Caldarelli, D., & Valvassori, G. (1977). The otologic manifestations of mandibulo-facial dystosis. *Transactions-American Academy of Ophthalmology and Otolaryngology, 84,* 520–528.

Jahrsdoerfer, R. A., & Jacobson, J. T. (1995). Treacher Collins syndrome: Otologic and auditory management. *Journal of the American Academy of Audiology, 6,* 95–102.

Janku, P., Robinow, M., Kelly, T., Bralley, R., Baynes, A., & Edgerton, M. T. (1980). The Van der Woude syndrome in a large kindred: Variability, penetrance, genetic risks. *American Journal of Medical Genetics, 5,* 117–123.

Jones, K. L. (2006). *Recognizable patterns of human malformation* (6th ed.). Philadelphia, PA: Elsevier Saunders.

Kamen, R. S., & Watson, B. C. (1991). Effects of long-term tracheostomy on spectral characteristics of vowel production. *Journal of Speech, Language, and Hearing Research, 34,* 1057–1065.

Knowlton, R. G., Weaver, E. J., Struyk, A. F., Knobloch, W. H., King, R. A., Norris, K., . . . Prockop, D. J. (1989). Genetic linkage analysis of hereditary arthro-ophthalmopathy (Stickler syndrome) and the type II procollagen gene. *American Journal of Human Genetics, 45,* 681–688.

Kondo, S., Schutte, B. C., Richardson, R. J., Bjork, B. C., Knight, A. S., Watanabe, Y., . . . Murray, J. C. (2002). Mutations in IRF6 cause Van der Woude and popliteal pterygium syndromes. *Nature Genetics, 32,* 2, 285–289.

Krieborg, S. (1981). Crouzon syndrome: A clinical and roentgencephalometric study. *Scandinavian Journal of Plastic and Reconstructive Surgery Supplement, 18,* 1–198.

Kreiborg, S., & Cohen, M. M., Jr. (1992). The oral manifestations of Apert syndrome. *Journal of Craniofacial Genetics and Developmental Biology, 12,* 41–48.

Kreiborg, S., & Dahl, E. (1993). Cranial base and face in mandibulofacial dysostosis. *American Journal of Medical Genetics, 47,* 753–760.

Kummer, A. W., Lee, L., Stutz, L. S., Maroney, A., & Brandt, J. W. (2007). The prevalence of apraxia characteristics in patients with velocardiofacial syndrome as compared with other cleft population. *Cleft Palate-Craniofacial Journal, 44,* 175–191.

LeBlanc, S. M., & Golding-Kushner, K. J. (1992). The effect of glossopexy on speech sound production in Robin sequence. *Cleft Palate-Craniofacial Journal, 29,* 239–245.

Lefebvre, A., Travis, F., Arndt, E. M., & Munro, I. R. (1986). A psychiatric profile before and after reconstructive surgery in children with Apert syndrome. *British Journal of Plastic Surgery, 39,* 310–313.

Liberfarb, R. M., & Goldblatt, A. (1986). Prevalence of mitral valve prolapse in the Stickler syndrome. *American Journal of Medical Genetics, 245,* 387–392.

Lindsay, J., Black, F., & Donnelly, W. (1975). Acrocephalosyndactyly (Apert syndrome): Temporal bone findings. *Annals of Otology, Rhinology & Laryngology, 84,* 174–178.

Luce, E., McGibbon, B., & Hoopes, H. (1977). Velopharyngeal insufficiency in hemifacial microsomia. *Plastic and Reconstructive Surgery, 60,* 602–606.

MacKenzie-Stepner, K., Witzel, M. A., Stringer, D. A., Lindsay, W. K., Munro, I. R., & Hughes, H. (1987). Abnormal carotid arteries in the velocardiofacial syndrome: A report of three cases. *Plastic and Reconstructive Surgery, 80,* 347–351.

Marques, I. L., Barbieri, M. C., & Bettiol, H. (1998). Etiopathogenesis of isolated Robin sequence. *Cleft Palate-Craniofacial Journal, 35,* 517–525.

Marino, B., Digilio, M. C., Toscano, A., Anaclerio, S., Gianotti, A., Feltri, C., . . . Dallapiccola, A. (2001). Anatomic patterns of conotruncal defects associated with deletion 22q11. *Genetics in Medicine, 3(1),* 45–48.

Marino, B., Digilio, M. C., Toscano, A., Giannotti, A., & Dallapiccola, B. (1999). Congenital heart defects in patients with DiGeorge/Velocardiofacial syndrome and del22q11. *Genetic Counseling, 10,* 25–33.

McCarthy, J. G. (2007). Craniofacial microsomia. In C.H. Thorne (Ed.), *Grabb and Smith's plastic surgery* (6th ed., pp. 248–255). Philadelphia, PA: Lippincott Williams & Wilkins.

McDonald-McGinn, D. M., Driscoll, D. A., Emanuel, B. S., Goldmuntz, E., Clark III, B. J., Cohen, M., . . . Zackai, E. H. (1997). Detection of a 22q11.2 deletion in cardiac patients suggests a risk for velopharyngeal incompetence. *Pediatrics, 99(5),* E9.

McDonald-McGinn, D. M., Kirschner, R., Goldmuntz, E., Sullivan, K., Eicher, P., Gerdes, M., . . . Zackai, E. H. (1999). The Philadelphia story: the 22q11.2 deletion: report on 250 patients. *Genetic Counsellors, 10,* 11–24.

Ming, J. E., McDonald-McGinn, D. M., Megerian, T. E., Driscooll, D. A., Elias, E. R., Russell, B. M., . . . Zackai, E. H. (1997). Skeletal anomalies and deformities in patients with deletions of 22q11. *American Journal of Medical Genetics, 72,* 200–215.

Moss, E. J., Batshaw, M. L., Solot, C., Gerdes, M., McDonald-McGinn, D. M., Driscoll, D., . . . Wang, P. (1999). Psychoeducational profile of the 22q11.2 microdeletion syndrome. *Journal of Pediatrics, 134,* 193–198.

Murphy, K. C., Jones, R. G., & Owen, M. J. (1999). High rates of schizophrenia in adults with velocardiofacial syndrome. *Archives of General Psychiatry, 56*, 940–945.

National Human Genome Research Institute. (2015). *Fluorescence in situ hybridization (FISH).* Retrieved from https://www.genome.gov/10000206

National Institutes of Health. National Human Genome Research Institute. (n.d.). *Talking glossary of genetic terms.* Retrieved from http://www.genome.gov/glossary/

Noetzel, M., Marsh, J., Palkes, H., & Gado, M. (1985). Hydrocephalus and mental retardation in craniosynostosis. *Journal of Pediatrics, 107*, 885–892.

Nowack, C. B. (1998). Genetics and hearing loss: A review of Stickler syndrome. *Journal of Communication Disorders, 31*, 437–454.

Nussbaum, R. L., McInnes, R. R., & Willard, H. F. (2004). *Thompson & Thompson genetics in medicine* (6th ed.). Philadelphia, PA: Saunders.

Oostlander, A. E., Meijer, G. A., & Ylstra, B. (2004). Microarray-based comparative genomic hybridization and its applications in human genetics. *Clinical Genetics, 66.* 488–495.

Orvidas, L. J., Fabry, L. B., Diacova, S., & McDonald, T. J. (1999). Hearing and otopathology in Crouzon syndrome. *Laryngoscope, 109*, 1372–1375.

Patton, M. A., Goodship, J., Hayward, R., & Landsdown, R. (1988). Intellectual development in Apert syndrome: A long term follow up of 29 patients. *Journal of Medical Genetics, 25*, 164–167.

Pergament, E. (2008). Cytogenetics. *Global Library of Women's Medicine.* doi:10.3843/GLOWM.10342

Perkins, J. A., Sie, K. C., Mitzcuk, H., & Richardson, M. A. (1997). Airway management in children with craniofacial anomalies. *Cleft Palate-Craniofacial Journal, 34*(2), 135–140.

Persson, C., Lohmander, A., Jönsson, R., Óskarsdottir, S., & Söderpalm, E. (2003). A prospective cross-sectional study of speech in patients with the 22q11 deletion syndrome. *Journal of Communication Disorders, 36*, 13–47.

Persson, C., Niklasson, L., Óskarsdottir, S., Johansson, S., Jönsson, R., & Söderpalm, E. (2006). Language skills in 5- to 8-year-old children with 22q11 deletion syndrome. *International Journal of Language and Communication Disorders, 41*, 313–333.

Peterson, S. J. (1973). Speech pathology in craniofacial malformations other than cleft lip and palate. In R. E. Wertz (Ed.), *Orofacial anomalies: Clinical and research implications.* ASHA Reports No. 111–131.

Peterson, S. J., & Pruzansky, S. (1974). Palatal anomalies in the syndromes of Apert and Crouzon. *Cleft Palate Journal, 11*, 394–402.

Peterson-Falzone, S. J. (1981). Impact of communicative disorders on otolaryngologic care of patients with craniofacial anomalies. *Otolaryngology Clinics of North America, 14*, 895–915.

Peterson-Falzone, S. J., & Figueroa, A. S. (1986). Longitudinal changes in cranial base angulation in mandibulofacial dysostosis. *Cleft Palate Journal, 26*, 14–22.

Peterson-Falzone, S. J., Hardin-Jones, M. S., & Karnell, M. P. (2010). *Cleft palate speech* (4th ed.). St. Louis, MO: Mosby.

Peterson-Falzone, S. J., & Pruzansky, S. (1976). Cleft palate and congenital palatopharyngeal incompetency in mandibulofacial dysostosis: Frequency and problems in treatment. *Cleft Palate Journal, 13*, 354–360.

Peterson-Falzone, S. J., Pruzansky, S., Parris, P. J., & Laffer, J. L. (1981). Nasopharyngeal dysmorphology in the syndromes of Apert and Crouzon. *Cleft Palate Journal, 18*, 237–250.

Peterson-Falzone, S. J., & Vallino, L. D. (1993). *A longitudinal perspective on communication development in 113 patients with 4 syndromes of craniofacial synostosis.* Presented at the Seventh International Congress on Cleft Palate and Related Craniofacial Anomalies, Queensland.

Phelps, P. D., Lloyd, G. A. S., & Poswillo, D. E. (1993). The ear deformities in craniofacial microsomia and oculo-auriculo-vertebral dysplasia. *Journal of Laryngology and Otology, 97*(11), 995–1005.

Phelps, P. D., Poswillo, D., & Lloyd, G. A. S. (1981). The ear deformity in mandibularofacial dysostosis (Treacher Collins syndrome). *Clinics in Otolaryngology, 6,* 15–28.

Philips, S. G., & Miyamoto, R. T. (1986). Congenital conductive hearing loss in Apert syndrome. *Otolaryngology-Head and Neck Surgery, 95,* 429–433.

Poswillo, D. E. (1973). The pathogenesis of the first and second branchial arch syndrome. *Oral Surgery, 35*(3), 302–328.

Printzlau, G., & Andersen, M. M. (2004). Pierre Robin sequence in Denmark: A retrospective population-based epidemiological study. *Cleft Palate-Craniofacial Journal, 41,* 47–52.

Pron, G., Galloway, C., Armstrong, D., & Posnick, J. (1993). Ear malformation and hearing loss in patients with Treacher Collins syndrome. *Cleft Palate-Craniofacial Journal, 30,* 97–103.

Proudman, T. X., Clark, B. E., Moore, M. H., Abbot, A. H., & David, D. J. (1995). Central nervous system imaging in Crouzon's syndrome. *Journal of Craniofacial Surgery, 6,* 401–405.

Rahbar, R., Robson, C. D., Mulliken, J. B., Schwartz, L., Dicanzio, J., Kenna, M. A., McGill, T. J., & Healy, G. B. (2001). Craniofacial, temporal bone, and audiologic abnormalities in the spectrum of hemifacial microsomia. *Archives of Otolaryngology-Head and Neck Surgery, 127*(3), 265–271.

Ranta, R., & Rintala, A. E. (1983). Correlations between microforms of the Van der Woude syndrome and cleft palate. *Cleft Palate Journal, 20,* 158–162.

Rarechromo.org Microarray-based comparative genomic hybridisation. (n.d.). Retrieved October 11, 2015.

Renier, D., Arnaud, E., Cinally, G., Sebag, G., Kerah, M. & Marchac, D. (1996). Prognosis for mental functioning in Apert syndrome. *Journal of Neurosurgery, 85,* 66–72.

Reyes, M. R. R., LeBlanc, E. M., & Bassila, M. K. (1999). Hearing loss and otitis media in velocardio-facial syndrome. *International Journal of Pediatric Otorhinolaryngology, 47,* 227–233.

Rintala, A. E., & Ranta, R. (1981). Lower lip sinuses: I. Epidemiology, microforms, and transverse sulci. *British Journal of Plastic Surgery, 34,* 26–30.

Rintala, A., Ranta, R., & Stegars, T. (1984). On the pathogenesis of cleft palate in the Pierre Robin syndrome. *Scandinavian Journal of Plastic and Reconstructive Surgery, 18,* 237–240.

Robin, N. H., Moran, R. T., Warman, M., & Ala-Kokko, L. (2011). In R. A. Pagon, T. C. Bird, & C. R. Dolan (Ed.), *GeneReviews* [Internet]. Seattle, WA: University of Washington. Stickler syndrome. 1993 Jun 9 [Updated 2011 Nov 3].

Robin, P. (1923). A drop of the base of the tongue considered as a new cause of nasopharyngeal respiratory impairment [in French]. *Bulletin De L Academie Nationale De Medecine, 89,* 37–41.

Rollnick, B. R., Kaye, C. I., Nagatoshi, K., Hauck, W., & Martin, A. O. (1987). Oculo-auriculovertebral dysplasia and variants: Phenotypic characteristics of 294 patients. *American Journal of Medical Genetics, 26,* 361–375.

Rommel, N., VanTrappern, G., Swillen, A., Devriendt, K., Feenstra, L., & Fryns, J. P. (1999). Retrospective analysis of feeding and speech disorders in 50 patients with velo-cardio-facial syndrome. *Genetic Counseling, 10*(1), 71–78.

Rose, P. S., Levy, H. P., Liberfarb, R. M., Davis, J., Szymko-Bennett, Y., Rubin, B. I., . . . Francomano, C. A. (2005). Stickler syndrome: Clinical characteristics and diagnostic criteria. *American Journal of Medical Genetics, 138A,* 199–207.

Ross, R. B. (1975). Lateral facial dysplasia (first and second branchial arch syndrome, hemifacial microsomia). *Birth Defects: Original Article Series, 11*(7), 51–59.

Ross, D. A., Witzel, M. A., Armstrong, D. C., & Thomson, G. H. (1996). Is pharyngoplasty a risk in velocardiofacial syndrome? An assessment of medically displaced carotid arteries. *Plastic and Reconstructive Surgery, 98*, 1182–1190.

Ruotolo, R. A., Veitia, N. A., Corbin, A., McDonough, J., Solot, C. B., McDonald-McGinn, D., . . . Kirschner, R. E. (2006). Velopharyngeal anatomy in 22q11.2 deletion syndrome: A three-dimensional cephalometric analysis. *Cleft Palate-Craniofacial Journal, 43*, 446–456.

Ryan, A. K., Goodship, J. A., Wilson, D. I., Philip, N., Levy, A., Seidel, H., . . . Scambler, P. J. (1997). Spectrum of clinical features associated with interstitial chromosome 22q11 deletions: A European collaborative study. *Journal of Medical Genetics, 34*, 798–804.

Saal, H. M. (2008). The genetic evaluation and common craniofacial syndromes. In A.W. Kummer (Ed.), *Cleft palate and craniofacial anomalies: Effects on speech and resonance* (2nd ed., pp. 86–118). Clifton Park, NY: Delmar Cengage.

Sando, I., Suehiro, S., & Wood, R. P. (1983). Congenital anomalies of the external and middle ear. In C. Blueston & S. Stool (Eds.), *Pedatirc Otoloaryngology.* (Vol. 1, pp. 309–346). Philadelphia, PA: Saunders.

Sarimski, K. (1998). Children with Apert syndrome: Behavioural problems and family stress. *Developmental Medicine and Child Neurology, 40*, 44–49.

Scherer, N. J., D'Antonio, L. L., & Kalbfleisch, J. H. (1999). Early speech and language development in children with velocardiofacial syndrome. *American Journal of Medical Genetics, 88*, 714–723.

Scherer, N. J., D'Antonio, L. L., & Rodgers, J. R. (2001). Profiles of communication disorder in children with velocardiofacial syndrome: Comparison to children with Down syndrome. *Genetics in Medicine, 3*, 72–78.

Schinzel, A., & Kläusler, M. (1986). The Van der Woude syndrome (dominantly inherited lip pits and clefts). *Journal of Medical Genetics, 23*, 291–294.

Schneider, E. L. (1973). Lip pits and congenital absence of second premolars: Varied expression of the lip pits syndrome. *Journal of Medical Genetics, 10*, 346–349.

Schutte, B. C., Sander, A., Malik, M., & Murray, J. C. (1996). Refinement of the Van der Woude gene location and construction of a 3.5-Mb YAC contig and STS map spanning the critical region in 1q32-q41. *Genomics, 36*, 507–514.

Seery, C. M., Pruett, R. C., Liberfarb, R. M., & Cohen, B. Z. (1990). Distinctive cataract in the Stickler syndrome. *American Journal of Ophthalmology, 110*, 143–148.

Selder, A. (1973). Hearing disorders in children. *ASHA Reports, #8: Orofacial anomalies: clinical and research implications* (pp. 95–110). Washington, DC: American Speech and Hearing Association.

Shaw, W. C., & Simpson, J. P. (1980). Oral adhesions associated with cleft lip and palate and lip fistulae. *Cleft Palate Journal, 17*, 127–131.

Shipster, C. (2004). Speech and language characteristics of children with craniosynostosis. In R. Hayward, B. Jones, D. Dunaway, & R. Evans (Eds.), *The clinical management of craniosynostosis* (pp. 270–298). London, UK: Mac Keith Press.

Shipster, C., Hearst, D., Dockrell, J. E., Kilby, E., & Hayward, R. (2002). Speech and language skills and cognitive functioning in children with Apert syndrome: A pilot study. *International Journal of Language and Communication Disorders, 37*, 325–343.

Shprintzen, R. J. (1988). Pierre Robin, micrognathia, and airway obstruction: The dependency of treatment on accurate diagnosis. *International Anesthesiology Clinics, 26*, 64–71.

Shprintzen, R. J. (1992). The implications of the diagnosis of Robin sequence. *Cleft Palate-Craniofacial Journal, 29*, 205–209.

Shprintzen, R. J. (2000). Velocardiofacial syndrome. *The Otolaryngologic Clinics of North America (Syndromic and Other Congenital Anomalies of the Head and Neck), 33*, 1217–1240.

Shprintzen, R. J. (2008). Velo-cardio-facial syndrome: 30 years of study. *Developmental Disability Research Review, 14*, 3–10.

Shprintzen, R. J., Croft, C. B., Berkman, M. D., & Rakoff, S. J. (1980). Velopharyngeal insufficiency in the facio-auriculo-vertebral malformation complex. *Cleft Palate Journal, 17*, 132–137.

Shprintzen, R. J., Goldberg, R. B., Golding-Kushner, K. J., & Marion, R. (1992). Late-onset psychosis in velo-cardio-facial syndromes [Letter]. *American Journal of Medical Genetics, 42*, 141–142.

Shprintzen, R. J., Goldberg, R. B., Lewin, M. L., Sidoti, E. J., Berkman, M. D., Argamaso, R.V. & Young, D. (1978). A new syndrome involving cleft palate, cardiac anomalies, typical facies, and learning disabilities: Velo-cardio-facial syndrome. *Cleft Palate Journal, 5*, 56–62.

Shprintzen, R. J., Goldberg, R. B., & Sidoti, E. J. (1980). The penetrance and variable expression of the Van der Woude syndrome: Implications for genetic counseling. *Cleft Palate Journal, 17*, 52–57.

Shprintzen, R. J., Goldberg, R., Young, D., & Wolford, L. (1981). The velo-cardio-facial syndrome: A clinical and genetic analysis. *Pediatrics, 67*, 167–172.

Siegel-Sadewitz, V., & Shprintzen, R. J. (1982). The relationship of communication disorders to syndrome identification. *Journal of Speech and Hearing Disorders, 47*, 338–354.

Skarżyński, H., Porowski, M., & Rodskarbi-Fayette, R. (2009). Treatment of ontological features of the oculoauriculovertebral dysplasia (Goldenhar syndrome). *International Journal of Pediatric Otorhinolaryngology, 73*, 915–921.

Smith, C. (1971). Recurrence risks for multifactorial inheritance. *American Journal of Human Genetics, 23*, 578–588.

Smith, C. A., Driscoll, D. A.,Emanuel, B. S., McDonald-McGinn, D. M., Zackai, E. H. & Sullivan, K. E. (1998). Increased prevalence of immunoglobulin A deficiency in patients with the chromosome 22q11.2 deletion syndrome (DiGeorge syndrome/velocardiofacial syndrome). *Clinical and Diagnostic Laboratory Immunology, 5*, 415–417.

Snead, M. P., & Yates, J. R. W. (1999). Clinical and molecular genetics of Stickler syndrome. *Journal of Medical Genetics, 36*(5), 353–359.

Solomon, L. M., Medenica, M., Pruzansky, S., & Kreiborg, S. (1973). Apert syndrome and palatal mucopolysaccharides. *Teratology, 8*, 287–292.

Solot, C. B., Gerdes, M., Kirschner, R. E., McDonald-McGinn, D. M., Moss, E., Wardin, M., . . . Want, P. P. (2001). Communications issues in 22q11.2 deletion syndrome: Children at risk. *Genetics in Medicine, 3*, 67–71.

Solot, C. B., Handler, S. D., Gerdes, M., McDonald-McGinn, D. M., Moss, E., Wang, P., . . . Droscoll, D. A. (2000). Communication disorders in the 22q11.2 microdeletion syndrome. *Journal of Communication Disorders, 33*(3), 187–204.

Sparks, S. N. (1984). *Birth defects and speech-language disorders*. San Diego, CA: College-Hill Press.

Spranger, J., Benirschke, K., Hall, J. G., Lenz, W., Lowry, R. B., Opitz, J. M., . . . Smith, D. W. (1982). Errors of morphogenesis: Concepts and terms. Recommendations of an International Working Group. *Journal of Pediatrics, 100*, 160–165.

Stickler, G. B., Belay, P. G., Farrell, F. J., Jones, J. D., Pugh, D. G., Steinberg, A. G., & Ward, L. E. (1965). Hereditary progressive arthro-ophthalmopathy. *Mayo Clinical Proceedings, 40*(8), 433–455.

Stickler, G. B., Hughes, W., & Houchin, P. (2001). Clinical features of hereditary progressive arthroophthalmopathy (Stickler syndrome): A survey. *Genetics in Medicine, 3*, 192–196.

Stickler, G. B., & Pugh, D. G. (1967). Hereditary progressive arthroophthalmopathy II. Additional observations on vertebral abnormalities: A hearing defect, and a report of a similar case. *Mayo Clinic Proceedings, 42*, 495–500.

Stoler, J. M., Rosen, H., Desai, U., Mulliken, J. B., Meara, J. G., & Rogers, G. F. (2009). Cleft palate in Pfeiffer syndrome. *Journal of Craniofacial Surgery, 20*, 1375–1377.

Sullivan, K. E., McDonald-McGinn, D., & Zackai, E. H. (2002). CD4(+) CD25(+)

T-cell production in healthy humans and in patients with thymic hypoplasia. *Clinical and Diagnostic Laboratory Immunology, 9,*1129–1131.

Swillen, A., Devriendt, K., Ghesquiere, P., & Fryns, J.-P. (2001). Children with a 22q11 deletion versus children with a speech-language impairment and learning disability: Behavior during primary school-age. *Genetic Counseling, 12,* 309–317.

Swillen, A., Devriendt, K., Legius, E., Eyskens, B., Dumoulin, M., Gewelling, M., & Fryns, J.-P. (1997). Intelligence and psychosocial adjustment in velocardiofacial syndreom (VCFS): A study of 37 children and adolescents with VCFS. *Journal of Medical Genetics, 34,* 453–458.

Swillen, A., Devriendt, K., Legius, E., Prinzie, P., Vogels, A., Ghesquiere, P., & Fryns, J.-P. (1999). The behavioral phenotype in velo-cardio-facial syndrome (VCFS): From infancy to adolescence. *Genetic Counseling, 10,* 79–88.

Szymko-Bennett, Y. M., Mastroianni, M. A., Shotland, L. I., Davis, J., Ondrey, F. G., Balog, J. Z., . . . Griffith, A. J. (2001). Auditory dysfunction in Stickler syndrome. *Archives of Otolaryngology-Head and Neck Surgery, 127,* 1061–1068.

Tan, T. Y., Kilpatrick, N., & Farlie, P. G. (2013). Developmental and genetic perspectives on Pierre Robin Sequence. *American Journal of Medical Genetics Part C (Seminars in Medical Genetics), 163C,* 295–305.

Theisen, A. (2008). Microarray-based comparative genomic hybridization (aCGH). *Nature Education, 1,* 45.

Thompson, D. N. P., & Britto, F. (2004). Classification and clinical diagnosis. In R. Hayward, B. Jones, D. Dunaway, & R. Evans (Eds.), *The clinical management of craniosynostosis.* London, UK: Mac Keith Press.

Trainor, P. A., Dixon, J., & Dixon, M. J. (2009). Treacher Collins syndrome: Etiology, pathogenesis and prevention. *European Journal of Human Genetics, 17,* 275–283.

Trainor, P. A., & Richtsmeier, J. T. (2015). Facing up to the challenges of advancing cra-niofacial research. *American Journal of Medical Genetics* A, *167,* 1451–1454.

Understanding chromosome disorders. Fluorescence in situ hybridization (FISH). (n.d.). Retrieved from Unique website: http://www.rarechromo.org/information/other/fish ftnw.pdf

Understanding chromosome disorders. Microarray-based comparative genomic hybridization. (n.d.). Retrieved from Unique website: http://www.rarechromo.org/information/other/arraycgh ftnw.pdf

Vallino-Napoli, L. D. (1996). Audiologic and otologic characteristics of Pfeiffer syndrome. *Cleft Palate-Craniofacial Journal, 33,* 524–529.

Vallino-Napoli, L. D. (2002). A profile of the features and speech in patients with mandibulofacial dysostosis. *Cleft Palate-Craniofacial Journal, 39,* 623–634.

Vallino, L. D., Peterson-Falzone, S. J., & Napoli, J. A. (2006). The syndromes of Treacher Collins and Nager. *Advances in Speech Language Pathology, 8,* 34–44.

Van der Woude, A. (1954). Fistula labii inferioris congenital and its association with cleft lip and palate. *American Journal of Human Genetics, 6,* 244–256.

Van Lierde, K. M., Van Cauwenberge, P., Stevens, I., & Dhooge, I. (2004). Language, articulation, voice, and resonance characteristics in 4 children with Goldenhar syndrome: A pilot study. *Folia Phoniatrica et Logopaedica, 56,* 131–143.

Vogels, A., & Fryns, J.-P. (2006). Pfeiffer syndrome. *Orphanet Journal of Rare Disorders, 1,* 19. Published online 2006 June 1. doi:10.1186/1750-1172-1-19

Weingeist, T. A., Hermsen, V., Hanson, J. W., Bumsted, R. M., Weinstein, S. L., & Olin, W. H. (1982). Ocular and systemic manifestations of Stickler's syndrome: A preliminary report. *Birth Defects: Original Article Series, 8,* 539–560.

Williams, M. A., Shprintzen, R. J., & Rkoff, S. J. (1987). Adenoid hypoplasia in the velo-cardio-facial syndrome. *Journal of Craniofacial Genetics and Developmental Biology, 7,* 23–26.

Young, D., Shprintzen, R. J., & Goldberg, R. B. (1980). Cardiac malformation in the velocardiofacial syndrome. *American Journal of Cardiology, 46,* 643–648.

Zaslav, A. L., Marino, M. A., Jurgens, C. Y., & Mercado, T. (2013). Cytogenetic evaluation: A primer for pediatric nurse practitioners. *Journal of Pediatric Health Care, 27*(6), 426–433.

Zemble, R., Luning Prak, E., McDonald, K., McDonald-McGinn, D., Zacka, E., & Sullivan, K. (2010). Secondary immunologic consequences in chromosome 22q11.2 deletion syndrome (DiGeorge syndrome/velocardiofacial syndrome). *Clinical Immunology, 136*(3), 409–418.

PART II

Birth to Age Three

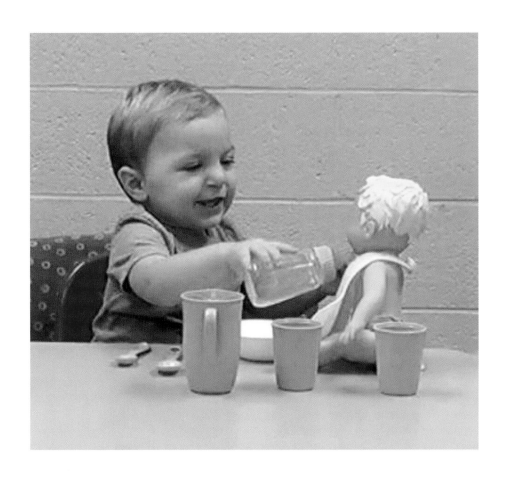

Arguably, the most important developmental period for the individual with an oral cleft is from birth to 3 years of age. Multiple medical and surgical treatment procedures may occur during this period that can significantly impact long-term growth and development. At birth, the immediate goal of the family is feeding the infant. This may be a formidable task depending on the type and severity of the cleft. Chapter 4, "Feeding the Newborn," describes the mechanics of both breastfeeding and bottle-feeding and strategies to promote the most natural and effective feeding method for mother and infant.

Depending on the philosophy of the craniofacial team, the infant—and family in many respects—may undergo relatively simple to complex orthopedic treatment prior to surgery to correct lip and palate deformities. Chapter 5, "Presurgical and Surgical Management," describes the purpose and application of many of these procedures. Chapter 5 also describes the typical timing and basic types of surgeries used to repair the lip and palate and special surgical procedures designed to relieve airway obstruction in infants with Pierre Robin sequence and micrognathia.

As described in Chapter 6, "Hearing and Otologic Management," infants born with cleft palate are highly likely to experience frequent bouts of otitis media with effusion. Although evidence is limited, chronic conductive hearing loss may be a factor in either speech or language delays in children with cleft palate. Chapter 6 provides an overview of hearing assessment techniques and the surgical insertion of ventilation tubes in the eardrums as a treatment strategy.

The final chapter in Part II, "Early Linguistic Development and Intervention," provides a discussion of early language and speech milestones through 3 years of age, and evidence-based assessment and intervention practices for children with cleft lip and palate. Nancy Scherer stresses that the speech goals for children this young should be to build consonant inventories, and that this occurs most effectively by stimulating vocabulary in naturalistic contexts to promote word attempts.

The information provided in Part II of the book is essential to help the speech-language pathologist provide effective services to children from birth to age 3. Knowledge of the type and timing of presurgical, surgical, hearing, speech, and language interventions during this period will also aid the speech-language pathologist in understanding the current condition and perhaps future needs of the older child.

4

Feeding the Newborn

INTRODUCTION

An infant with intact oral structures and normal neurological processes will instinctively seek out and suckle at the mother's breast. A coordinated pattern of sucking, swallowing, and breathing will soon develop, guided by innate reflexes. This initial feeding experience fosters bonding between mother and child. Perhaps no other maternal activity will be as important relative to the long-term physical and psychological well-being of an infant as early feeding experiences.

The natural activity of feeding by an infant may be severely disrupted by an oral cleft. If a complete cleft of the primary palate is present (i.e., lip and alveolus), the infant may be unable to form a secure lip seal around the nipple to initiate the feeding process. If a complete cleft of the secondary palate is present (i.e., hard and soft palate), the infant may be unable to generate positive and negative pressures that are integral to breastfeeding. Reflux of milk or formula into the nasal cavity, prolonged feeding times, fatigue, excessive intake of air into the stomach, and coughing or gagging may be common problems that occur when a palatal cleft is present, for either breastfeeding or bottle-feeding.

These problems are likely to disrupt feeding efficiency, result in poor weight gain, and lead to frustration of both the mother and infant.

This chapter describes the mechanical feeding behaviors of the infant, effects of oral clefts on those behaviors, and some of the common strategies to overcome feeding problems. As described below, typical feeding intervention consists of maternal education, use of modified bottles and nipples, and instruction on specific feeding techniques. The overall approach is designed to help the infant and mother overcome the physical challenges and frustrations to feeding in the presence of an oral cleft. As with most aspects of care for infants with craniofacial anomalies, there is no clear consensus on strategies and little empirical evidence to guide specific interventions.

INITIAL MATERNAL REACTIONS

The typical reaction of the mother and father to the birth of a child with a cleft deformity, even if a prenatal diagnosis was made, is shock. Oral clefts, especially bilateral clefts involving the primary palate, can be quite disfiguring. Initial shock is likely to be followed by anger or guilt. Anger is a natural response to the loss of an expected intact child. Guilt may occur if the mother questions if she did something before or during pregnancy to cause the cleft (e.g., alcohol, drug, or tobacco use). In the midst of such emotions, a mother may take solace in the act of feeding and bonding with the infant. Because the feeding activity is likely to be disrupted by the cleft, a vicious cycle of negative emotions may ensue.

Often, a mother's greatest desire is to breastfeed her infant born with a palatal cleft. Unfortunately, some will encounter health care professionals (e.g., nurses, lactation consultants, speech-language pathologists) whose message is simple and severe—that it is impossible to breastfeed an infant with a cleft. Although this is indeed the case for most infants with palatal clefts, it should not be taken as an absolute. In general, we believe that clinicians should be cautious in using words such as "impossible" or "never" when communicating with parents. If the cleft is confined to just the soft palate, it may be possible for some infants to breastfeed. As noted later in this chapter, at least one hospital has reported success in promoting exclusive breastfeeding in some infants with even complete cleft lip and palate.

INFANT FEEDING MECHANICS

At birth, the infant is primed anatomically and physiologically to feed. The architecture of the upper airway of the infant is designed to facilitate feeding. As illustrated in Figure 4–1, the tongue is positioned relatively forward and occupies most of the volume of the oral cavity. The larynx is relatively high, and the epiglottis approximates the soft palate. This configuration—along with a tongue that largely occludes the oral cavity—essentially limits the infant to be an obligatory nasal breather. Conditions that restrict nasal breathing, therefore, such as *posterior choanal atresia*, are life threatening to the infant and require immediate medical attention.

Reflexes of the newborn include the *rooting* and *sucking* reflexes. The rooting reflex is elicited by the mother and involves tactile stimulation of the skin around the infant's mouth (Woolridge, 1986). As noted by Ito (2015), facial skin is densely innervated with cutaneous mechanoreceptors compared to other parts of the body, with the corners of the mouth being the most densely innervated region of the face (Johansson, Trulsson, Olsson, & Abbs, 1988; Nordin & Hagbarth, 1989). When stimulated by the mother's breast, the infant will turn his or her head to the source of stimulation and open the mouth in anticipation of the nipple. The rooting reflex is present at birth and typically disappears by 4 months of age as it comes under voluntary control (Odent, 1977). The sucking reflex occurs in response to an object being placed in the infant's mouth. It has been observed in the fetus as early as 15 to 18 weeks' gestation, elicited by fingers in the mouth (Humphrey, 1964; Ianniruberto & Tajani, 1981). Woolridge (1986) states that the mother's nipple elicits the sucking reflex during breastfeeding by tactile stimulation of the palate, not the tongue. He notes that this is a "highly adaptive" behavior as the primary activity of the tongue during sucking is to generate compressive forces on the nipple as described next.

Sucking consists of rhythmic oral movements that create *positive* and *negative* pressures that are responsible for fluid flow. Woolridge (1986) described the

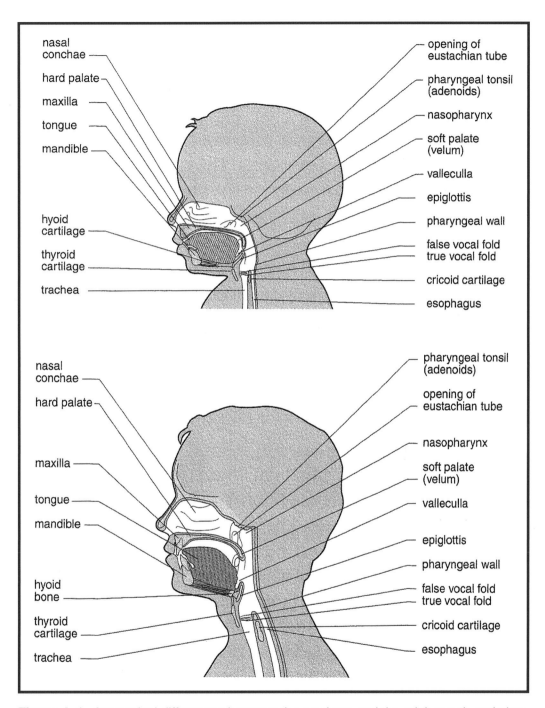

Figure 4–1. Anatomical differences between the newborn and the adult mouth and pharynx. From *Pre-Feeding Skills: A Comprehensive Resource for Mealtime Development, Second Edition* (p. 52), by Suzanne Evans Morris, Marsha Dunn Klein 2000, Austin, TX: PRO-ED. Copyright 2000 by PRO-ED, Inc. Reprinted with permission.

mechanics of sucking during breastfeeding based on cineradiographic films provided by Ardran, Kemp, and Lind (1958a). According to Woolridge, suction pressure is needed to draw out the nipple to approximately three times its length at rest, with the nipple typically extended back to the junction of the hard and soft palate. The base of the nipple is sealed with the upper gum ridge and tongue (Figure 4–2A). The sucking cycle begins with upward movement of the anterior tongue and lower jaw against the nipple (Figure 4–2B). The tongue continues to compress the nipple along its length in a "roller-like peristaltic wave" extending past the tip of the nipple and against the soft palate (Figure 4–2C–E). Tongue compressions end at the posterior base of the tongue followed by lowering of the tongue and jaw to enlarge the oral cavity and create negative pressure to once again pull the nipple into the mouth (Figure 4–2F).

Woolridge (1986) emphasized that sucking is a dynamic process and that compression pressure by the tongue is the primary force that expels milk from the nipple. Although suction or negative pressure is clearly at play, Woolridge noted that its primary role is to draw the nipple into the mouth and fill the nipple with milk in preparation for compressive or stripping action by the tongue. To be sure, Ellison, Vidyasagar, and Anderson (1979) reported that sucking behavior in the newborn during the first 5 minutes of life is characterized primarily by compression pressure with infants quickly learning to incorporate suction by the end of the first hour of life. It should be noted, however, that suction pressure might be more primary during bottle-feeding. Ardran, Kemp, and Lind (1958b), for example, reported that if

the material of a bottle nipple is too stiff, the infant might not be able to effectively constrict the base of the nipple to prevent milk from flowing back into the bottle during compression. As discussed later in the chapter, some commercially available bottles designed for infants with cleft palate incorporate one-way flow valves to circumvent this problem during feeding.

Typically, infants quickly learn to coordinate sucking, swallowing, and breathing behaviors. Studies have reported that by 2 months of age, swallows occur more frequently during expiration as compared to inspiration or between respiratory phases (Kelly, Huckabee, Jones, & Frampton, 2007a, 2007b). Although an expiratory pattern of swallowing is typical of adults, Kelly et al. (2007a) noted that this pattern was present even in newborn infants, suggesting "an adult-like feature of breathing-swallowing coordination even from birth" (p. 150).

Impact of Oral Clefts

Wide clefts involving the lip may impede the infant in achieving a complete seal around the nipple to initiate feeding. Clefts that extend into the alveolar ridge may further impede sealing the nipple. Because of the lack of alveolar bone, the infant may not be able to efficiently compress the base of the nipple against a hard surface. This may be especially difficult when the infant has a bilateral cleft of the primary palate and lacks substantial bone area.

Clefts of the secondary palate, especially complete clefts involving the soft and hard palates, severely limit the generation of positive and negative pressures required for breastfeeding and bottle-

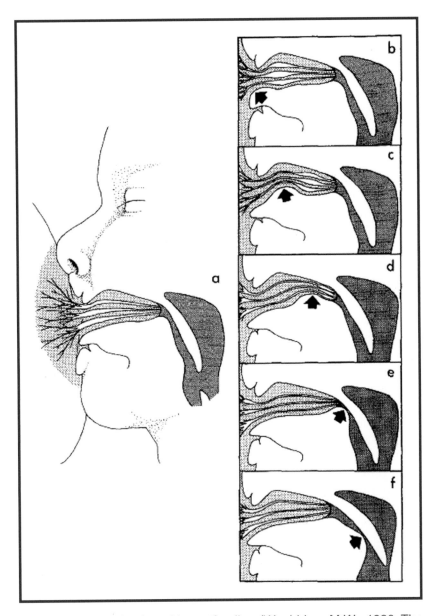

Figure 4–2. Mechanics of breastfeeding (Woolridge, M.W., 1986. The "anatomy" of infant sucking. *Midwifery*, *2*, 164–171. Used with permission.)

feeding. Because of the lack of palatal bone, the infant is unable to compress the nipple against the hard palate to expel milk. Similarly, because of the open communication between the oral and nasal cavities, the infant cannot generate negative pressure by enlarging the oral cavity during sucking behavior. Attempts at sucking, therefore, typically result in the intake of large volumes of air into the stomach, leading to fussy babies and poor weight gain. Reflux of milk and formula into the open nasal cavity commonly occurs, especially if the infant is fed in a prone position.

In addition to oral-stage feeding problems, infants with cleft lip and palate (CLP) may have pharyngeal stage difficulties (Masarei, Wade, Mars, Sommerlad, & Sell, 2007). Masarei et al. studied two groups of infants with unilateral CLP. One group was fitted with presurgical orthopedic appliances (see Chapter 5), and the other group did not use appliances. All infants were followed longitudinally with measures of sucking efficiency obtained during bottle-feedings. In addition, a subset of infants underwent videofluoroscopic evaluations of swallowing. Masarei et al. reported that 19 of 21 infants triggered a swallow after the bolus had left the valleculae, rather than before or at the valleculae as reported for infants without cleft palate. Similarly, Nagaoka and Tanne (2007), in an electromyographic study, showed that adults with repaired CLP exhibited prolonged pharyngeal but shortened oral phases of swallowing. Although the reasons for pharyngeal timing differences in individuals with CLP, if extant, are not known, Masarei et al. (2007) suggested that it may be related to structural anomalies that affect sensory feedback. Indeed, initiation of a swallow is dependent on precisely timed feedback from oral structures including the faucial pillars, uvula, soft palate, and posterior tongue (Miller, 1986).

In summary, clefts of the secondary palate disrupt feeding due to inefficient sucking, prolonged feeding times, fatigue, excessive air intake, and nasal reflux. These disruptions can lead to poor weight gain in the infant and frustration of both the infant and mother.

FEEDING STRATEGIES FOR INFANTS WITH CLEFT PALATE

Maternal education and reassurance are the primary strategies regarding infant feeding. The mother needs to understand infant feeding mechanics and learn ways to circumvent the infant's limitations in generating sucking pressures. Above all else, the mother needs to be reassured that successful feeding can be achieved, and the infant will gain weight and be healthy. Typically, the initial role of feeding instruction will fall to either the hospital nurse, lactation consultant, or speech-language pathologist who specializes in feeding. At most major tertiary hospitals, one of these health care providers will be well trained and experienced to assist mothers of the newborn with a cleft palate. Regardless of the health care provider involved, the primary objective is to instruct the mother in feeding techniques that will result in successful feeding and weight gain for the infant, with the least stress experienced by the infant and family (Goyal, Chopra, Bansal, & Marwaha, 2014).

Special Bottles and Nipples

Given the inefficient sucking behavior of the infant with a cleft, bottles and nipples are used that maximize the flow of formula. There are several commercially available bottles specifically designed for feeding the infant with cleft palate. As described below, these bottles employ nipples that either (a) deliver an increased rate of formula flow to the infant, or (b) allow the feeder to manually assist the infant by squeezing.

Haberman Feeder

As the saying goes, "Necessity is the mother of invention." Mandy Haberman, a mother in England whose daughter was born with congenital anomalies including cleft palate, was frustrated with the lack of effective ways to feed her daughter. As a result, she researched and developed the Haberman Feeder, currently marketed as the Medela Special Needs Feeder (Figure 4–3). The feeder is designed to take advantage of the mechanics of breastfeeding that, as reviewed above, relies more on "pumping" or compression than sucking. The Haberman feeder uses a large nipple with a slit opening housed at the end of a reservoir. A one-way valve is placed between the nipple/reservoir and bottle to prevent formula from re-entering the bottle. Compression of the nipple by the tongue or gums opens the slit and allows formula to flow into the infant's mouth. Because of the slit configuration of the nipple, it can be positioned within the infant's mouth to provide different rates of flow. When the slit is positioned perpendicular to the force of compression, it opens maximally. When the slit is positioned parallel to the force of compression, it opens minimally. The slit configuration also closes the nipple following release of compression to stop flow and allow the baby to swallow. An additional feature of the Haberman is that the mother can manually assist the infant by squeezing the reservoir. Compressions applied manually, however, must be timed to the natural rhythm of the infant and periodically stopped to allow for swallowing (see Figure 4–10). Cost of the Haberman is relatively high as compared to regular nipples and bottles, and this may be a concern for some parents.

Pigeon Bottle

The Pigeon nipple and bottle also use a one-way valve and special nipple design (Figure 4–4). The nipple, however, is shorter in length than the Haberman, has no reservoir, and is Y-cut. The nipple is also stiffer on one side than the other. The stiff side of the nipple is to be positioned toward the palate during feeding to help provide a stable surface for compressions by the tongue. Some parents prefer the Pigeon to the Haberman as the Pigeon looks more like a regular bottle. Similar to the Haberman, however, cost of the Pigeon is also more expensive than regular nipples and bottles.

Enfamil Cleft Palate Nurser

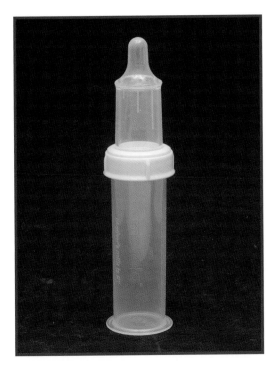

Figure 4–3. Haberman feeder. The long soft nipple is slit cut. The reservoir is squeezable. Note flow rate indicators on reservoir.

This bottle, produced by Mead Johnson, is a low-cost alternative to both the Haberman and Pigeon (Figure 4–5). It has a soft,

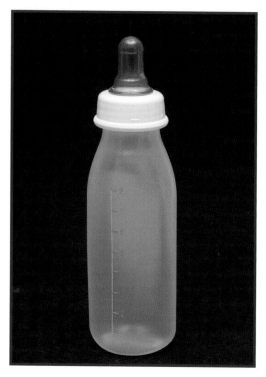

Figure 4–4. Pigeon feeder. Back half of nipple (*toward right in photo*) is stiffer than front half to facilitate compression by infant.

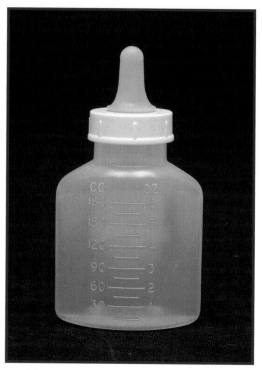

Figure 4–5. Mead Johnson Cleft Palate Nurser. Nipple is crosscut. Bottle is soft and squeezable.

long nipple that is crosscut and attaches to a squeezable bottle. Unlike the Haberman and Pigeon, however, there is no one-way valve to help keep formula in the nipple during feeding.

Dr. Brown's Natural Flow Bottle

This bottle, although not specifically designed for infants with cleft palate, has become popular with many mothers (Figure 4–6). The bottle has a unique internal venting system that eliminates nipple collapse and promotes positive flow, more like breastfeeding according to the manufacturer. The venting feature also reduces air intake during feeding. This claim, if valid, is especially appealing to mothers of infants with cleft palate. Clear silicone

nipples are available in different sizes and flow rates to be used with the bottle.

Modified Regular Nipples

Some craniofacial centers advocate the use of regular nipples and bottles and simply instruct the mother on how to make modifications that will facilitate feeding. The Cleft and Craniofacial Team at Children's Hospital of New Orleans has produced an educational video that describes step-by-step instructions for modifying any regular nipple (see http://www.neworleanscleftteam.org\video .html). As described in this video, a regular nipple is simply crosscut to provide increased flow once compressed by the infant. A significant advantage of this

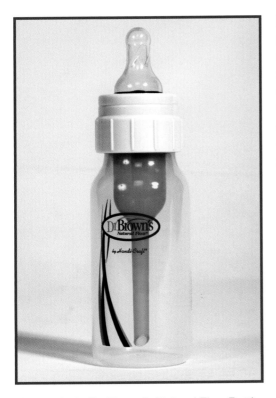

Figure 4–6. Dr. Brown's Natural Flow Bottle.

approach is that parents can use less expensive nipples that are readily available in any local store or market. Many health care providers recommend the use of commercially available bottles, but we must note that there is essentially no well-designed research to show that these are any more effective than simple modifications to regular nipples.

Feeding Instructions

The successful use of any nipple or bottle is largely dependent on clear and concise instructions given to the mother. The feeding specialist should strive to convey a sense of optimism in feeding the infant. Regardless of the bottle used, the mother should be instructed to (a) hold the bottle

in a vertical position, (b) keep the infant somewhat upright, at least at a 45° to 60° angle, and (c) frequently burp the infant during and after feeding. A vertically positioned bottle will allow gravity to assist in providing formula flow while a slightly upright-positioned infant will decrease the likelihood of reflux of formula into the nasal cavity. Frequent burping is important to eliminate excessive intake of air into the stomach that may occur. Finally, when feeding an infant with a unilateral cleft of the primary palate, the mother should position the nipple under the noncleft side of the palate to facilitate compression pressure by the tongue.

Obturator Nipples and Feeding Plates

Obturator Nipples

Beginning in the 1960s, obturator nipples were recommended to facilitate feeding. An obturator nipple has a half-hood attached to the base of a regular nipple (Figure 4–7). The hood is designed to cover the cleft (i.e., function as an artificial palate) and thus promote normal sucking. An advantage over feeding plates (discussed next) is that an impression of the cleft does not have to be taken. Obturator nipples have fallen into disfavor due to difficulty with actual use and limited closure of the cleft provided by a one-size-fits-all design. Even if complete coverage of the cleft were obtained, sucking efficiency may not improve given the hood is rather flexible and does not provide a hard surface to facilitate nipple compression.

Feeding Plates

Feeding plates are recommended by some craniofacial centers to facilitate feeding

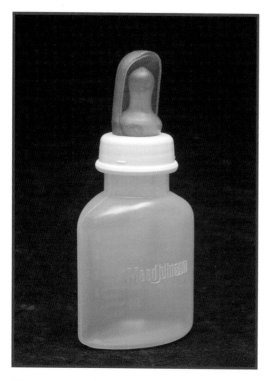

Figure 4–7. Obturator nipple. Half hood functions as artificial palate.

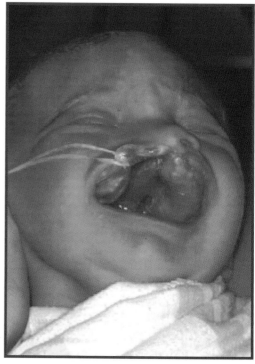

Figure 4–8. Infant with feeding plate. (Hansen, P. A., Cook, N. B., & Ahmad, O., 2015. Fabrication of a feeding obturator for infants. *Cleft Palate-Craniofacial Journal.* Advance online publication. Used with permission.)

(Figure 4–8). A feeding plate functions as an artificial palate with a rigid surface. Use of a feeding plate requires the services of a pediatric dentist or orthodontist to take an impression of the cleft area and fabricate the plate (Hansen, Cook, & Ahmad, 2015). Masarei et al. (2007) summarized the proposed advantages of feeding appliances as: (a) providing a stable surface for compression of the nipple, (b) reducing the likelihood of painful ulceration of the exposed nasal septum by the nipple, (c) correcting abnormal tongue positioning which may improve patency of the airway, (d) helping the infant to generate negative oral pressure during sucking, and (e) minimizing the occurrence of food

residue in the cleft and/or nasal reflux of food. As discussed later in the chapter, there is little empirical evidence to support any of these claims. Feeding plates are also costly and require modification as the infant grows (Agarwal, Rana, & Shafi, 2010; Hansen et al., 2015). Given the lack of evidence, expense, and need for adjustments, relatively few centers advocate the use of feeding plates.

Nasoalveolar Molding Appliances

Some centers offer nasoalveolar molding (NAM) therapy for infants prior to lip and palate surgery (Figure 4–9). Although the primary purpose of a NAM appliance is

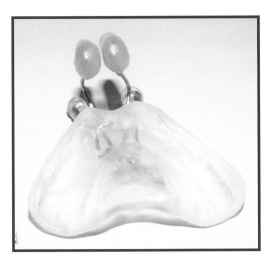

Figure 4–9. Nasoalveolar molding (NAM) appliance. Hard plate facilitates nipple compression. The extensions lift and shape the nostrils (see Chapter 5).

to align the maxillary segments prior to surgery (see Chapter 5), a secondary benefit is that the appliance essentially functions as a feeding plate. Some parents have anecdotally reported improved feeding with a NAM appliance. As discussed next, however, there is little research to support these claims.

Evidence to Support Feeding Appliances. Choi, Kleinheinz, Joos, and Komposch (1991) studied five infants with unrepaired cleft palate who were fitted with orthopedic feeding plates. They reported that use of feeding plates failed to generate any negative oral pressures during feeding. This finding should not be too surprising given that orthopedic appliances are not designed to cover the entire cleft area. Perhaps more surprising, Masarei et al. (2007) reported that presurgical orthopedic appliances did not promote positive compression pressures in infants with CLP. Recall that Masarei et al. studied a group of infants with unilateral CLP who wore

orthopedic appliances and a group who did not have appliances. Masarei et al. reported no difference between the groups regarding positive compression pressures during bottle-feeding. A possible reason for this finding may be that only infants with unilateral CLP were studied, and mothers are typically instructed to position the nipple on the noncleft side during feeding. This may have resulted in similar compression pressures in both groups of infants.

Zajac, van Aalst, Pimenta, and Santiago (2014) studied an infant with unrepaired *bilateral* cleft lip and palate at 4 weeks of age before being fitted with a NAM appliance and again at 6 weeks of age with the appliance. The investigators used a miniature, fiberoptic pressure transducer inserted into a bottle to record positive compression pressure during feeding. They reported that compression pressure was significantly higher with NAM (7 cm H_2O) than without the appliance (2 cm H_2O). A control infant without cleft lip or palate was also studied at two similar time points. The control infant generated stable positive pressures of approximately 14 cm H_2O over both time points. These findings indicate that the infant with cleft lip and palate benefited from the NAM appliance during bottle-feeding. It must be noted, however, that the infant achieved compression pressure that was approximately half of that achieved by the control infant. Of interest, the infant with cleft lip and palate was fed using a Haberman bottle with the mother squeezing the reservoir to assist with feeding. Figure 4–10 shows approximately 2 minutes of feeding by the infant without the NAM appliance during which the mother initially provides manual compressions and then stops. As shown in the figure, there is a dramatic

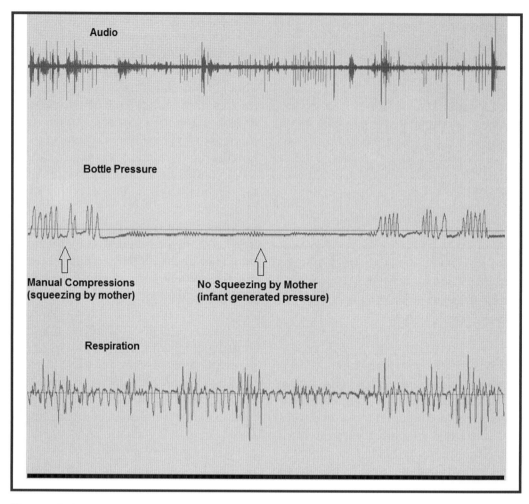

Figure 4–10. Audio (neck microphone), bottle pressure, and respiration (nasal cannula) during feeding of an infant with unrepaired bilateral CLP using the Haberman feeder without a NAM appliance. The infant generated relatively little compression pressure when mother stopped manual squeezing.

reduction in compression pressure when the mother stops squeezing the reservoir and the infant compresses the nipple.

Breastfeeding

Some mothers are intent on breastfeeding their infants with cleft palate. If the cleft is confined to just the soft palate, then the infant may be able to breastfeed to some extent (Goyal et al., 2014). In such cases, the hard palate is intact and this will enable nipple compression by the tongue. In addition, the infant may learn to use the posterior tongue to effectively seal the oral cavity. This adaptation, however, may reduce overall efficiency of the pulsatile compression wave generated by the tongue. Regardless, we have encountered some mothers of infants with clefts of only the soft palate who were able to breastfeed. One mother experienced prolonged feeding times and due to weight gain concerns of the infant, she was subsequently advised to switch to bottle-feeding. As a bottom line, we believe that if a mother is intent to try breastfeeding—even with an infant who has a complete cleft of the secondary palate—she should be allowed in a supportive environment. If she and the baby experience undo feeding difficulty and frustration, then alternative recommendations will be more willingly accepted, as in the case above, and a good relationship with the health care provider will ensue.

As mentioned at the beginning of the chapter, breastfeeding may be possible even with infants who have complete clefts of the lip and palate. Pathumwiwatana, Tongsukho, Naratippakorn, Pradubwong, and Chusilp (2010) reported an encouraging study done in Thailand. They instructed 20 mothers of infants born with complete clefts of the lip and palate on exclusive breastfeeding techniques and followed the mothers and infants for 6 months. The mothers were instructed to use either the cross-cradle or football position to hold their infants with one hand while they used the other hand to manually squeeze the breast to express milk for the infants. Pathumwiwatana et al. reported that all 20 infants breastfed exclusively at 1-week and 1-month follow-ups with normal weight gains. At 3- and 4-month follow-ups, four infants were breastfed exclusively with 16 infants using bottle supplements, due to work obligations of the mothers. At the 6-month follow-up, only two infants were still breastfed exclusively. Pathumwiwatana et al. noted that the mothers of these two infants were financially well off and were stay-at-home mothers who could continue exclusive breastfeeding.

Future Directions

Given the importance of feeding and the challenges faced by mothers and their infants with oral clefts, systematic research is needed to guide effective intervention. Reid (2004) reviewed the published literature on feeding intervention and reported a paucity of well-designed data-driven studies. Specifically, Reid found that of 55 published articles on feeding intervention between 1955 and 2002, only two were randomized controlled trials, and 50 (91%) were expert opinion.

Although at least one randomized study has investigated feeding intervention in infants with palatal clefts since that time (e.g., Masarei et al., 2007), additional studies are needed. As pointed out by Reid (2004), future studies must (a) clearly identify the nature of feeding difficulties, the infants most at risk, and the predictors of poor feeding, (b) explore how various feeding interventions work and how they impact overall feeding efficiency, and (c) control for multiple intervention approaches that might impact results. Relative to this last point, Goyal et al. (2014) emphasized that a single feeding intervention may not be optimal for all infants with cleft palate. They called for more research that combined the use of palatal obturators, special nipples and bottles, and feeding education to determine best clinical practice.

CHAPTER SUMMARY

Feeding is the essential activity of the newborn, and successful feeding is vital for development of physical, social, and emotional health. Newborn infants with intact oral structures and neurological processes use innate reflexes to seek the mother's breast and suckle efficiently. Rhythmic movements of the tongue create both positive and negative pressures to express milk from the nipple. Infants with oral clefts, especially involving the hard and soft palates, have difficulty compressing the nipple and creating negative pressure to feed efficiently. Mothers typically use special nipples and bottles designed to maximize fluid flow. Breastfeeding is especially problematic for infants with cleft lip and palate. Some mothers, through training in positioning of the infant and manual expression of breast milk, may be able to effectively breastfeed.

REFERENCES

Agarwal, A., Rana, V., & Shafi, S. (2010). A feeding appliance for a newborn baby with cleft lip and palate. *National Journal of Maxillofacial Surgery, 1*(1), 91–93.

Ardran, G. M., Kemp, F. H., & Lind, J. (1958a). A cineradiographic study of breast feeding. *British Journal of Radiology, 31*, 156–162.

Ardran, G. M., Kemp, F. H., & Lind, J. (1958b). A cineradiographic study of bottle feeding. *British Journal of Radiology, 31*, 11–22.

Choi, B. H., Kleinheinz, J., Joos, U., & Komposch, G. (1991). Sucking efficiency of early orthopaedic plate and teats in infants with cleft lip and palate. *International Journal of Oral and Maxillofacial Surgery, 20*(3), 167–169.

Ellison, S. L., Vidyasagar, G., & Anderson, C. (1979). Sucking in the newborn infant during the first hour of life. *Journal of Nurse-Midwifery, 24*, 18–25.

Goyal, M., Chopra, R., Bansal, K., & Marwaha, M. (2014). Role of obturators and other feeding interventions in patients with cleft lip and palate: A review. *European Archives of Paediatric Dentistry, 15*, 1–9.

Hansen, P. A., Cook, N. B., & Ahmad, O. (2015). Fabrication of a feeding obturator for infants. *Cleft Palate-Craniofacial Journal.* Advance online publication.

Humphrey, T. (1964). Some correlations between the appearance of human fetal reflexes and the development of the nervous system. *Progress in Brain Research, 4*, 199–205.

Ianniruberto, A., & Tajani, E. (1981). Ultrasonographic study of fetal movements. *Seminars in Perinatololgy, 5*, 175–181.

Ito, T. (2015). Orofacial cutaneous function in speech motor control and learining. In M. A. Redford (Ed.), *The handbook of speech production* (pp. 248–266). Malden, MA: Blackwell.

Johansson, R. S., Trulsson, M., Olsson, K. Z., & Abbs, J. H. (1988). Mechanoreceptor afferent activity in the infraorbital nerve in man during speech and chewing movements. *Experimental Brain Research, 72*, 209–214.

Kelly, B. N., Huckabee, M. L., Jones, R. D., & Frampton, C. M. A. (2007a). The early impact of feeding on infant breathing-swallowing coordination. *Respiratory Physiology and Neurobiology, 156*(2), 147–153.

Kelly, B. N., Huckabee, M. L., Jones, R. D., & Frampton, C. M. A. (2007b). The first year of human life: Coordinating respiration and nutritive swallowing. *Dysphagia, 22*(1), 37–43.

Masarei, A. G., Wade, A., Mars, M., Sommerlad, B. C., & Sell, D. (2007). A randomized control trial investigating the effect of presurgical orthopedics on feeding in infants with cleft lip and/or palate. *Cleft Palate-Craniofacial Journal, 44*(2), 182–193.

Miller, A. J. (1986). Neurophysiologic basis of swallowing. *Dysphagia, 1*, 91–100.

Morris, S. E., &. Klein, M. D. (2000). *Pre-feeding skills: A comprehensive resource for mealtime development* (2nd ed.). Austin, TX: Pro-Ed.

Nagaoka, K., & Tanne, K. (2007). Activities of the muscles involved in swallowing in patients with cleft lip and palate. *Dysphagia, 22*, 140–144.

Nordin, M., & Hagbarth, K. E. (1989). Mechanoreceptive units in the human infra-orbital nerve. *Acta Physiologica Scandinavica, 135*, 149–161.

Odent, M. (1977). The early expression of the rooting reflex. *Proceedings of the 5th Interna-*

tional Congress of Psychosomatic Obstetrics and Gynaecology, Rome 1977 (pp. 1117–1119). London, UK: Academic Press.

Pathumwiwatana, P., Tongsukho, S., Naratippakorn, T., Pradubwong, S., & Chusilp, K. (2010). The promotion of exclusive breastfeeding in infants with complete cleft lip and palate during the first 6 months after childbirth at Srinagarind Hospital, Khon Kaen Province, Thailand. *Journal of the Medical Association of Thailand, 93*(Suppl. 4), S71–S77.

Reid, J. (2004). A review of feeding interventions for infants with cleft palate. *Cleft Palate-Craniofacial Journal, 41*, 268–278.

Woolridge, M. W. (1986). The "anatomy" of infant sucking. *Midwifery, 2*, 164–171.

Zajac, D., van Aalst, J., Pimenta, L., & Santiago, P. (2014). *Compression pressure during bottle feeding of an infant with a nasal-alveolar molding appliance.* Poster presented at the American Speech Language Hearing Association Annual Convention, November, Orlando, FL.

5

Presurgical and Surgical Management

INTRODUCTION

An infant born with an oral cleft faces multiple medical and surgical procedures during his or her life, especially during the first 12 to 14 months. Parents are naturally eager to have the birth defect repaired. If the cleft involves the lip only (i.e., an isolated and incomplete cleft of the primary palate), usually one operation will be required. If the infant has both cleft lip and palate, a second operation will follow to repair the palate. Infants born with cleft palate, with or without involvement of the lip, will likely require an additional surgical procedure called *myringotomy* with insertion of ventilation tubes into the tympanic membranes. This is usually done at the time of either lip or palate surgery (see Chapter 6). In addition, some infants with clefts of the lip and palate may undergo presurgical procedures designed to reduce the width of the cleft and align the maxillary segments prior to lip repair. The use of presurgical procedures varies, depending on the severity of the cleft and the experience and philosophy of the treating craniofacial team. Infants with clefts of the lip *and* alveolar

ridge (i.e., a complete cleft of the primary palate) will require another surgery to correct the bone defect. This surgery, known as the *alveolar bone graft*, is most often done in late childhood (see Chapter 12) but may be done as early as the first year of life at some centers. Finally, infants born with Pierre Robin sequence may undergo additional surgical procedures to manage airway obstruction prior to palate repair.

Given the potential impact multiple procedures have on facial growth, aesthetics, dentition, hearing, and speech development, it is not surprising that controversies exist regarding the actual need of some procedures and the timing of others. In the United States, for example, there is no consensus regarding the need for presurgical management of cleft deformities. Likewise, there is also controversy regarding the timing of common procedures such as cleft lip and cleft palate repair. Typically, the individual surgeon will determine the timing of surgeries based on a number of factors including overall health of the infant, evidence-based practice, and personal preference. Although most surgeons in the United States will repair the lip at 2 to 3 months of age followed by the palate at 8 to 14 months of age, some surgeons may offer parents a single surgery to repair both the lip and palate in the early neonatal period. Denk and Magee (1996), for example, reported their experience with neonatal lip and palate surgery, with some infants undergoing repair as early as the first week of life before discharge from the hospital. Neonatal repair, however, is relatively uncommon, and long-term outcomes have not yet been reported.

The reason for such disparate approaches to surgical timing is based upon competing goals for the infant. Early surgery may satisfy parental desire and possibly better functional outcome, particularly for speech, but may yield poor outcome regarding facial growth and aesthetic appearance. Later surgery may allow for improved facial growth and aesthetic outcome but at the risk of poorer speech outcome. Unfortunately, there are few well-controlled, randomized studies that have used objective outcome measures to shed light on the question of optimal timing for palate surgery.

This chapter reviews (a) presurgical treatments available to the infant, (b) timing and types of surgeries required for cleft lip and palate reconstruction, (c) surgical insertion of ventilation tubes, (d) surgical procedures to relieve airway obstruction in cases of Pierre Robin sequence, and (e) the controversy regarding the optimal time for palate repair. The speech-language pathologist (SLP) should be aware that hospitalizations and surgeries are major stressors of parents that may impede effective communication. Although at this time, the primary role of the SLP may be limited to feeding intervention, he or she can begin dialogue with parents regarding speech develop-

ment and to facilitate an understanding of presurgical and surgical treatment goals. Such involvement prior to surgery allows parents to develop a relationship and a bond with the SLP at an early age, which can carry forward during the months and years following palate repair surgery.

PRESURGICAL MANAGEMENT

Presurgical management, also called *presurgical orthopedics*, is often recommended for infants who have severe clefts of the lip and palate. When clefts are wide or bilateral, the initial lip repair is technically more difficult compared to a cleft that is narrow or unilateral. Also, in cases of complete bilateral cleft lip, the premaxilla may significantly protrude and further complicate lip surgery. Presurgical procedures are designed to (a) reduce the extent (width) of the cleft, (b) align the maxillary segments, and (c) in cases of bilateral clefts, reposition the premaxilla posteriorly to align with the maxillary segments.

There are a variety of presurgical procedures that run the gamut from simple and relatively noninvasive to highly complex that require general anesthesia. There is controversy regarding the long-term effectiveness of presurgical orthopedics, especially the use of intraoral devices. Successful presurgical orthopedics may facilitate initial lip repair, reduce lip tension across the cleft following surgery, and promote overall better aesthetic outcome (Billmire, 2008; Grayson & Maull, 2004; McComb, 1985). Another advantage may be socioemotional involvement of the parents, with many parents feeling that they are actively participating in the treatment of their child by following presurgical treatment protocols. Some authors, however, have noted no improvement of dental arch alignment in the permanent dentition (Huddart, North, & Davis, 1966; Ross, 1970); others have actually claimed that maxillary growth is disrupted (Berkowitz, 1996; Berkowitz, Mejia, & Bystrik, 2004). The frequent visits and additional cost of presurgical orthopedic therapy may increase the burden of care for the family of an infant born with cleft lip and palate. Although detailed coverage of presurgical orthopedics is beyond the scope of this chapter, we briefly summarize some of the treatments to familiarize SLPs with the varied approaches.

Taping of the Lip

The easiest of presurgical procedures is simply applying tape across the cleft segment(s) of the upper lip (Figure 5–1). This will help to bring the segments together to reduce the width of the cleft or reposition a protruding premaxilla. Taping can be done using standard surgical tape (e.g., Steri-Strips, Micropore) or special tape designed and marketed for infants with cleft lip and palate. Some special tapes also help lift and shape a collapsed nose similar to nasoalveolar molding appliances described in the next section.

Passive Intraoral Appliances

These devices are placed in the oral cavity to guide growth of the maxillary segments and prevent collapse or narrowing of the maxillary arch. A pediatric dentist or orthodontist takes an impression of the infant's cleft, and the impression is used to fabricate an oral appliance. The appliance is usually held in place by means of external taping that also acts to bring the cleft segments together. The appliance may cause gum irritation. Therefore, both the appliance and the oral cavity need to be cleaned and monitored regularly.

Some passive appliances also incorporate extensions to lift and shape the nostril. These devices are called *nasoalveolar molding* (NAM) appliances (Figure 5–2A). NAM appliances—which also require oral impressions to fabricate—are placed soon

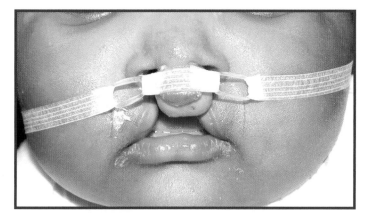

Figure 5–1. Lip taping of an infant with bilateral complete cleft lip and palate. (Courtesy of Joseph A. Napoli, MD, DDS, Plastic, Maxillofacial, and Craniofacial Surgery, Alfred I. duPont Hospital for Children, Wilmington, DE.)

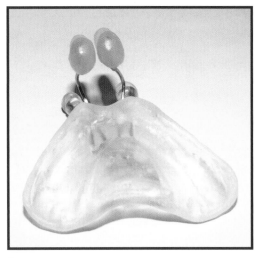
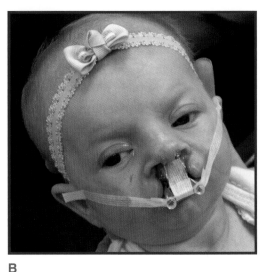

A   B

Figure 5–2. A. Nasoalveolar molding (NAM) appliance made for an infant with unrepaired bilateral cleft lip and palate. Extensions lift and shape the nostrils. **B.** Infant wearing the NAM appliance shown in **A**.

after birth at 2 to 3 weeks of age and are typically worn by the infant until time of lip repair. The NAM appliance shown in Figure 5–2A was made for an infant with complete bilateral cleft lip and palate. Initially, the infant wore the appliance without the two nasal extensions. An orthodontist added the extensions after several weeks. The extensions are designed to lift the collapsed alar rims of the nose and stretch the columella (Figure 5–2B). Figure 5–3 shows a different infant with a wide unilateral cleft lip and palate before, during, and after NAM therapy. NAM was highly effective in reducing the width of the cleft and the collapse of the nostril prior to surgery leading to an exceptional aesthetic outcome after surgery. Some advocates of NAM suggest that failure to correct the nasal cartilage deformity may result in the need for multiple surgical revisions for aesthetics when the child is older (Grayson & Garfinkle, 2014).

NAM devices are labor intensive not only relative to initial construction and fitting, but also because frequent adjustments must be made due to growth before lip repair. Typically, weekly visits to the orthodontist are required for monitoring and adjustments. Proponents of NAM view it as an essential component of habilitation of the infant with a cleft. Opponents, however, express the view that NAM appliances are elective and highly dependent on the compliance of the family and the availability of dental specialists who are well trained in fabricating and fitting the device.

Active Intraoral Appliances

These devices are similar to passive molding appliances but use active force to align the maxillary segments. Active devices need to be placed under general

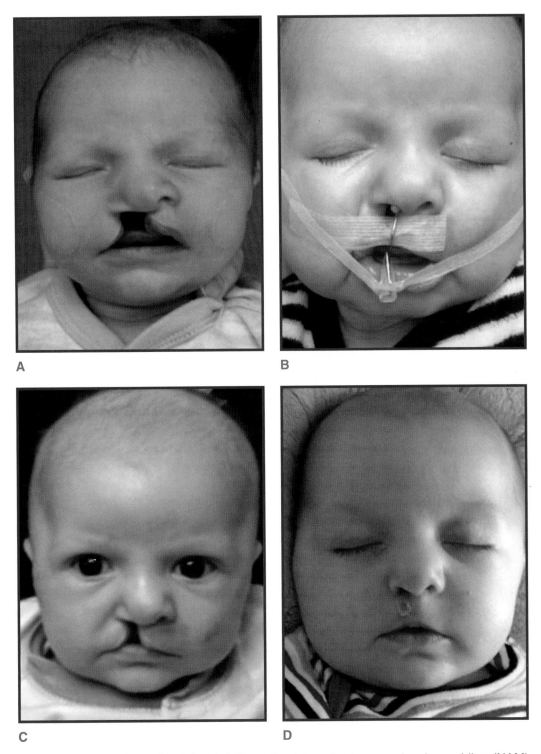

Figure 5–3. A. Infant with right cleft lip and palate prior to nasoalveolar molding (NAM) therapy. Note wide cleft and nostril collapse. **B.** Same infant with NAM appliance. **C.** Same infant without NAM appliance prior to lip surgery. Note reduced width of cleft and collapse of nostril. **D.** Same infant following lip surgery.

anesthesia as pins are inserted into the maxillary segments to hold the appliance. The pins are inserted on an oblique angle to avoid damaging tooth buds (Latham, 1980). Springs or screws are attached to the appliance and used to bring the maxillary segments together over a 3- to 5-week period or more (Figure 5–4). Use of active devices has been reported to effectively reduce cleft width in infants with unilateral cleft lip and palate prior to lip repair (Allareddy, Ross, Bruun, Lee, & Shusterman, 2015).

Lip Adhesion

Finally, some surgeons will perform a lip adhesion prior to lip repair when a cleft is wide (Figure 5–5). Essentially, this is a two-staged surgical procedure that typi-cally involves a simple straight-line repair of the cleft lip at approximately 6 weeks of age followed by definite lip surgery when the infant is 3 to 4 months of age (Billmire, 2008). The lip adhesion functions to bring cleft segments together and apply pressure to the premaxilla similar to nonsurgical techniques. A disadvantage of lip adhesion is that, depending on the type, scarring may make dissection and mobilization of tissue more difficult during the definitive lip repair (Noordhoff & Kuo-Ting Chen, 2006).

Summary

Presurgical procedures are designed to reduce the width of the cleft, align segments, and retroposition the premaxilla in cases of bilateral cleft lip and palate. Table 5–1 summarizes the various procedures.

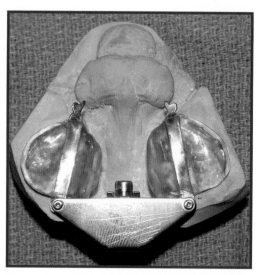

A

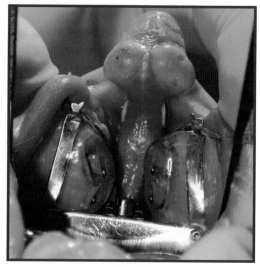

B

Figure 5–4. A. Latham-type orthopedic appliance shown on a model. The two arms are screwed open to expand the cleft maxillary segments. **B.** Latham-type appliance in an infant with bilateral cleft lip and palate. Extensions attached to the premaxilla pull it back into alignment with the cleft maxillary segments. The appliance is pinned into the maxillary segments. (Courtesy of Joseph A. Napoli, MD, DDS, Plastic, Maxillofacial, and Craniofacial Surgery, Alfred I. duPont Hospital for Children, Wilmington, DE.)

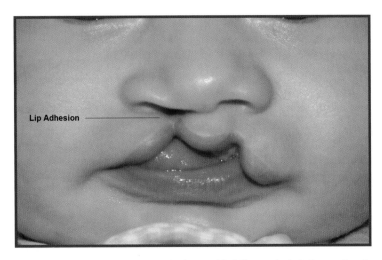

Figure 5–5. Lip adhesion. Infant with bilateral cleft lip and palate, complete on the right and incomplete on the left (same infant as in Chapter 2, Figure 2–6). (Courtesy of Joseph A. Napoli, MD, DDS, Plastic, Maxillofacial, and Craniofacial Surgery, Alfred I. duPont Hospital for Children, Wilmington, DE.)

Table 5–1. Presurgical Procedures: Approximate Ages and Functions

Procedure	Approximate Age	Function(s)
Lip taping	1–2 weeks to lip repair	Reduce cleft width; align segments; retroposition premaxilla
Passive orthopedic appliances	2–3 weeks to lip repair	Reduce cleft width; align segments; retroposition premaxilla; may assist with feeding
Active orthopedic appliances	2–3 weeks to lip repair	Reduce cleft width; align segments; retroposition premaxilla
Lip adhesion	6 weeks	Reduce cleft width; retroposition premaxilla

SURGICAL MANAGEMENT

Lip and Nose Reconstruction

If a cleft is confined to just the lip (i.e., an incomplete cleft of the primary palate), then a single surgery is typically required to correct the tissue and muscle defect. If the cleft is a complete cleft of the primary palate that extends into or through the alveolar ridge, then a second surgery will be required to repair the bony defect to support eruption of permanent teeth. This second surgery, called an *alveolar bone graft,* is typically done when the child is 7 to 9 years of age and in the stage of mixed dentition (see Chapter 12). The SLP needs to be aware that the unrepaired alveolar cleft can be a source of nasal reflux of foods and liquids, nasal air emission, or contribute to articulation difficulty. Backing of alveolar consonants, for example, may be due to structural anomalies associated with an alveolar cleft such as oronasal fistulas and narrowing of the maxillary segments (see Chapter 8).

Timing of Lip and Nose Surgery

Most surgeons will repair a cleft of the lip when the infant is about 3 months of age. This timing has its roots in the "rule of 10s" advocated by Wilhelmsen and Musgrave (1966). The rule of 10s states that an infant should be at least 10 weeks of age, weigh at least 10 pounds, and have a hemoglobin count of at least 10 grams prior to surgery. This rule not only ensures the safety of the infant during surgery but also allows time for the diagnosis of other potentially complicating medical conditions in the infant.

Some surgeons advocate early repair of the lip and palate. Denk and Magee (1996) reported on a series of 17 infants who underwent both lip and palate repair in the neonatal period. All of the infants received surgery within 30 days of birth with some as early as the first week of life. Denk and Magee pointed out that because of advancements in medicine and anesthesia since the 1960s, the rule of 10s might be an unnecessary burden to the infant and family. In their series of infants, Denk and Magee reported no deaths and postsurgical complication rates that were comparable to rates when surgeries were performed later. The controversy of early palate surgery is discussed later in the chapter.

Lip Repair Techniques

The goal of cleft lip surgery (also called *cheiloplasty*) is to provide structural integrity of the upper lip with adequate vertical length and symmetry, repair the underlying orbicularis oris muscle, and correct the nasal deformity (Ruiz & Costello, 2009). Early surgical approaches used straight-line lip repairs. Essentially, this means that incisions were made along the edges of the cleft lip and muscle and tissue were simply sutured together, resulting in a straight-line scar. Although straight-line techniques typically achieved the goal of reconstruction of the upper lip, aesthetic outcomes were often less than desirable. To enhance aesthetic outcomes, surgical techniques were developed to reduce the visible effects of scarring such as the Tennison triangular-flap (Bardach, 1994; Randall, 1959) and the Millard rotation-advancement flap procedure (Millard, 1964a, 1964b; Trier, 1985). As noted by Billmire (2008), techniques were developed that attempted "to place the scars in normally occurring lines and anatomical breaks, such as the philtral ridges" (p. 512).

Currently, most surgeons will perform lip repair using the Millard technique or some variation of it (Ruiz & Costello, 2009). The Millard technique places an initial incision along the philtral ridge on the cleft side of the upper lip. Instead of continuing a straight-line incision, the surgeon makes a curved incision along the base of the nose (Figure 5–6). This incision frees the upper lip to be rotated down to approximate the lip on the opposite side. The rotation of tissue on the cleft side leaves a gap beneath the nose that is filled with tissue that is advanced from an incision made on the opposite side. Billmire (2008) notes that the Millard procedure

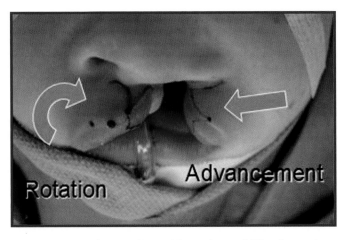

Figure 5–6. Surgical markings for a Millard rotation-advancement lip repair. (Courtesy of John van Aalst, MD, Pediatric Surgery, Cincinnati Children's Medical Center.)

is "perhaps the most anatomical of the repairs" given its attempt to follow normal anatomical landmarks (p. 512).

Primary Alveolar Bone Grafting and Gingivoperiosteoplasty

A complete cleft of the primary palate involves a bony defect in the alveolar ridge that will require bone grafting to repair. Although most centers will delay alveolar bone grafting to when the child is in the mixed dentition at roughly 7 to 9 years of age (see Chapter 12), some centers may advocate for early repair by 1 year of age, called *primary alveolar bone grafting*. The rationale for late repair of the alveolar cleft is to limit maxillary growth restriction due to surgical scarring and allow eruption of the permanent teeth. Advocates of early alveolar bone grafting, however, believe that once lip repair is done, medial pressure exerted on the unrepaired maxillary segments may cause collapse and restricted growth (Rosenstein, Monroe, Kernahan, Jacobson, Griffith, &

Bauer, 1982; Wood, 1970). To counteract medial pressure resulting from lip repair, early bone grafting is advocated to establish a unified maxillary arch. In support of this approach, Wood (1970) noted that the incidence of maxillary collapse and *pseudo-prognathism* in children who had not undergone early bone grafting was 66%, and it was only 15% in children who had received early bone grafting.

Primary alveolar bone grafting is controversial. Proponents believe that early repair and stabilization of the maxillary arch are essential to promoting growth and preventing maxillary collapse (e.g., Wood, 1970), but opponents counter that just the opposite may occur due to scarring from early surgery that restricts maxillary growth both laterally and anterior-posteriorly (e.g., Koberg, 1973). Because of this ongoing debate and the relative lack of evidence to support early alveolar bone grafting, most craniofacial centers in the United States favor late alveolar cleft repair, also called *secondary* alveolar bone grafting. SLPs, therefore, need to be aware that most of the early school-aged children with repaired cleft lip and palate whom they encounter will not yet have had alveolar bone grafting. Consequently, these children may have oral-nasal fistula of varying sizes and locations that may affect speech. If maxillary collapse or dental anomalies are present, then articulation of tongue tip-alveolar sounds may be adversely affected. Indeed, as reviewed in Chapter 8, evidence is emerging that maxillary arch collapse may directly contribute to certain articulation errors such as palatalized stops (Zajac, Cevidanes, Shah, & Haley, 2011).

Finally, some surgeons may perform *gingivoperiosteoplasty* (GPP) in cases where presurgical orthopedics has successfully aligned the cleft maxillary arches. GPP, typically done at the time of lip repair, closes the alveolar clefts by elevating flaps of gingival tissue and periosteum, a fibrous membrane covering bone. Advocates of GPP feel that in addition to providing a stable maxillary arch, it may also stimulate the growth of bone, thus avoiding the need for alveolar bone grafting.

Surgery to Repair the Palate

The primary goal of palate surgery is to restore velar muscle continuity and physically close the cleft deformity to allow for normal development of speech. Most palatal surgeries performed in the United States are one-stage repairs. This means that the soft and hard palates—if both are affected—are repaired at the same time. At some centers (mostly in Europe), two-stage palatal surgeries may be done. This means that the soft palate is repaired first and the hard palate is repaired later during another surgery. As discussed later, the rationale for two-stage palatal surgeries is to give the infant time to grow without scarring of the hard palate that may inhibit facial growth.

Timing of Secondary Palatal Surgery

Surgery to repair a cleft of the secondary palate typically is done between 8 and 14 months of age at most centers in the United States. A review of recent surgeries done at the Craniofacial Center at the University of North Carolina at Chapel Hill revealed a mean age of 10 months for palate repair with the earliest done at 8 months. It must be emphasized that all of these infants were diagnosed with nonsyndromic cleft palate and were in good physical health. For infants diagnosed with syndromes, especially those associated with respiratory disorders and cardiac conditions, palatal surgery may be delayed to 18 months of age or later.

Palate Repair Techniques

Similar to cleft lip surgery, early attempts at cleft palate repair typically involved relatively simple, straight-line repairs. That is, the surgeon would simply make incisions along the edges of the two cleft segments and suture the palatal segments together at midline. Although this technique might be adequate to physically separate the oral and nasal cavities, it does not restore the velar musculature required for normal velopharyngeal function. It was not until the 1960s that surgeons began to realize the need for velar muscle reconstruction, called *intravelar veloplasty*, to achieve satisfactory speech outcomes (Brown, Cohen, & Randall, 1983; Kriens, 1969, 1970; Ruding, 1964).

As noted above, early surgical procedures did not attempt to reconstruct the velar musculature. Recall that the paired levator veli palatini muscles originate from the right and left sides of the cranial base and insert into the midline of the velum, thereby creating a sling (see Chapter 1, Figure 1–8). The primary function of the levator sling is to elevate and retract the soft palate during oral speech sounds. When a cleft of the soft palate occurs, levator veli palatini and palatopharyngeus muscles insert onto the posterior hard palate, a condition called the *cleft muscle of Veau*. This abnormal configuration essentially inhibits efficient elevation and retraction of the velum. Ruding (1964) suggested that normal function of the velum can only occur by detaching the levator from the hard palate to create a normal levator sling. Brown et al. (1983) further supported the need to detach the levator from the hard palate as part of routine palate repair. Brown et al. retrospectively evaluated speech outcomes of 45 children who underwent reconstruction of the levator sling as part of palatoplasty and 40 children who did not undergo levator reconstruction. The children were considered to have normal speech if no hypernasality or nasal air escape was detected by an SLP who was blind to the type of surgery. Brown et al. reported that 47% of the children who received intravelar veloplasty exhibited normal speech 2 years following surgery compared to 30% of children who did not receive intravelar veloplasty. The difference between groups, however, was not statistically significant. Brown et al. noted that when only children with Veau type II clefts (complete clefts of the secondary palate) were considered, 60% of the children who received intravelar veloplasty had normal speech. Brown et al. concluded that detachment of levator did not add morbidity to the surgery and resulted in better speech outcomes for some children. It should be noted that the lack of significant results in this study might have been due to its retrospective nature and the apparent fact that an unspecified number of surgeons were involved. Regardless, most surgeons today consider intravelar veloplasty an integral part of palate surgery for the infant with cleft palate.

Although specific surgical techniques vary greatly from surgeon to surgeon, two general procedures are commonly used to repair clefts of the secondary palate. The first is the *two-flap palatoplasty* (Bardach, 1990). This involves making lateral relaxing incisions along the hard palate and raising bilateral tissue flaps to be sutured at the midline (Figure 5–7A). As seen in Figure 5–7B, the lateral open, denuded areas of the palate are left to close on their own by a process known as healing by secondary intention. This procedure produces a straight-line scar in the mid-palate. As noted above, most surgeons will also perform an intravelar veloplasty as part of this procedure.

A second frequently used procedure is the *double-opposing Z-plasty* (DOZ) (Furlow, 1986). This is a relatively complicated surgery that incorporates intravelar veloplasty. The surgeon first makes incisions within the soft palate in a Z-shaped orientation (see Chapter 11, Figure 11–5). Oral tissue flaps are elevated while nasal tissue flaps are rotated and closed. The oral flaps are then rotated and closed. DOZ, also called Furlow repair, is a popular procedure because it simultaneously reconstructs the levator sling while lengthening the soft palate using the principles of a Z-plasty, a technique originally designed to lengthen tissue and revise scars. As reviewed in Chapter 11, DOZ is also used as a secondary surgical procedure to lengthen the soft palate when velopharyngeal inadequacy is diagnosed in older

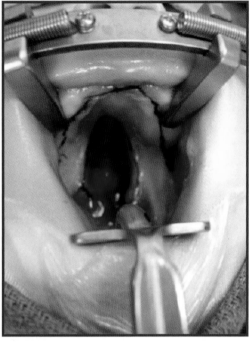 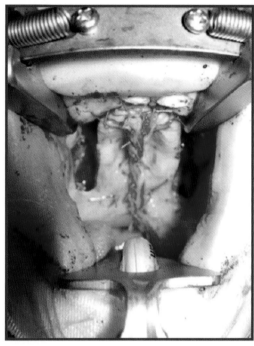

A   B

Figure 5–7. A. Surgical markings for a two-flap palatoplasty procedure. **B.** Midline repair of hard palate defect. (Courtesy of John van Aalst, MD, Pediatric Surgery, Cincinnati Children's Medical Center.)

children, especially those who have previously undergone two-flap, straight-line procedures.

Myringotomy and Insertion of Ventilation Tubes

Myringotomy involves making a surgical incision in the tympanic membrane(s), suctioning out fluid from the middle ear(s), and inserting ventilation tube(s). Because eustachian tube dysfunction is almost universal in infants with unrepaired cleft palate (see Chapter 6), most infants will undergo myringotomy with tube placement either at the time of lip or palate repair. At the Craniofacial Center at the University of North Carolina at

Chapel Hill, myringotomies are done at the time of palate repair, or sooner if otitis media with effusion is present. Ventilation tubes are placed to aerate the middle ear, equalize pressure between the middle ear and atmosphere, and drain fluids if present. Essentially, ventilation tubes perform the functions of the nonworking eustachian tubes. Ventilation tubes can remain functional from 6 to 12 months on average depending upon the type. Typically, the tubes are extruded from the tympanic membranes over time and fall into the external ear canals. The tubes are replaced as needed if otitis media with effusion persists. At times, the tubes may fall into the middle ear. In these cases, the tubes must be removed surgically. It is common for a child with cleft palate to have multiple sets of ventilation tubes during infancy and early childhood. Typically, the need for myringotomy and ventilation tubes subsides beginning at 6 years of age or older.

Glossopexy and Mandibular Lengthening by Distraction Osteogenesis

As described in Chapter 3, micrognathia is the primary feature of Pierre Robin sequence (PRS). Infants with this condition may experience episodes of upper airway obstruction caused by posterior displacement of the tongue (glossoptosis). In moderate to severe cases, the infant may experience poor feeding and respiratory distress with associated failure to thrive, prompting the need for tracheotomy. In this section, several surgical options are described that may prevent the need for tracheotomy in infants with Pierre Robin sequence.

Tongue-lip adhesion (TLA) or glossopexy is a procedure designed to relieve obstruction of the upper airway (Resnick, Dentino, Katz, Mulliken, & Padwa, 2015). The anterior tip of the tongue is fused to the inner surface of the lower lip (Figure 5–8). The goal of this procedure is to prevent the tongue from falling back and blocking the airway.

Infants who have undergone TLA with successful management of the airway can usually have the tongue-lip adhesion divided at the time of the cleft palate repair. Complications of TLA include scar formation, dehiscence (failure of the tongue to adhere to the lip), and failure to secure a stable airway.

Another surgical option in the management of airway obstruction in severe micrognathia is mandibular lengthening by distraction osteogenesis (MLDO). In this procedure, osteotomies (bone cuts) are created on both sides of the mandible and distraction hardware is attached to the mandible allowing it to be gradually

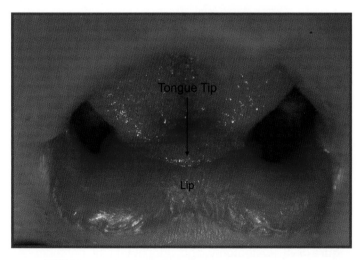

Figure 5–8. Tongue-lip adhesion in an infant with micrognathia. (Courtesy of Joseph A. Napoli, MD, DDS, Plastic, Maxillofacial, and Craniofacial Surgery, Alfred I. duPont Hospital for Children, Wilmington, DE.)

lengthened over a period of a few days to a few weeks (Figure 5–9). Lengthening the mandible and moving it forward also brings the tongue forward because it has attachments to the inner surface of the anterior mandible. MLDO, therefore, increases the air space between the posterior pharyngeal wall and the tongue base. Figure 5–10A shows a side view of an infant with distraction hardware following surgery. Figure 5–10B shows a radiograph of the same infant. The cleft palate is repaired once the airway is secured.

MLDO is intended for those infants who experience airway obstruction and increased effort in breathing that is not readily managed by conservative treatment. Complications may include damage to developing tooth buds, injury to the inferior alveolar nerve, malunion of the bone, and fracture or loosening of the hardware.

Infants with Pierre Robin sequence should undergo a thorough assessment of the airway as part of the decision-making process regarding management before selecting and proceeding with a surgical procedure to secure the airway. It is important to note that if laryngeal or tracheal abnormalities contribute to airway compromise, MLDO may not be successful and a tracheotomy may be necessary to provide a secure airway during infancy. Finally, it is important to note that some infants with even severe micrognathia may achieve normal mandibular growth by early childhood. Figure 5–11 shows a girl with Pierre-Robin sequence as an infant and again at 4 years of age. The child did not have MLDO and experienced catch-up mandibular growth.

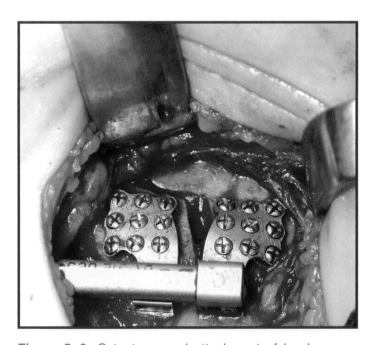

Figure 5–9. Osteotomy and attachment of hardware as part of mandibular lengthening by distraction osteogenesis (MLDO) in an infant with micrognathia. (Courtesy of Joseph A. Napoli, MD, DDS, Plastic, Maxillofacial, and Craniofacial Surgery, Alfred I. duPont Hospital for Children, Wilmington, DE.)

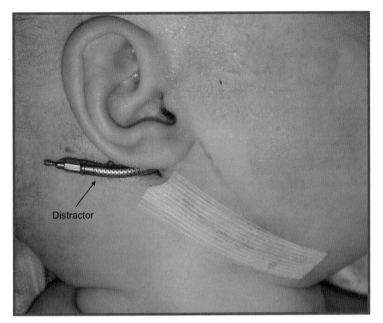

A

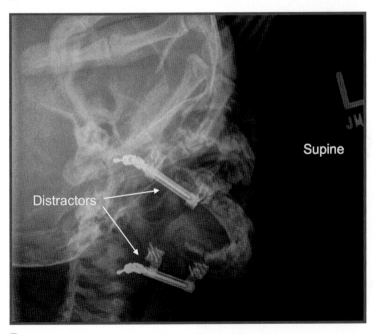

B

Figure 5–10. A. Side view of infant following MLDO. **B.** Radiograph of same infant in **A** showing placement of bilateral distractor hardware on mandible. (Courtesy of Joseph A. Napoli, MD, DDS, Plastic, Maxillofacial, and Craniofacial Surgery, Alfred I. duPont Hospital for Children, Wilmington, DE.)

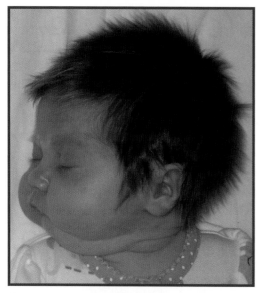

A

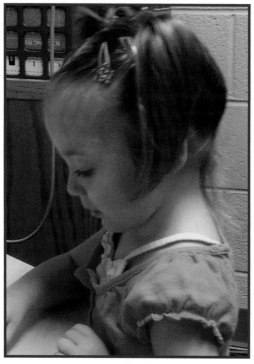

B

Figure 5–11. A. Girl with Pierre Robin sequence and severe micrognathia as an infant. **B.** Same girl at 4 years of age with normal mandibular growth. *Note.* MLDO was not done.

Summary of Surgical Procedures

Table 5–2 summarizes the types and timing of surgical procedures that an infant with cleft lip and palate may undergo during the first 12 to 14 months of life.

CONTROVERSY OF PALATE REPAIR TIMING

A brief history of team care for infants born with cleft lip and palate may facilitate understanding of the controversy surrounding the optimal age for palate repair. Cleft lip and palate are congenital birth defects that affect the infant and family at multiple levels of function including medical/dental, emotional, psychological, social, and communicative. Because of the multiple aspects of the condition, it has long been recognized that an interdisciplinary team is best suited to provide and coordinate long-term care for the infant and family. The first recognized attempt at team care was initiated at the Lancaster, Pennsylvania, cleft palate clinic in 1938 by Herbert Cooper. He was an orthodontist and early advocate for federal resources for individuals with cleft conditions (Moller, 2009). Through the efforts of Cooper and other dental specialists, the Academy of Cleft Palate Prosthesis was formed in 1943 in Pittsburgh, Pennsylvania. A major concern of the academy was the effects of surgery on facial growth and development of infants with repaired cleft palate (Moller, 2009). This academy was the forerunner of the present-day American Cleft Palate-Craniofacial Association (ACPA). ACPA is a multidisciplinary group whose major focus is the development of universal parameters of care for individuals with cleft lip and palate. In 2014, of more than 2,500 members of

Table 5–2. Surgical Procedures: Approximate Ages

Procedure	Approximate Age
Lip/nose reconstruction	2–3 months* (up to 5–6 months if presurgical appliances used)
Primary alveolar bone grafting	12 months (some centers)
Gingivoperiosteoplasty	At time of lip repair (some centers)
Palate repair	8–14 months*
Myringotomy/tubes	At time of palate repair (earlier if needed)
Glossopexy	1–2 weeks (infants with Pierre Robin)
Mandibular lengthening by distraction osteogenesis	1–2 months (infants with Pierre Robin)

Note. *Neonatal period, occasionally.

ACPA, approximately 30% were orthodontists and oral maxillofacial surgeons, 27% were plastic surgeons, and 14% were SLPs. Although ACPA fosters interdisciplinary education among members, it is nevertheless an organization influenced greatly by dental and medical concerns.

In light of the history of ACPA, it should not be surprising that facial growth and aesthetics took precedence over speech and communication when determining the optimal age for palate surgery. To be sure, there are many reasons for this. First, the surgeon forms a special bond with the family. With this special bond comes a natural trust and reliance on the knowledge and skills of the surgeon. Regardless of the surgeon's preference relative to age of palate repair, the family will understandably accept this timing as being the best for their child.

Second, surgery in the neonatal or early period of infancy (i.e., up to 2 months of age) has been viewed historically as having increased risk. The rule of 10s advocated in the 1960s was followed to reduce surgical risks involving excessive blood loss, anesthesia, and postsurgical healing complications. As noted previously, however, advances have occurred in medical care and anesthesia since the 1960s. As reported by Denk and Magee (1996), there appears to be no increased risk to medically healthy infants who undergo early versus late palate repair.

Third, there was a general lack of knowledge regarding the importance of early babbling behavior by the infant. Surgeons and other members of the cleft team believed that meaningful speech did not begin until the child was about 18 to 24 months of age and using multiple words (see Chapter 7 for a review of the importance of early babbling).

Finally, and perhaps most important, creation of scar tissue as a result of surgery

impedes growth of the maxillofacial complex. Surgeons in the early part of the
20th century tended to delay closure of
the secondary palate until the child was
2 years of age due to growth concerns.
The most rapid growth of the hard palate
occurs during the first 24 months of life
(Vorperian et al., 2009). Thus, by waiting
until this age, the surgeon allowed unimpeded growth during a critical period. In
addition, it was technically easier to repair
a narrower cleft in a larger oral cavity due
to natural growth of the infant.

If waiting until 2 years of age for palate repair was advantageous for facial
growth, then why not wait until 4 or 5
years of age to increase the benefit? Some
surgeons advocated this exact approach
(Schweckendiek, 1978; Slaughter & Pruzansky, 1954). Typically, surgeons would
repair the soft palate by 18 months of age
but not the hard palate until 4 or 5 years
of age. During the time between surgeries, an appliance was surgically pinned
into the hard palate to obturate the cleft.
Advocates of this approach believed that
the child benefited from (a) facial growth
unimpeded by scar tissue on the hard
palate, (b) a natural reduction in width
of the cleft due to growth, and (c) normal
speech acquisition in that the soft palate
was repaired early and the hard palate
was obturated. This "delayed hard palate
repair" was largely abandoned because
both speech and facial growth outcomes
were less than expected (Bardach, Morris,
& Olin 1984; Cosman & Falk, 1980; Jackson, McLennan, & Scheker, 1983). It should
be noted, however, that some centers still
employ a modification of this approach.
We have seen some children who had
early soft palate repair by 9 to 12 months
of age followed by hard palate repair at 15
to 18 months of age. No palatal appliance,
however, was used between surgeries.

Compromise "Early" Palate Repair

Largely because of poor speech outcomes
and marginal maxillofacial growth benefits associated with either late or delayed
hard palate repair protocols, there was a
shift to "early" one-stage palate surgeries in the latter half of the 20th century.
This shift was accelerated by longitudinal
research on facial growth in individuals with repaired cleft lip and palate. In
a landmark study, Ross (1987) examined
1,600 cephalometric radiographs of 538
males born with unilateral cleft lip and
palate from birth through skeletal maturity. Ross found that facial growth was
least restricted in those individuals who
never had surgery to repair the hard palate or if palate repair occurred as a teenager. These findings were consistent with
prevailing beliefs on the negative effects
of palate surgery on facial growth. Ross,
however, also reported unexpected findings. Specifically, Ross found that facial
growth was only marginally affected when
palate repair occurred *before* 11 months of
age but was most affected when it occurred
after 20 months of age (but before the teenage years), including delayed hard palate
repairs. These and other findings stimulated a shift to performing palate surgery
by 11 to 12 months of age as an "early"
compromise.

At least one speech study provided
support for the paradigm shift to early
palatal closure. Dorf and Curtin (1990)
followed 131 children with cleft palate at
3-month intervals from approximately 6
to 30 months of age. They divided the children into "early" and "late" palate repair
groups using 12 months of age as an arbitrary dividing point for surgery. Dorf and
Curtin reported a dramatic difference in
the percentage of children who developed
compensatory articulations based upon

age of surgery. Although nearly 90% of children who had late palate repair developed compensatory articulations, this occurred in less than 5% of children who had early surgery. Dorf and Curtin suggested that it was "the child's stage of phonemic development, or articulation age, at the time of palatal reconstruction" that appeared to determine postsurgical speech patterns (p. 347).

Optimal Age for Palate Repair?

Coinciding with research on maxillofacial growth in the 1980s, there was also longitudinal research on early speech and language development of infants with cleft palate. These studies showed that (a) prior to palate repair, infants exhibit limited phonetic inventories largely devoid of stop consonants, and (b) even following palate repair, emergence of stop consonants was often delayed and protracted (see Chapter 7 for a review). These findings prompted SLPs to question if "early" palate repair by 11 to 12 months of age was actually too late relative to facilitating normal speech acquisition. As suggested by Dorf and Curtin (1990), articulation versus chronological age seemed to be an important variable relative to at least the development of compensatory articulations. Kemp-Fincham, Kuehn, and Trost-Cardamone (1990) tackled the issue of optimal age for palate repair in a comprehensive review of speech and motor development in infants without cleft palate. Kemp-Fincham et al. concluded that, based on known developmental processes, palate repair should be completed between 2 and 4 months postnatally to optimize speech development. They did not recommend this age, however, because "the risk factors associated with surgery at this early age may again outweigh socioemotional and developmental considerations" (p. 743). Rather, Kemp-Fincham et al. recommended "surgery between 4 and 6 months of age be viewed as the target age for primary palatoplasty" (p. 744).

We need to note that the reluctance of Kemp-Fincham et al. (1990) to recommend surgery before 4 months of age was based upon medical risks that subsequent, albeit limited, research suggested is no greater than risks associated with surgery at older ages (Denk & Magee, 1996). It should be further noted that lip surgery at 2 to 3 months of age has been accepted as standard. Even though lip repair may be a less extensive surgery than palate repair in most cases, it is nonetheless a major surgery. There may be little reason, therefore, for an isolated cleft of the soft palate —which typically requires less extensive surgery than a complete cleft of the secondary palate—not to be repaired between 2 to 4 months of age, consistent with the optimal age for palate repair acknowledged by Kemp-Fincham et al. (1990).

Might there be social-emotional and developmental benefits from early palate repair in that feeding, mother-infant bonding, hearing, and speech may be improved? Does the potential of multiple psycho-social-communicative benefits outweigh the risks of medical/dental concerns? Obviously, these are not easy questions to answer, and the answers depend on sound scientific evidence that, unfortunately, currently does not exist. We have evaluated children, however, who underwent neonatal lip and palate surgery. Although some of these children had maxillary deficiency, all had speech without any maladaptive compensatory articulations. Until definitive data to the contrary are available, SLPs must be more vocal in expressing the view that from a speech and language standpoint, early palate surgery is to be preferred when the infant is not at increased medical risk.

CHAPTER SUMMARY

An infant born with cleft lip and palate may face multiple dental and medical procedures during the first year of life. Presurgical orthopedics is designed to narrow the width of the cleft and align maxillary segments prior to initial lip repair. There are multiple procedures that range from simple taping of the lip to intraoral appliances that actively bring cleft segments together. Surgery to repair the lip typically occurs between 2 to 3 months of age, and surgery to repair the palate typically occurs between 8 to 14 months of age. There is no consensus on timing of palate repair, and it is affected by multiple factors including health of the infant, concerns for facial growth and aesthetics, and philosophy of the cranio-facial team. Based on known developmental processes and trajectories, palate repair by 4 months of age may promote the most favorable outcomes for speech and language.

REFERENCES

Allareddy, V., Ross, E., Bruun, R., Lee, M. K., & Shusterman, S. (2015). Operative and immediate postoperative outcomes of using a Latham-type dentomaxillary appliance in patients with unilateral complete cleft lip and palate. *Cleft Palate-Craniofacial Journal, 52*(4), 405–410.

Bardach, J. (1990). Cleft palate repair: Two flap palatoplasty, research philosophy, technique and results. In J. Bardach & H. L. Morris (Eds.), *Multidisciplinary management of cleft lip and palate* (pp. 352–365). Philadelphia, PA: W.B. Saunders.

Bardach, J. (1994). Unilateral cleft lip. In M. Cohen (Ed.), *Mastery of plastic and reconstructive surgery. Volume 1.* Boston, MA: Little, Brown.

Bardach, J., Morris, H. L., & Olin, W. H. (1984). Late results of primary veloplasty: The Marburg project. *Plastic and Reconstructive Surgery, 73*, 207–215.

Berkowitz, S. (1996). A comparison of treatment results in complete bilateral cleft lip and palate using a conservative approach versus Millard-Latham PSOT procedure. *Seminars in Orthodontics, 2*(3), 169–184.

Berkowitz, S., Mejia, M., & Bystrik, A. (2004). A comparison of the effects of the Latham-Millard procedure with those of a conservative treatment approach for dental occlusion and facial aesthetics in unilateral and bilateral complete cleft lip and palate: Part I. Dental occlusion. *Plastic and Reconstructive Surgery, 113*(1), 1–18.

Billmire, D. A. (2008). Surgical management of clefts and velopharyngeal dysfunction. In A. W. Kummer (Ed.), *Cleft palate and craniofacial anomalies: Effects on speech and resonance* (2nd ed., pp. 508–540). Clifton Park, NY: Thomson Delmar Learning.

Brown, A. S., Cohen, M. A., & Randall, P. (1983). Levator muscle reconstruction: Does it make a difference? *Plastic and Reconstructive Surgery, 72*(1), 1–8.

Cosman, B., & Falk, A. S. (1980). Delayed hard palate repair and speech deficiencies: A cautionary report. *Cleft Palate Journal, 17*, 27–33.

Denk, M. J., & Magee, W. P., Jr. (1996). Cleft palate closure in the neonate: Preliminary report. *Cleft Palate-Craniofacial Journal, 33*(1), 57–61.

Dorf, D. S., & Curtin, J. W. (1990). Early palate repair and speech outcome: A ten-year experience. In J. Bardach & H. L. Morris (Eds.), *Multidisciplinary management of cleft lip and palate* (pp. 341–348). Philadelphia, PA: W.B. Saunders.

Furlow, L. T. (1986). Cleft palate repair by double opposing Z-plasty. *Plastic and Reconstructive Surgery, 78*, 724–736.

Grayson, B. H., & Garfinkle, J. S. (2014). Early cleft management: The case for nasoalveolar molding. *American Journal of Orthodontics and Dentofacial Orthopedics, 145*(2), 134–141.

Grayson, B. H., & Maull, D. (2004). Nasoalveolar molding for infants born with clefts of the lip, alveolus, and palate. *Clinics in Plastic Surgery, 31,* 149–158.

Huddart, A. G., North, J. F., & Davis, M. E. (1966). Observations on the treatment of cleft lip and palate. *Dental Practitioner and Dental Record, 16*(7), 265–274.

Jackson, I. T., McLennan, G., & Scheker, L. (1983). Primary veloplasty or primary palatal plasty: Some preliminary findings. *Plastic and Reconstructive Surgery, 72,* 153–157.

Kemp-Fincham, S. L., Kuehn, D. P., & Trost-Cardamone, J. (1990). Speech development and the timing of primary palatoplasty. In J. Bardach & H. L. Morris (Eds.), *Multidisciplinary management of cleft lip and palate,* (pp. 736–745). Philadelphia, PA: W.B. Saunders.

Koberg, W. R. (1973). Present view on bone grafting in cleft palate. (A review of the literature). *Journal of Maxillofacial Surgery, 1*(4), 185–193.

Kriens, O. B. (1969). An anatomical approach to veloplasty. *Plastic and Reconstructive Surgery, 43*(1), 29–41.

Kriens, O. B. (1970). Fundamental anatomic findings for an intravelar veloplasty. *Cleft Palate Journal, 7,* 27–36.

Latham, R. A. (1980). Orthopedic advancement of the cleft maxillary segment: A preliminary report. *Cleft Palate Journal, 17,* 227–233.

McComb, H. (1985). Primary correction of unilateral cleft lip nasal deformity: A 10-year review. *Plastic and Reconstructive Surgery, 75,* 791–799.

Millard, D. R., Jr. (1964a). Rotation-advancement principle in cleft lip closure. *Cleft Palate Journal, 1*(2), 246–252.

Millard, D. R., Jr. (1964b). Refinements in rotation-advancement cleft lip technique. *Plastic and Reconstructive Surgery, 33,* 26–38.

Moller, K. T. (2009). Interdisciplinary team approach: Issues and procedures. In K. T. Moller & L. E. Glaze (Eds.), *Cleft lip and palate: Interdisciplinary issues and treatment* (2nd ed., pp. 3–37). Austin, TX: Pro-Ed.

Noordhoff, M. S., & Kuo-Ting Chen, P. (2006). Unilateral cheiloplasty. In S. J. Mathes (Ed.), *Plastic surgery: Volume 4: Pediatric plastic surgery* (pp. 165–215). Philadelphia, PA: Saunders Elsevier.

Randall, P. (1959). A triangular flap operation for the primary repair of unilateral clefts of the lip. *Plastic and Reconstructive Surgery, 23,* 331–347.

Resnick, C. M., Dentino, K., Katz, E., Mulliken, J. B., & Padwa, B. L. (2015). Effectiveness of tongue-lip adhesion for obstructive sleep apnea in infants with Robin sequence measured by polysomnography. *Cleft Palate-Craniofacial Journal.* Advance online publication.

Rosenstein, S. W., Monroe, C. W., Kernahan, D. A., Jacobson, B. N., Griffith, B. H., & Bauer, B. S. (1982). The case for early bone grafting in cleft lip and palate. *Plastic and Reconstructive Surgery, 70*(3), 297–307.

Ross, R. B. (1970). The clinical implications of facial growth in cleft lip and palate. *Cleft Palate Journal, 7,* 37–47.

Ross, R. B. (1987). Treatment variables affecting facial growth in complete unilateral cleft lip and palate. *Cleft Palate Journal, 24,* 54–77.

Ruding, R. (1964). Cleft palate: Anatomic and surgical considerations. *Plastic and Reconstructive Surgery, 33,* 132–147.

Ruiz, R. L., & Costello, B. J. (2009). Repair of the unilateral cleft lip: A comparison of surgical techniques. In T. A. Turvey (Ed.), *Oral and maxillofacial surgery, Volume III* (2nd ed., pp. 735–758). St. Louis, MO: Saunders Elsevier.

Schweckendiek, W. (1978). Primary veloplasty: Long-term results without maxillary deformity. *Cleft Palate Journal, 15,* 268–274.

Slaughter, W. B., & Pruzansky, S. (1954). The rationale for velar closure as a primary procedure in the repair of cleft palate defects. *Plastic and Reconstructive Surgery, 13*(5), 341–357.

Trier, W. C. (1985). Repair of unilateral cleft lip: The rotation-advancement operation. *Clinics in Plastic Surgery, 12*(4), 573–594.

Vorperian, H. K., Wang, S., Chung, M. K., Schimek, E. M., Durtschi, R. B., Kent, R. D., . . . Gentry, L. R. (2009). Anatomic development of the oral and pharyngeal portions of the vocal tract: An imaging study. *Journal of the Acoustical Society of America, 125*(3), 1666–1678.

Wilhelmsen, H. R., & Musgrave, R. H. (1966). Complications of cleft lip surgery. *Cleft Palate Journal, 3,* 223–231.

Wood, B. G. (1970). Control of the maxillary arch by primary bone graft in cleft lip and palate cases. *Cleft Palate Journal, 7,* 194–205.

Zajac, D. J., Cevidanes, L., Shah, S., & Haley, K. L. (2011). Maxillary arch dimensions and spectral characteristics of children with cleft lip and palate who produce middorsum palatal stops. *Journal of Speech Language Hearing Research, 55*(6), 1876–1886.

6

Hearing and Otologic Management

INTRODUCTION

Hearing loss is prevalent in cleft palate and craniofacial anomalies. A hearing loss compounds the already existing challenges imposed upon this population. The functional, social, and economic impact of hearing loss can be great (World Health Organization, 2015). The obvious functional impact is the potential for delayed speech and language and the inability to communicate with others. For some, hearing impairment can affect social interactions and academic performance, and later vocational opportunities (Joint Commission on Infant Hearing, 2007). Early detection and intervention of hearing loss and vigilant monitoring are essential elements in the total audiologic and otologic care of individuals with cleft and craniofacial anomalies.

We begin this chapter with a brief overview of the structure and function of the hearing mechanism. Ear and hearing problems most commonly associated with cleft and craniofacial anomalies will be discussed. Audiologic assessment of hearing and the treatment of hearing loss will be presented. In the final section, we will discuss the role of the speech-language pathologist (SLP) in providing information to caregivers about ear problems and hearing loss associated with cleft and craniofacial anomalies. Information about hearing that is important for the SLP to know prior to undertaking speech therapy will be given.

OVERVIEW OF THE STRUCTURE AND FUNCTION OF THE EAR

Understanding normal structure and function of the ear is fundamental to understanding the impact of ear pathology on hearing. The ear is made up of three main sections: the outer, middle, and inner ear (Figure 6–1).

The *outer* ear is divided into the pinna, or auricle, and the external auditory canal (EAC). The pinna is made up of cartilage (Figure 6–2). It serves as a collector of sound and aids in localization and provides an efficient means for directing high-frequency sounds to the ear canal. The external auditory canal (EAC) is an extension of the pinna. The first third of the EAC is made of cartilage, and the inner two thirds are bony or osseous. The

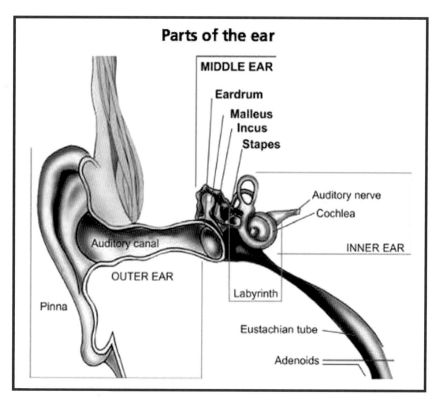

Figure 6–1. Diagram of the outer, middle, and inner ear. (Credit: Photo courtesy of the National Institutes of Health, Department of Health and Human Services).

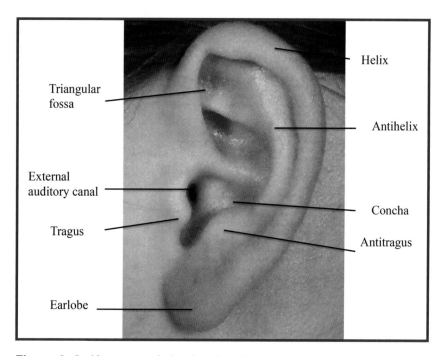

Figure 6–2. Key anatomic landmarks of a normal left pinna.

function of the EAC is to direct sound waves to the eardrum.

The *middle ear* consists of the tympanic membrane (TM) or eardrum, three ossicles, two muscles, and the eustachian tube (described separately). The TM lies at the end of the EAC and separates the outer and middle ears (see Figure 6–1). It is a thin, stiff, semitransparent membrane that vibrates when the sound transmitted through the EAC hits it. The middle ear is an air-filled cavity that contains three small bones or ossicles: the malleus, the incus, and the stapes. The malleus is attached to the fibrous portion of the tympanic membrane. When the tympanic membrane vibrates in response to sound, the vibration is carried to the malleus then transferred to the incus and then to the stapes. There are two muscles in the middle ear: the tensor tympani and stapedial muscle. The tensor tympani is attached to the handle (manubrium) of the malleus and responds to nonauditory stimulation. The stapedius attaches to the stapedial bone and contracts in response to loud noise.

The *inner* ear is located in the petrous portion of the temporal bone and contains a complex labyrinth consisting of the cochlea and semicircular canals (see Figure 6–1). The cochlea is the auditory center of the inner ear, and the semicircular canals are responsible for balance. The inner ear is innervated by the auditory nerve (cranial nerve VIII). This is a sensory nerve that transfers information from the cochlea to the auditory cortex for receptive auditory comprehension.

All of auditory structures must be intact for normal hearing. A disorder can occur anywhere along the auditory pathway resulting in one of three types of hearing loss: conductive, sensorineural, or mixed. A conductive loss occurs as a result of a problem in the outer or middle ear that interferes with the way sound is transmitted from the middle ear to reach the inner ear. A sensorineural hearing loss is caused by damage or malformation to the inner ear (e.g., cochlea or auditory nerve) or neural pathways of hearing—there is no problem with the outer and middle ear. A mixed loss occurs as a result of the conditions causing both a conductive and sensorineural hearing loss.

NATURE OF HEARING LOSS IN CLEFT AND CRANIOFACIAL ANOMALIES

Hearing loss can be categorized as acquired or congenital. An acquired hearing loss is one that can occur after birth as a result of a medical condition or injury. Examples of conditions that cause an acquired hearing loss are middle ear fluid and perforated eardrum. A congenital hearing loss is one that is present at birth. Examples of conditions that cause a congenital hearing loss are structural malformations of the outer and middle ear.

Conductive hearing loss is the most common type of hearing loss associated with cleft palate and craniofacial anomalies. Sensorineural and mixed hearing losses can and do occur, but do so with lesser frequency. A hearing loss can take on any number of features. It can be unilateral or bilateral, vary in configuration, and range in severity from slight to profound. Conditions can cause a hearing loss that is fluctuating, permanent, or progressive in nature.

Causes of Hearing Loss

Hearing loss in children with cleft and craniofacial anomalies most often occurs as a result of structural malformations of the outer and middle ear, or secondary to middle ear fluid. Inner ear defects are less common. The types of ear malformations and associated hearing loss are described in the next sections.

Anomalies in Front of the Outer Ear

Preauricular tags and ear pits occur in front of the external or outer ear. A preauricular tag is a small tag in front of the pinna (Figure 6–3) that can present with variation in shape and size. An ear pit appears as a small hole located in the front of the ear (Figure 6–4).

An ear tag or ear pit in isolation does not cause hearing loss, but the presence of either one may be associated with other congenital anomalies (i.e., oculo-auriculo-vertebral spectrum [OAVS]) and malformations of the middle and inner ear (Bartel-Friedrich & Wulke, 2007). If an infant has ear tags or ear pits and a malformation not yet identified, the child should be referred for further physical, genetic, and audiologic examinations.

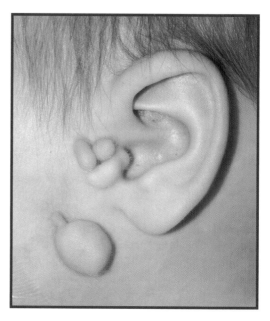

Figure 6–3. Preauricular tag in a child with oculoauriculovertebral spectrum (OAVS). (Photo courtesy of Joseph A. Napoli, MD, DDS, Plastic, Maxillofacial, and Craniofacial Surgery, Alfred I. duPont Hospital for Children, Wilmington, DE.)

Outer Ear Anomalies

A common congenital deformity of the pinna is microtia. It is a salient feature of a number of branchial arch anomalies (see Chapter 3). *Microtia* is a term used to refer to a small or underdeveloped pinna (Figure 6–5). The extent of microtia may vary from person to person and sometimes between the ears in the same person. The pinna may be small, it may consist only of a cartilaginous remnant, or the pinna may be completely absent (anotia). Microtia can cause a conductive hearing loss, the severity of which is dependent upon the extent of the pinna anomaly.

The external auditory canal (EAC) may be stenotic or narrow, the degree to which can vary (Figure 6–6). In the more severe form, the canal may be under-developed or absent, a condition referred to as *atresia*.

Atresia of the EAC often co-occurs with microtia. As a matter of fact, stenosis or atresia of the EAC and microtia are quite common in Treacher Collins Syndrome (TCS) (Pron, Galloway, Armstrong, & Posnick, 1993) and OAVS. In a less severe form, stenosis of the ear canal can cause a mild conductive hearing loss. On the other hand, severe stenosis and atresia of the ear canal can cause a moderate to moderately severe hearing loss.

Middle Ear Anomalies

Ossicular deformities including malformed ossicles, ossicular chain fixation, and stapes fixation are common findings among a number of craniofacial condi-

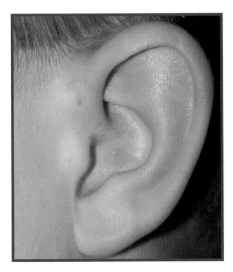

Figure 6–4. Photo of an ear pit. (Photo courtesy of Joseph A. Napoli, MD, DDS, Plastic, Maxillofacial, and Craniofacial Surgery, Alfred I. duPont Hospital for Children, Wilmington, DE.)

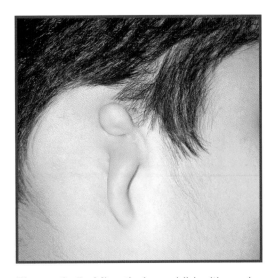

Figure 6–5. Microtia in a child with oculo-auriculoverterbral spectrum (OAVS). (Photo courtesy of Joseph A. Napoli, MD, DDS, Plastic, Maxillofacial, and Craniofacial Surgery, Alfred I. duPont Hospital for Children, Wilmington, DE.)

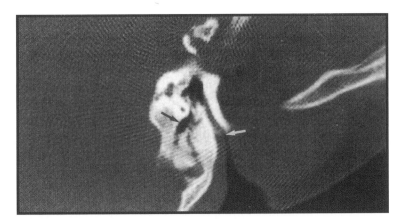

Figure 6–6. Coronal computed tomography (CT) scan of the temporal bone showing severe stenosis of both the cartilaginous and bony portions of the external auditory canal (*white arrow*) and hypoplastic middle ear cavity (*black arrow*). ("Audiologic and otologic characteristics of Pfeiffer syndrome" by L. D. Vallino-Napoli, 1996, *Cleft Palate-Craniofacial Journal, 33*, 327. Copyright 1996 by American Cleft Palate Craniofacial Association. Reprinted with permission.)

tions (see Chapter 3). Figure 6–7 shows an ossicular chain abnormality in a child with Pfeiffer syndrome.

In addition, the middle ear cavity may be hypoplastic and the middle ear cavity enlarged (Vallino-Napoli, 1996).

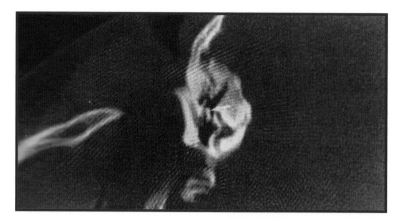

Figure 6–7. Coronal CT scan showing hypoplastic ossicular chain fused to the lateral tympanic wall (*white arrow*). ("Audiologic and otologic characteristics of Pfeiffer syndrome" by L. D. Vallino-Napoli, 1996, *Cleft Palate-Craniofacial Journal, 33*, 328. Copyright 1996 by American Cleft Palate Craniofacial Association. Reprinted with permission.)

Middle ear anomalies may or may not occur with outer ear anomalies.

The abnormalities of the middle ear cause a conductive hearing loss that typically ranges from moderate to moderately severe. Figure 6–8 shows an audiogram of a 9-year-old with oculo-auriculo-vertebral spectrum (OAVS). He has a moderately severe right unilateral conductive hearing loss and normal hearing in the left ear. Findings on a 3-dimensional CT scan showed an absent external auditory canal and hypoplastic ossicles and normal inner ear structures. The outer, middle, and inner ear structures are normal in the left ear.

Figure 6–9 shows a child with Treacher Collins syndrome who has bilateral middle ear atresia. Her unaided audiogram shows a moderately severe conductive hearing loss bilaterally.

Inner Ear Anomalies

As mentioned earlier, congenital malformations of the inner ear in cranio-facial syndromes are less common than outer or middle ear anomalies. When present, they can include dilated vestibules, malformed lateral canals, and cochlear dysplasia (Zhou, Schwartz, & Gopen, 2009), as well as enlarged vestibular aqueducts and hypoplastic cochlea (Hennersdorf et al., 2014). These abnormalities can cause severe to profound sensorineural hearing loss.

Abnormalities of the outer or middle ear (conductive) may co-occur with abnormalities of the inner ear (sensorineural), causing a mixed hearing loss. Figure 6–10 shows an audiogram of a child with Stickler syndrome and a bilateral moderate to mild mixed hearing loss.

THE EUSTACHIAN TUBE

The eustachian tube (ET) plays an important role in middle ear function and hearing in cleft palate and abnormal craniofacial structures. Therefore, it has been given separate consideration.

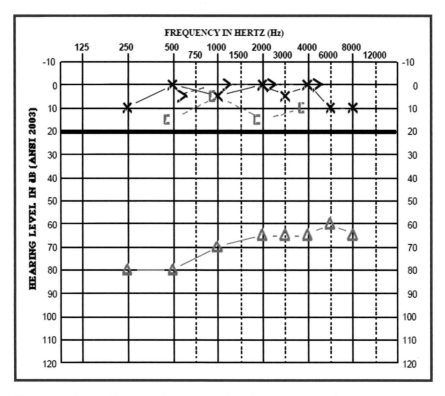

Figure 6–8. Audiogram of a 9-year-old with oculoauriculoverterbral spectrum (OAVS) showing a moderately severe conductive hearing loss from 250 through 8000 Hz in the right ear and normal hearing from 250 through 8000 Hz in the left ear.

The ET extends from the middle ear to the nasopharynx (see Figure 6–1). Its function is to ventilate the middle ear space, protect the middle ear from nasopharyngeal secretions, and drain fluids out of the middle ear space (Bluestone & Doyle, 1988). Anatomically, the ET in infants and toddlers is shorter, narrower, and more horizontal than the adult (Bluestone & Klein, 1990). Under normal conditions, the ET is closed and opens when we swallow, chew, or yawn.

The two primary muscles associated with ET function are the tensor veli palatini (TVP) and the levator veli palatini (LVP) (see Chapter 1). The function of the TVP is to open or dilate the eusta-

chian tube, which keeps the pressure in the middle ear space equal to atmospheric pressure, allowing fluids to drain out of the middle ear. The levator veli palatini elevates the palate to separate the nasal and oral cavities necessary for normal resonance, and to prevent reflux or oral secretions and food into the nasopharynx during swallowing (Drake & Swibel Rosenthal, 2013). In children with cleft palate, the course and insertion of the tensor veli palatini muscle are disrupted, failing to dilate the eustachian tube, causing it not to open easily (Bluestone, 1971; Doyle, Cantekin, & Bluestone, 1980).

There are other conditions present in children with cleft and craniofacial anom-

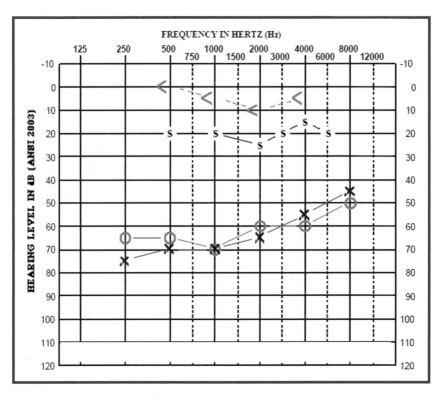

Figure 6–9. Audiogram of a 12-year-old with Treacher Collins syndrome. Unaided responses to pure tone show a moderate to severe conductive hearing loss bilaterally. When wearing a bone conduction hearing aid, responses to stimuli presented in soundfield (S) are in the normal range.

alies that can impede the opening of the ET. The ET may fail to function as a result of an intrinsic (inside) or extrinsic (outside) mechanical obstruction. ET dysfunction due to intrinsic mechanical obstruction is caused by swelling in the mucous lining of or around the ET as a result of an upper respiratory tract infection or allergies. Extrinsic mechanical obstruction can be caused by enlarged adenoids or a narrow nasopharyngeal space that impedes the opening of the ET.

When the ET fails to function, air is prevented from getting into the middle ear, causing negative middle ear pressure and retraction (inward pushing) of the tympanic membrane. If the obstruction persists, fluid accumulates in the middle ear space behind the eardrum, resulting in a condition called otitis media with effusion (OME).

OTITIS MEDIA WITH EFFUSION IN CHILDREN WITH CLEFT LIP AND PALATE

Otitis media with effusion (OME) is a buildup of fluid behind the eardrum most often caused by eustachian tube dysfunction. This fluid is typically not infected, nor does it cause discomfort or pain. OME causes a mild to moderate fluctuating conductive hearing loss. Long-term middle ear effusion can produce patho-

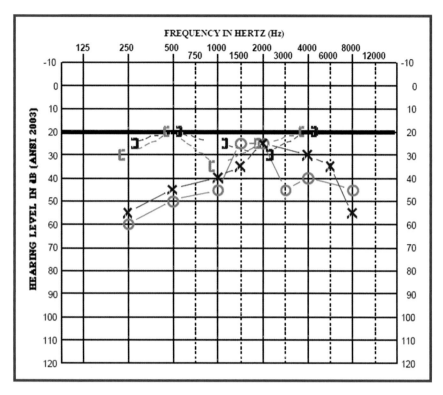

Figure 6–10. Audiogram of a 10-year-old with Stickler syndrome showing a moderate to mild mixed hearing loss bilaterally.

logic changes in the mucosa of the middle ear and the ossicular chain (Orchik, Schumaier, Shea, & Ge, 1995; Paparella et al., 1984). Where the loss may have initially been temporary, these structural changes can result in a permanent hearing loss. Figures 6–11 and 6–12 each show an audiogram of a conductive hearing loss caused by OME.

OME develops in nearly all infants with unrepaired cleft palate (Paradise, Bluestone, & Felder, 1969; Ponduri et al., 2009; Stool & Randall, 1967). Infants and children with submucous cleft palate and congenital velopharyngeal inadequacy are also predisposed to OME (Shehan et al., 2004). It has been suggested that children with cleft lip are at little risk for middle ear disease (Kwan, Abdullah,

Liu, van Hasselt, & Tong, 2011; Sheahan, Miller, Sheahan, Earley, & Blayney, 2003). However, there are reports to the contrary (Deedler et al., 2011; Reugg et al., 2015; Vallino, Zuker, & Napoli, 2008). The prevalence of the disease is lower in cleft lip than cleft palate, but occurs at a higher rate than in children who do not have a cleft.

In their study of ear disease in 95 3-year-old children with CL with or without cleft of the alveolus (CL/A), Vallino et al. (2008) reported that 33% experienced one or more episodes of OME during their first three years. Based on the results of a parent survey, Deedler et al. (2011) also reported that 33% of 161 children with CL/A had a history of acute otitis media and 41% had repeated episodes. In a recent study, Reugg et al. (2015) cited a rate of middle ear disease in children with cleft lip that was similar to those previously reported (Deedler et al., 2011; Vallino et al., 2008). Given these findings, both Vallino et al. (2008) and Deedler et al. (2011) recommended that ear status in children with CL/A should be monitored routinely.

In the general population, about 50% of infants will develop OME during the first year of life. The episodes generally resolve spontaneously within 3 months (Kuo, Lien, Chu, & Shio, 2013). In contrast, nearly 90% of children with cleft will have experienced OME by their first birthday (Ponduri et al., 2009), of which not all will resolve spontaneously in 3 months. Some individuals will experience recurrent episodes of OME throughout childhood (Flynn, Möller, Jönsson, & Lohmander, 2009) and few may also present with the condition in adolescence and adulthood (Flynn & Lohmander, 2014; Moller, 1975; Sheahan, Miller, Sheahan, Ealy, & Blayney, 2004).

Although there can be a reduction in middle ear pathology after the cleft palate is repaired, palatoplasty does not guarantee improvement in eustachian tube function and elimination of middle ear disease in all children. In children who experience recurrent OME, Tatum and Senders (1993) suggested that the tensor veli palatini muscle, which is responsible for active opening of the eustachian tube, continues to be misaligned even after appropriate reinsertion of the levator veli palatini muscle to form a sling necessary for adequate separation of the oral and nasal cavities for speech. As a result, eustachian tube dysfunction persists causing impaired ventilation of the middle ear and a buildup of fluid behind the eardrum.

There is ample evidence to suggest that OME improves with increasing age (Doyle et al., 1980; Handzic-Cuk, Cuk, Risavi, Katusic, & Stanjer-Katusic, 1996; Möller, 1981; Sheahan et al., 2003; Smith, DiRuggiero, & Jones, 1994). Timmons, Poorten, Desloovere, and DeBruyne (2006) examined middle ear status of 20 children with cleft palate between the ages of 10 and 15 years and found a decrease in OME from 50% at 3 years to 13% after age 10. Flynn and Lohmander (2014) reported that OME decreased from 89% at age 1 year to 10% in the young adult. In their longitudinal study of 23 children with CLP at ages 3, 4, and 5 years, Zavala, Morlet, Napoli, and Vallino (2013) reported that although there was a decline in the rate of OME from 3 to 5 years old, the condition persisted in nearly 60% of the children at age 5. With these data, it is reasonable then to consider that it may take some time for the eustachian tube to recover normal function after the cleft palate repair. Smith et al. (1994) reported that the average time to recovery of the eustachian tube following surgery is about 6 years (range: 1.0 to 10.3 years). It may take longer. There may be other yet unknown independent variables that can have an impact on this recovery.

In most children with CLP, hearing improves as they get older. This more often than not coincides with the decrease in OME. In their cohort of 44 3-year-old children, Rynnel-Dagöö, Linberg, Bagger-Sjöback, and Larson (1992) reported that 82% of the 3 and 4-year-old children studied had normal hearing after cleft palate repair. In a recent study, Skuladottir, Sivertsen, Assmus, Remme, Dahle, and Vindenes (2015) examined hearing outcomes of 317 patients with CLP and CP at ages 4, 6, and 15 years. Pure tone averages (PTA) were calculated using 15 dBHL and 20 dBHL cutoffs for normal

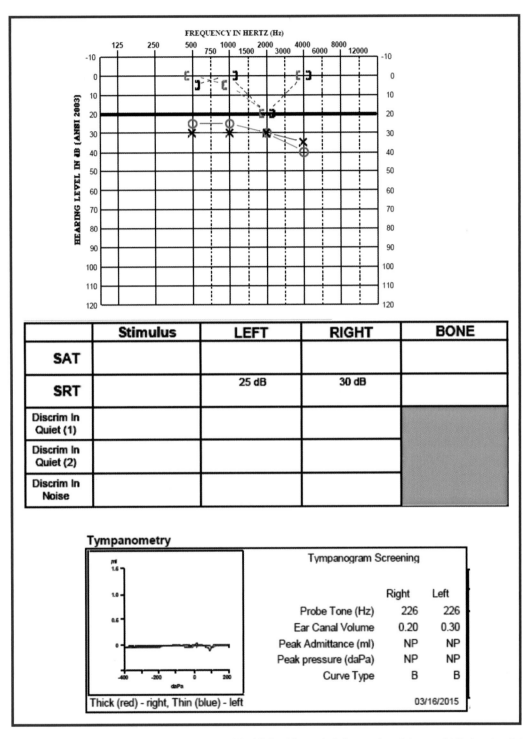

Figure 6–11. Audiogram of a 6-year-old child with a cleft lip and palate and bilateral mild conductive hearing loss. Note air-bone gaps from 500 to 4,000 Hz. Speech reception thresholds (SRTs) are consistent with pure tone averages. Flat tympanometric configurations confirm the presence of otitis media with effusion.

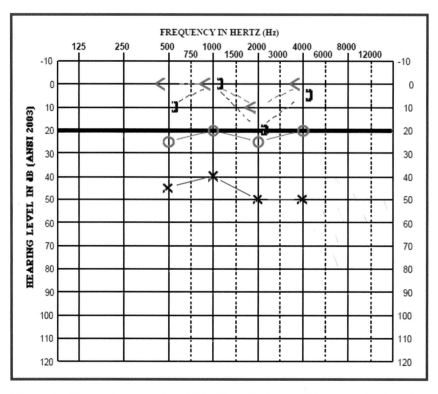

Figure 6–12. Audiogram of a child with a slight to mild conductive hearing loss in the right ear and a moderate conductive hearing loss in the left ear.

hearing. There was a significant improvement with age in both groups. For CLP, the median PTA was 16 dBHL at 4 years, 13 dBHL at 6 years, and 9 dBHL at 15 years. Similarly, the median PTA for CP was 15 dBHL, 12 dBHL, and 9 dBHL at 4, 6, and 15 years, respectively. Interestingly, children who had palate repair at 18 months had a better PTA at age 15 when compared with patients who had palate repair at 12 months.

Zavala et al. (2013) examined frequency-specific pure-tone thresholds in 23 children at ages 3, 4, and 5 years. They tested hearing at 500, 1,000, 2,000, and 4,000 Hz using a 15dB HL cutoff threshold. As shown in Figure 6–13, there was a trend for hearing to improve with increasing age. However, a slight loss at 500 Hz and 1,000 Hz persisted at age 5 years, a finding that cannot be identified using PTA. This may coincide with the persistence of OME at this age. The effects of the loss have yet to be explained.

In summary, there is a high prevalence of OME among children with cleft palate. Although the rate of OME is lower in CL than it is in CP, it is higher than in the general population. OME causes a fluctuating conductive hearing loss. There is evidence to support reduction in OME and improvement with increasing age, yet for some children, OME can persist into the school years. Diligent monitoring of ear disease and hearing in children with CLP is imperative.

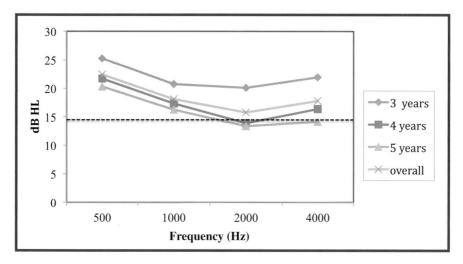

Figure 6–13. Frequency-specific mean thresholds of children with cleft lip/palate at ages 3, 4, and 5 years. The cutoff for normal hearing was 15 dB HL.

AUDIOLOGIC ASSESSMENT

Every child with a cleft lip/palate and craniofacial anomaly needs and should receive longitudinal otologic and audiologic monitoring and follow up (American Cleft Palate-Craniofacial Association, 2009). Identifying a hearing loss and cause is paramount to appropriate management.

NEWBORN HEARING SCREENING

Universal newborn hearing screening has been valuable in identifying infants who are likely to have hearing impairment. Cleft palate and craniofacial anomalies are risk factors for hearing loss and are targeted during the screening process (Joint Commision on Infant Hearing, 2007). Passing a hearing screening does not mean that the child with CLP has normal hearing and is unlikely to develop a hearing loss. As shown by several studies, the majority of infants with cleft palate often do pass their newborn hearing screening because either the middle ear fluid has not yet accumulated enough to cause hearing loss, or the loss is borderline or so mild that it goes undetected during screening (Chen, Messner, & Curtin, 2008; Jordan & Sidman, 2014; Szabo, Langevin, Schoem, & Mabry, 2010). From the foregoing discussions we know that OME inevtably develops in most children with cleft palate resulting in a hearing loss.

A craniofacial anomaly increases the likelihood that an affected infant will have a hearing loss that will be detected during newborn screening. However, there will be some hearing impaired infants that will be missed even with a targeted risk factor screening. Hence, even if a newborn with cleft palate or craniofacial anomaly passes a newborn neonatal hearing screening, he or she should be scheduled for a diagnostic hearing evaluation by at least 6 months with routine monitoring of hearing at designated intervals thereafter.

ASSESSING HEARING

Every child who has a CLP and craniofacial anomaly requires longitudinal otological and audiologic assessment, monitoring, and follow up (American Cleft Palate-Craniofacial Association [ACPA], 2009). The purpose of this assessment is to measure hearing sensitivity, determine the nature and degree of hearing loss, establish baseline for future monitoring, and determine best treatment options.

The audiologic assessment typically includes otoscopy, tympanometry, otoacoustic emissions (OAEs) screening, pure-tone audiometry, and speech audiometry. Auditory brainstem audiometry (ABR) may also be conducted. These tests will be briefly described.

Otoscopy

Otoscopy is the procedure used to visualize the tympanic membrane and external auditory canal. A normal tympanic membrane is translucent and moves when air is blown through the otoscope causing a pressure change. In contrast, when OME is present, the tympanic membrane is opaque yellow and typically retracted with limited mobility in response to pressure change.

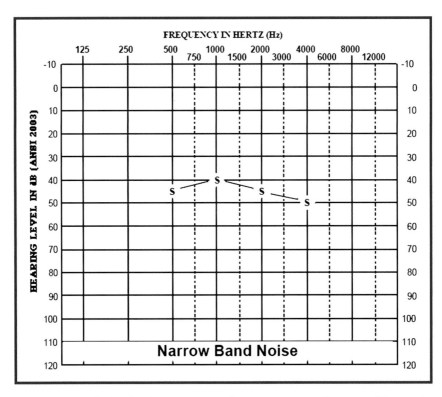

Figure 6–14. Behavioral response audiometry test results on an 11-month-old child with cleft palate and otitis media with effusion. Soundfield thresholds (S) suggest a moderate hearing loss from 500 to 4000 Hz for at least the better ear.

Tympanometry

Tympanometry is an objective measurement of middle ear function and is used in conjunction with standard audiometric tests. Tympanometry can be performed with infants using a high-frequency probe tone, and after 6 months, the conventional 226-Hz probe tone can be used. Tympanometry provides useful information about the presence of middle ear fluid, patency of PE tubes, eardrum perforations, middle ear mobility, and ear canal volume (see Figure 6–11).

Otoacoustic Emissions (OAEs)

OAEs are low-level sounds produced primarily by the outer hair cells (sensory hair cells) when the cochlea is stimulated by an auditory signal. When the sound stimulates the cochlea, outer hair cells begin to vibrate, and this in turn sends back a very soft, almost inaudible sound back to the middle ear, which can be measured (Kramer & Guthrie, 2008). OAEs that are present suggest that the outer ear, middle ear, and outer hair cells in the cochlea are functioning within normal limits. If OAEs are absent, this could represent either a conductive hearing loss, cochlear hearing loss, or mixed hearing loss, and further testing would be needed to determine the type and severity of the loss. OAEs are present in individuals with normal hearing. They can be absent in those with OME who have a conductive hearing loss of 30 dB HL or greater.

Pure Tone Audiometry and Speech Audiometry

From about a developmental age of 6 or 7 months to 2 years of age, children can be assessed using behavioral techniques including visual response audiometry and behavioral response audiometry (Sirimanna, 2004). These assessments are conducted in soundfield without headphones. Because the two ears cannot be tested separately, thresholds for the better ear are reported (Figure 6–14). As a child matures, he or she is able to wear headphones to allow for each ear to be tested separately. Pure tone air and bone conduction thresholds are obtained at selected frequencies ranging from 500 to 4,000 Hz; providing information about hearing loss (see Figures 6–11 and 6–12).

Conventionally, the hearing level (HL) considered to be normal is 20 db HL or less. However, in a child, even a slight loss in hearing sensitivity may have an effect on a child who is acquiring language (DeBonis & Donohue, 2008). It has been suggested that a 15 dB HL in a child with a cleft or craniofacial condition is detrimental to language learning (Gould, 1990; Lewis, 1976). Tunçbilek, Özgür, and Belgin (2003) stated that a 15 dB HL loss may be "potentially threatening" (p. 307) to a child with cleft palate who is already at risk for speech and language difficulties. To illustrate this point, consider the young child for whom puretone air conduction hearing thresholds are obtained at 15 dB HL at 500 Hz, 1000 Hz, and 2000 Hz, and bone conduction hearing thresholds are obtained at 0 dB HL at these frequencies. The air-bone gap is 15 dB HL, consistent with a conductive hearing loss.

Speech audiometry is also an important component of the assessment protocol because it provides information about the degree of hearing communication handicap. The most commonly used speech audiometry tests are speech recognition thresholds and word recognition testing (see Figure 6–11).

Auditory Brainstem Response Audiometry (ABR)

ABR testing is used in newborn hearing screening, on children less than 6 months of age, children who are difficult to test or unable to cooperate for conventional testing, or children for whom reliable test results have not yet been obtained (Sirimana, 2004). Using clicks or tones ABR can estimate hearing threshold sensitivity from the 2000 to 4000 Hz range. Based on waveform patterns, information about conductive, sensorineural, and retrocochlear hearing losses can be identified and distinguished. Although an infant with cleft palate is more likely to have a fluctuating conductive hearing loss attributed to OME, it is nonetheless important to obtain thresholds during ABR. Because it is possible that an underlying sensorineural hearing loss can coexist, the information obtained from ABR can be used to rule out or confirm this impairment.

TREATING OTITIS MEDIA WITH EFFUSION

Management using antibiotic therapy to treat OME has limited benefit (Roberts et al., 2004). Because middle ear fluid is persistent, the most common treatment approach is myringotomy with insertion of ventilation tubes (also called pressure-equalization (PE) tubes, tympanostomy tubes, and grommets) (Figure 6–15). In some children, these tubes may stay in place for as long as a couple of years.

Myringotomy is a surgical procedure in which an incision is made in the eardrum to relieve the pressure built up behind it and to drain the accumulated fluid from the middle ear. The tubes are then inserted into the eardrum to allow air to enter the middle ear cavity directly and prevent fluid from reaccumulating. When OME is resolved, hearing is restored. Figure 6–16 shows an audiogram of a child with cleft lip and palate before and after tube insertion. Note the improved hearing afterward.

For years, otolaryngologists managed OME with ventilation tube insertion as a prophylactic treatment with the idea that it would resolve the sequelae of OME and associated hearing loss

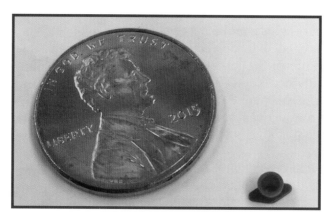

Figure 6–15. Duravent ventilation tube. (Photo courtesy of Dr. Amelia Drake, University of North Carolina, Department of Otolaryngology.)

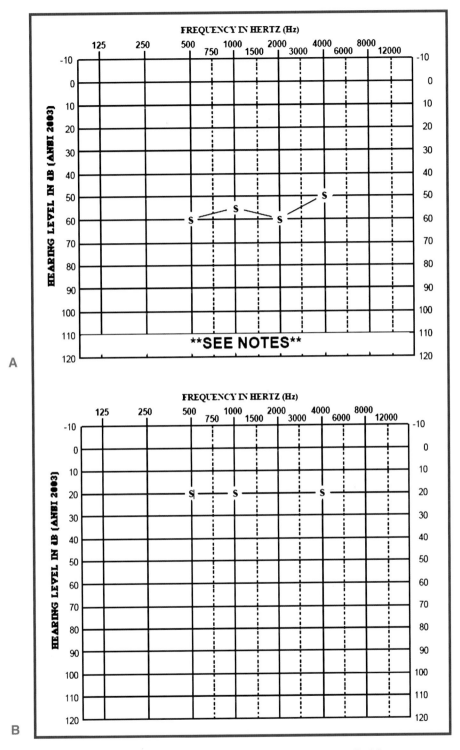

Figure 6–16. A. Audiogram of a 5-month-old with Pierre Robin sequence. Responses to stimuli presented in soundfield (S) shows a moderate hearing loss for at least the better ear. **B.** 2 week postoperative audiogram of the same child who had ventilation tubes inserted at the time of cleft palate repair at 12 months. Findings show normal hearing for at least the better ear.

(Paradise & Bluestone, 1974). This meant that tubes would be inserted at the time of cleft lip or cleft palate repair, even if OME was not present (Ponduri et al., 2009). The reasons behind this regimen were to ensure and maintain optimal hearing for speech and language development (Broen, Moller, Carlstrom, Doyle, Devers, & Keenan, 1995; Paradise, 1975). The short-term gain is positive in that with the tubes in place, hearing improves (Paradise & Bluestone, 1974; Ponduri et al., 2009). Yet, even after palatoplasty, many of the children with CLP will experience recurrent OME and require another set (or more) of tubes.

There is currently appreciable evidence to suggest that repeated insertion of ventilation tubes is associated with complications including otorrhea or ear discharge, tympanic membrane perforations, retracted eardrum, tympanosclerosis, and cholesteatoma (Curtin, Messner, & Change, 2009; Goudy, Lott, Canady, & Smith, 2006; Spilsbury, Ha, Semmens, & Lannigan, 2013), any of which can cause a conductive hearing loss. These pathologies are often observed in the older school-age child and teenager.

As a result of these complications, clinicians are now considering a more conservative approach to the management of OME in children with cleft palate called "watchful waiting." It is a selective approach in which tubes are inserted when symptomatic ear effusion develops and is present for at least 2 or 3 months (Kwan et al., 2011; Phua, Salkeld, & de Chalain, 2009; Robson et al., 1992). As an outcome of "watchful waiting," the rate at which universal insertion of tubes in children with cleft palate and mild hearing loss has been reduced. To be clear, ventilation tubes would still be used as a treatment of choice to treat persistent OME but only after thoughtful consider-

ation of the otologic and audiologic information. The proponents of the conservative approach support the insertion of ventilation tubes in children with persistent and unrelenting OME and moderate hearing loss (Gani, Kinshuck, & Sharma, 2012; Kwan et al., 2011). Sometimes this means inserting the tubes prior to palate repair.

A hearing aid is another conservative alternative to managing a moderate hearing loss associated with OME (Flanagan et al., 1996; Jardine, Griffiths, & Midgley, 1999; Maheshwar, Milling, Kumar, Clayton, & Thomas, 2002; Zavala, personal communication, 2015). It can be used until the condition is resolved and hearing improves, or until tubes are inserted at the time of cleft palate repair. Although it is reasonable to use a conventional behind the ear hearing aid, a bone conduction hearing aid on a soft band is usually recommended over the conventional air conduction hearing aid that can be difficult to program with a hearing loss that potentially fluctuates due to fluid and OME (Zavala, personal communication). Hearing aids are described in the following section.

MANAGING HEARING LOSS IN CRANIOFACIAL ANOMALIES

A congenital ear deformity associated with a craniofacial anomaly causes a permanent hearing loss. However, OME can co-occur. If present, ventilation tubes are inserted but because of the more permanent nature of the hearing loss in these disorders, tubes alone do not improve hearing.

Because the hearing loss is present at birth, early amplification is integral to speech and language development and later, to academic outcomes of children with hearing loss. An infant can be fit with a hearing aid as young as 3 months of age.

The purpose of a hearing aid is to improve the person's ability to hear and to prevent or reduce communication problems related to the hearing loss. A person with either a unilateral or bilateral loss can benefit from a hearing aid. The type of hearing aid depends on the nature and extent of the hearing loss.

Hearing Aids

A person with a craniofacial anomaly is usually a candidate for one of two categories of hearing aids: air conduction and bone conduction. The selection of the type of hearing aid is determined by the type and degree of hearing loss. The *conventional air conduction hearing aid* is most appropriate for the person who has an intact pinna and open ear canal. This type of hearing aid is suitable for all degrees of hearing loss from mild to profound. The most common type of air conduction hearing aid is a behind-the-ear (BTE) in which

the aid hooks over the ear and rests behind the ear and a tube connects to an earmold that fits in the ear canal (Figure 6–17).

Infants and children with sensorineural hearing loss often benefit from an air conduction hearing aid. For those with severe or profound losses, a cochlear implant may be helpful in providing some sense of sound.

Candidates for *bone conduction hearing aids* are those with conductive or mixed hearing loss attributable to congenital outer or middle ear malformations such as microta, atresia, or auditory canal anomalies, as is often the case with Treacher Collins syndrome and oculoauriculo-vertebral spectrum. Because of chronic middle ear drainage, some children may not be able to wear the earmold that comes with the air condition hearing aid. Instead, they might benefit from a bone conduction hearing aid.

The most common type of bone conduction aid consists of a bone vibrator that is connected to a headband and sits on the mastoid process (Figure 6–18). In younger children the hearing aid is held

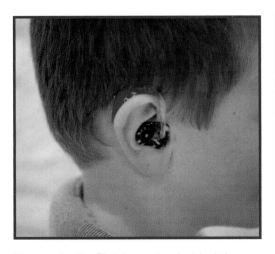

Figure 6–17. Child wearing behind-the-ear hearing aid (Photo courtesy of Sarah Zavala, AuD, Clinical Audiologist, Alfred I. duPont Hospital for Children, Wilmington, DE.)

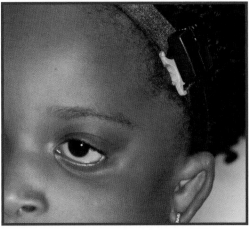

Figure 6–18. Young girl with Treacher Collins syndrome wearing a bone conduction hearing aid. Note microtia of the left ear.

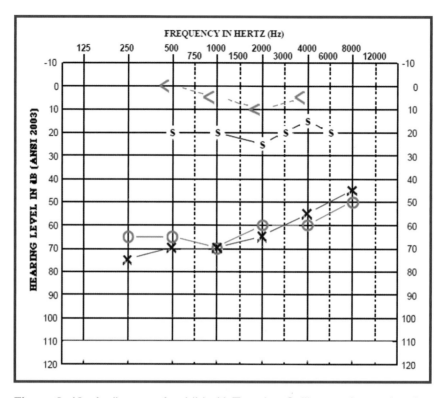

Figure 6–19. Audiogram of a child with Treacher Collins syndrome showing a bilateral moderately severe conductive hearing loss. Her aided responses to tones (S) wearing a bone conduction hearing aid fall within the range of normal hearing.

on using a soft band. The sound vibrations are transmitted directly to the inner ear, bypassing the outer and middle ears, directly stimulating the cochlea. If the auditory nerve is intact, the person who wears a bone conduction hearing aid usually experiences normal or near normal hearing. Figure 6–19 shows the auditory responses of a child before and after wearing a bone conduction hearing aid. Note that aided responses are within the range of normal limits.

As a child gets older, he or she often finds the look of the bone conduction hearing aid unattractive and uncomfortable. A popular option is the bone-anchored hearing aid (BAHA), an implantable bone conduction device. This requires a surgical procedure in which the receiver of the hearing aid is implanted in the temporal bone behind the ear, and through an external screw the sound processor is attached.

Other Assistive Listening Options

A child who has a hearing loss, whether it is permanent or fluctuating, unilateral or bilateral, can benefit from any number other assistive listening options that will maximize auditory input in the classroom and in speech-language therapy. This can include preferential seating toward the front of the classroom or a seat in a part of a room that attenuates extraneous noise or reverberations (i.e., windows). A wireless personal frequency modulation (FM) system that directly transmits the speech from the speaker's microphone to the receiver worn by the listener can be beneficial. The FM system can be used with a hearing aid or as a stand-alone for those who do not wear a hearing aid but who, for example, have a fluctuating mild hearing loss and might need to hear speech (i.e., instructions) within the classroom. The speech-language pathologist can often assist the classroom teacher with these arrangements.

Reconstructive Surgery for Microtia

Some patients with microtia and external auditory canal atresia may be candidates for reconstructive surgery. The pinna can be reconstructed with either rib (costal) cartilage (Brent, 1980, 1992; Tanzer, 1959, 1971) or prosthetic material (Reinisch & Lewin, 2009). In patients with external auditory atresia, those with favorable anatomy may be candidates for external auditory canal reconstruction to improve hearing.

THE ROLE OF THE SPEECH-LANGUAGE PATHOLOGIST

When counseling parents of infants and children about the impact of cleft palate on speech and language, it is incumbent upon the SLP to also talk about the nature of OME and its potential effect on hearing and early speech and language development, and offer strategies to enhance communication and listening. These strategies include instructing the caregiver to focus on the child's face and speak clearly,

maintain the child's attention throughout the interaction, and minimize distracting background noises when talking to the child.

Community SLPs who treat children with cleft palate and craniofacial conditions also need to be aware of the impact of fluctuating or permanent hearing loss on communication and academic performance. Many of these children will have bilateral losses, but others, like those with OAVS, will have a unilateral loss and so too may be at risk for language and academic difficulties (Lieu, 2004; Lieu, Tye-Murray, Karzon, & Piccirillo, 2010).

To plan appropriately for assessment and treatment, the speech-language pathologist should know about the following (Rosenfeld et al., 2004):

- Results from most recent hearing test. If an audiologic evaluation has not been done in the past 6 month, refer for testing.
- Type and degree of hearing loss and laterality (i.e., unilateral or bilateral). For questions about hearing, contact the treating audiologist.
- History and duration of OME and the conditions that might exacerbate it (i.e., allergies, upper respiratory infection, day care environment).
- Hearing aid. If the child wears a hearing aid, begin each therapy session by checking the earmold for fit and testing the batteries and aid to see that they are working.

CHAPTER SUMMARY

Hearing loss is a major complication of cleft palate and craniofacial anomalies. However mild or transient, a hearing loss can have an adverse effect on speech and language development and consequential effects on other aspects of a child's life. The loss can be temporary or permanent, mild or severe. In any and all cases, the speech language pathologist should have a complete understanding of the loss and its etiology. Standard care includes routine otologic and audiologic monitoring and follow-up. Caregivers should be counseled about the otopathologic condition affecting their child's hearing and its impact on function. When treating a child with a cleft, the speech-language pathologist should know the child's hearing history and current ear and hearing status, and refer for testing if or when concerns arise.

REFERENCES

American Cleft Palate-Craniofacial Association (2009). *Parameters for the evaluation and treatment of patients with cleft lip/palate or other craniofacial anomalies.* Retrieved October 20, 2015 from http://www.acpa-cpf.org/uploads/site/Parameters_Rev_2009.pdf

Bartel-Friedrich, S., & Wulke, C. (2007). Classification and diagnosis of ear malformations. *GMS Current Topics in Otorhinolaryngology, Head and Neck Surgery, 6,* Doc05.

Bluestone, C. D. (1971). Eustachian tube obstruction in the infant with cleft palate. *Annals of Otology, Rhinology & Laryngology, 80,* 1–3.

Bluestone, C. D., & Doyle, W. J. (1988). Anatomy and physiology of eustachian tube and middle ear related to otitis media. *Journal of Allergy and Clinical Immunology, 81*(5, Pt. 2), 997–1003.

Bluestone, C. D., & Klein, J. O. (1990). Otitis media, atelectasis and eustachian tube dysfunction. In Bluestone, C. D., Stool, S. E., & Sheetz, M. D. (Eds.), *Pediatric otolaryngology* (2nd ed., pp 320–486). Philadelphia, PA: W.B. Saunders.

Brent, B. (1980). The correction of microtia with autogenous cartilage grafts II: Atypical and complex deformities. *Plastic and Reconstructive Surgery, 66,* 13–21.

Brent, B. (1992). Auricular repair with autogenous rib cartilage grafts: Two decades of experience with 600 cases. *Plastic and Reconstructive Surgery, 90,* 355–374.

Broen, P. A., Moller, K. T., Carlstrom, J., Doyle, S. S., Devers, M., & Keenan, K. M. (1996). Comparison of the hearing histories of children with and without cleft palate. *Cleft Palate-Craniofacial Journal, 33,* 127–133.

Carvalho, G. J., Song, C. S., Vargervik, K., & Lalwani, A. K. (1999). Auditory and facial nerve dysfunction in patients with hemifacial microsomia. *Archives of Otolaryngology-Head and Neck Surgery, 125,* 209–212.

Chen, J. L., Messner, A. H., & Curtin, G. (2008). Newborn hearing screening in infants with cleft palates. *Otology & Neurotology, 29,* 812–815.

Corey, J. P., Caldarelli, D. D., & Gould, H. J. (1987). Otopathology in cranial facial dysostosis. *American Journal of Otology, 8,* 14–17.

Curtin, G., Messner, A. H., & Cheng, K. W. (2009). Otorrhea in infants with tympanostomy tubes before and after surgical repair of a cleft palate. *Archives of Otolaryngology-Head and Neck Surgery, 135,* 748–751.

DeBonis, D. A., & Donohue, C. L. (2008). *Survey of audiology. Fundamentals for audiologists and health professions* (2nd ed.). Boston, MA: Pearson Education.

Deedler, J. D., Breugem, C. C., de Vries, I. A., de Bruin, M., Mink van der Molen, A. B., & van der Horst, C. M. (2011). Is an isolated cleft lip an isolated anomaly? *Journal of Plastic Reconstructive and Aesthetic Surgery, 64,* 754–758.

Doyle, W. J., Cantekin, E. I., & Bluestone, C. D. (1980). Eustachian tube function in cleft palate children. *Annals of Otology, Rhinology and Laryngology Supplement, 89*(3), 34–40.

Drake, A. F., & Swibel Rosenthal, L. H. (2013). Otolaryngologic challenges in cleft/craniofacial care. *Cleft Palate-Craniofacial Journal, 50,* 734–743.

Flannagan, P. M., Knight, L. C., Thomas, A., Browning, S., Aymat, A., & Clayton, M. I.

(1996). Hearing aids and glue ear. *Clinical Otolaryngology and Allied Science, 21*, 297–300.

Flynn, T., & Lohmander, A. (2014). A longitudinal study of hearing and middle ear status in individuals with UCLP. *Otology & Neurotology, 35*, 989–996.

Flynn, T., Möller, C., Jönsson, R., & Lohmander, A. (2009). The high prevalence of otitis media with effusion in children with cleft lip and palate as compared to children without clefts. *International Journal of Pediatric Otorhinolaryngology, 73*, 1441–1446.

Goudy, S., Lott, D., Canady, J., & Smith, R. J. H. (2006). Conductive hearing loss and otopathology in cleft palate patients. *Otolaryngology-Head and Neck Surgery, 134*, 946–948.

Gould, H. J. (1990). Hearing loss and cleft palate: The perspective of time. *Cleft Palate Journal, 27*, 36–39

Handzic-Cuk, J., Cuk, V., Risavi, R., Katusic, D., & Stajner-Katusic, S. (1996). Hearing levels and age in cleft palate patients. *International Journal of Pediatric Otorhinolaryngology, 37*, 227–242.

Hennersdorf, F., Friese, N., Löwenheim, H., Tropitzch, A., Ernemann U., & Bisdas, S. (2014). Temporal bone changes in patients with Goldenhar syndrome with special emphasis on inner ear abnormalities. *Otology & Neurotology, 35*, 826–830.

Jardine, A. H., Griffiths, M. V., & Midgley, E. (1999). Acceptance of hearing aids for children with otitis media with effusion. *Journal of Laryngology and Otology, 113*, 314–317.

Joint Commission on Infant Hearing. (2007). Year 2007 position statement: Principles and guidelines for early hearing detection and intervention programs. *Pediatrics, 120*, 898–921.

Jordan, V. A., & Sidman, J. D. (2014). Hearing outcomes in children with cleft palate and referred newborn hearing screen. *Laryngoscope, 124*, E384–E388. doi:10.1002/lary.24727

Kramer, S., & Guthrie, L. A. (2008). *Audiology workbook*. San Diego, CA: Plural.

Kuo, C. L., Lien, C. F., Chu, C. H., & Shioa, A. S. (2013). Otitis media with effusion in children with cleft lip and palate: A narrative review. *International Journal of Pediatric Otorhinolaryngology, 77*, 1403–1409.

Kwan, W. M., Abdullah, V.J., Liu, K., van Hasselt, C.A. & Tong, M. C. (2011). Otitis media with effusion and hearing loss in Chinese children with cleft lip and palate. *Cleft Palate-Craniofacial Journal, 48*, 684–689.

Lewis, N. (1976). Otitis media and linguistic incompetence. *Archives of Otolaryngology-Head and Neck Surgery, 102*, 387–390.

Lieu, J. E. (2004). Speech-language and educational consequences of unilateral hearing loss in children. *Archives of Otolaryngology-Head and Neck Surgery, 130*, 524–530.

Lieu, J. E., Tye-Murray, N., Karzon, R. K., & Piccirillo, J. F. (2010). Unilateral hearing loss is associated with worse speech-language scores in children. *Pediatrics, 125*, e1348–e1355.

Maheshwar, A. A, Milling, M. A., Kumar, M., Clayton, M. A., & Thomas, A. (2002). Use of hearing aids in the management of children with cleft palate. *International Journal of Pediatric Otorhinolaryngology, 21*, 55–62.

Moller, P. (1975). Long-term otologic features of cleft palate patients. *Archives of Otolaryngology, 101*, 605–607.

Moller, P. (1981). Hearing, middle ear pressure, and otopathology in a cleft palate population. *Acta Otolaryngologica, 92*, 521–528.

Orchik, D. J., Schumaier, D. R., Shea, J. J., Jr., & Ge, X. (1995). Middle ear and inner ear effects on clinical bone-conduction threshold. *Journal of the American Academy of Audiology, 6*, 256–260.

Paparella, M. R., Morizono, T., Le, C. T., Mancini, F., Sipila, P., Cook, Y. B., Kiden, G., & Kim, C. S. (1984). Sensorineural hearing loss in otitis media. *Annals of Otology, Rhinology & Laryngology, 93*, 623–629.

Paradise, J. L. (1975). Middle ear problems associated with cleft palate. *Cleft Palate Journal, 12*, 17–22.

Paradise, J. L., & Bluestone, C. D. (1974). Early treatment of the universal otitis media of infants with cleft palate. *Pediatrics, 53*, 48–54.

Paradise, J. L., Bluestone, C. D., & Felder, H. (1969). The universality of otitis media in 50 infants with cleft palate. *Pediatrics, 44*, 35–42.

Phua, Y. S., Salkeld, L. J., & de Chalain, T. M. (2009). Middle ear disease in children with cleft palate: Protocols for management. *International Journal of Pediatric Otorhinolaryngology, 73*, 307–313.

Ponduri, S., Bradley, R., Ellis, P. E., Brookes, S. T., Sandy, J. R., & Ness, A. R. (2009). The management of otitis media with early routine insertion of grommets in children with cleft palate—A systematic review. *Cleft Palate-Craniofacial Journal, 46*, 30–38.

Pron, G., Galloway, C., Armstrong, D., & Posnick, J. (1993). Ear malformation and hearing loss in patients with Treacher Collins syndrome. *Cleft Palate-Craniofacial Journal, 30*, 97–103.

Reinisch, J. F., & Lewin, S. (2009). Ear reconstruction using a porous polyethylene framework and temporoparietal fascia flap. *Facial Plastic Surgery, 25*, 181–189.

Roberts, J., Hunter, L., Gravel, J., Rosenfield, R., Berman, S., Haggard, M., . . . Wallace, I. (2004). Otitis media, hearing loss, and language learning: Controversies and recent research. *Journal of Developmental Behavioral Pediatrics, 25*, 110–122.

Robson, A. K., Blanshard, J. D., Jones, K., Albery, E. H., Smith, I. M., & Maw, A. R. (1992). A conservative approach to the management of otitis media with effusion in cleft palate. *Journal of Laryngology and Otology, 196*, 788–792.

Rosenfeld, R. M., Culpepper, L., Doyle, K. J., Grundfast, K. M., Hoberman, A., Kenna, M. A., . . . Yawn, B. (2004). Clinical practice guideline: Otitis media with effusion. *Otolaryngology-Head and Neck Surgery, 130*, S95–S118.

Ruegg, T. A., Cooper, M. E., Leslie, E. J., Ford, M. D., Wehby, G. L., Deleyiannis, F. W. B., . . . Weinberg, S. M. (2015). Ear infection in isolated cleft lip: Etiological implications. *Cleft Palate-Craniofacial Journal*. Advance online publication. doi:10.1597/15-010

Rynnel-Dagöö, B., Linberg, K., Bagger-Sjöback, D., & Larson, O. (1992). Middle ear disease in cleft palate children at three years of age. *International Journal of Pediatric Otorhinolaryngology, 23*, 201–209.

Sheahan, P., Miller, I., Sheahan, J. N., Ealey, M. J., & Blayney, A. W. (2003). Incidence and outcome of middle ear disease in cleft lip and/or cleft palate. *International Journal of Pediatric Otorhinolaryngology, 67*, 785–793.

Sheahan, P., Miller, I., Sheahan, J. N., Ealey, M. J., & Blayney, A. W. (2004). Middle ear disease in children with congenital velopharyngeal insufficiency. *Cleft Palate-Craniofacial Journal, 41*, 364–367.

Sirimanna, T. (2004). Hearing problems in children with craniosynostosis. In Haywood, R., Jones, B., Dunaway, D., & Evans, R. (Eds.), *The Clinical Management of Craniosynostosis* (pp. 299–310). London, UK: Mac Keith Press.

Skuladottir, H., Sivertsen, A., Assmus, J., Rommetveit Remme, A., Dahlen, M., & Vindenes, A. (2015). Hearing outcomes in patients with cleft lip and palate. *Cleft Palate-Craniofacial Journal, 52*, e23–e31.

Smith, T. L., DiRuggiero, D. C., & Jones, K. R. (1994). Recovery of eustachian tube function and hearing outcome in patients with cleft palate. *Otolaryngology-Head and Neck Surgery, 111*, 423–429.

Spilsbury, K., Ha, J. F., Semmens, J. B., & Lannigan, F. (2013). Cholesteatoma in cleft lip and palate: A population-based follow-up study of children after ventilation tubes. *Laryngoscope, 123*, 2024–2029.

Stool, S. E., & Randall, P. (1967). Unexpected ear disease in infants with cleft palate. *Cleft Palate Journal, 4*, 99–103.

Szabo, C., Langevin, K., Schoem, S., & Mabry, K. (2010). Treatment of persistent middle ear effusion in cleft palate patients. *International Journal of Pediatric Otolaryngology, 74*, 874–877.

Tanzer, R. C. (1959). Total reconstruction of the external ear. *Plastic and Reconstructive Surgery and the Transplantation Bulletin, 23*, 1–15.

Tanzer, R. C. (1971). Total reconstruction of the auricle: The evolution of a plan of treatment. *Plastic and Reconstructive Surgery, 47*, 523–533.

Tatum, S., & Senders, C. (1993). Perspectives on palatoplasty. *Facial Plastic Surgery, 9*, 225–231.

Timmermans, K., Wander Poorten, V., Desloo-vere, C., & Debruyne, F. (2006). The middle ear of cleft palate patients in their early teens: A literature study and preliminary file study. *B-ENT, 2*(Suppl. 4), 95–101.

Tunçbilek, G., Özgür, F., & Belgin, E. (2003). Audiologic and tympanometric findings in children with cleft lip and palate. *Cleft Palate-Craniofacial Journal, 40*, 304–309.

Vallino, L. D., Zuker, R., & Napoli, J. A. (2008). A study of speech, language, hearing, and dentition in children with cleft lip only. *Cleft Palate-Craniofacial Journal, 45*, 485–493.

World Health Organization (WHO). (2015). *Deafness and hearing loss.* Fact sheet, No. 300. Geneva, Switzerland: Author.

Zavala, S. Personal communication. September 2, 2015.

Zavala, S., Morlet, T., Napoli, J. A., & Vallino, L. D. (2013). *Otological and audiological outcomes of children with cleft lip/palate from 3, 4 and 5 years.* International Congress on Cleft Lip/Palate and related craniofacial anomalies. Orlando, FL, May 5–10.

Zhou, G., Schwartz, L. T., & Gopen, Q. (2009). Inner ear anomalies and conductive hearing loss in children with Apert syndrome: An overlooked otologic aspect. *Otology and Neurotology, 30*, 184–189.

7

Early Linguistic Development and Intervention

Nancy J. Scherer

INTRODUCTION

Early intervention for children with cleft lip and palate (CLP) has the potential to address early speech and language delays that result from having an insufficient oral mechanism to support early speech and language production prior to palate repair and to prevent the emergence of compensatory articulation patterns. This chapter will present a discussion of early language and speech milestones up through 3 years of age, and evidence-based assessment and intervention practices for children with CLP.

EARLY SPEECH AND LANGUAGE MILESTONES

Early Vocalization and Gesture

Around 6 months of age, children begin to combine vowels and consonants in strings that are word like (e.g., mama, bubu). This canonical babbling milestone marks a crit- ical transition in the complexity of early vocalizations. For many children with CLP, this milestone is delayed in onset, complexity and composition regardless of cleft type or early obturation of the palate (Chapman 1991; Chapman, Hardin-Jones, & Schulte, 2001; Hardin-Jones, Chapman, & Schulte, 2003; Scherer, D'Antonio, & Kalbfliesch, 1999; Scherer, D'Antonio, & McGahey, 2008). Most children with CLP in the United States have their palates repaired between 10 and 12 months of age. So the early delay in the onset of canonical babbling is not surprising given the status of the child's oral mechanism during a period associated with the emergence of babbling (6+ months of age). Prior to palate repair, children with CLP are unable to implode oral air pressure to differentiate nasal consonants from high-pressure consonant (stops, fricatives, affricates) and results in small consonant inventories consisting of nasals, glides, and glottals with few alveolars or palatals (Chapman, 1991; Chapman et al., 2001; Scherer, Williams, & Proctor-Williams, 2008). Given the limitations in early sound development, how do young children with CLP communicate? Studies have shown that despite their limited consonant inventories, young children with CLP vocalize as frequently as noncleft children (Chapman et al., 2001; Scherer, Williams, & Proctor-Williams, 2008). When all components of early communication acts are examined—gesture, vocalizations, and eye gaze—all components show rates similar to noncleft children prior to the onset of words (Scherer, Boyce, & Martin, 2013. When the onset of words was factored in, there was a significant difference between children with CLP and noncleft peers in the age at which they made the transition to words. Children with CLP continued to rely on vocalization and gesture longer than noncleft peers.

Onset of First Words and Vocabulary Expansion

One of the most notable characteristics of many children with CLP is delayed onset of words (Broen, Devers, Doyle, Prouty, & Moller, 1998; Hardin-Jones & Chapman, 2014; Scherer, D'Antonio, & Kalbfliesch, 1999). There are a number of factors that contribute to the etiology of these early delays. Children with CLP are without a normal oral mechanism for most of the first year of life until the palate is repaired, which limits the ability to implode oral air pressure for the production of most oral consonants. The consonant inventories then consist of sounds that do not require oral pressure (i.e., nasals, glides, and glottals) or have place of articulation at the extremes of the vocal tract (i.e., labials, velars, glottals) (Estrem & Broen, 1989; Hardin-Jones & Chapman, 2014; Willadsen, 2013). Children are more likely to produce words with these limited consonant inventories, which may further limit speech sound acquisition.

The Relationship Between Early and Later Speech and Language Development

Studies have shown some significant relationships between prelinguistic and early sound development and later language use. Scherer, Boyce, and Martin (2013) found children with CLP who had more canonical vocalizations at 18 months had more advanced vocabulary development at 30 months. In another study, Chapman (2004) found a significant correlation between stop consonant production immediately following palate repair and language development at 39 months of age. These studies showed continuity between speech and language development over short periods of time, but studies examining predictive factors over longer periods of time have shown a different pattern. Chapman (2004) and Scherer, D'Antonio, and McGahey (2008) found that children who had a larger consonant inventory and vocalization rates prior to palate surgery had poorer language development at 30 to 39 months of age. Although these studies appear to be in conflict, a closer look suggests that because of the substantial change in speech and language development that can occur following palate repair, we cannot predict later development from performance very early on. Therefore, our best ability to predict later development begins following palate repair (Jones, Chapman, & Hardin-Jones, 2003).

The critical predictors of later speech and language following palate repair are the number and variety of stop consonant production, vocalization rate, and the number of communicative acts per minute (Hardin-Jones & Chapman, 2014; Scherer et al., 2013). The number of stop consonants produced after surgery provides an initial indication that the child can achieve palate closure, which is a good prognostic sign for future acquisition of high-pressure consonants. The number of communicative acts per minute is a measure that includes gesture, eye gaze, and vocalizations used in a communicative way. This measure reflects the child's engagement in interaction that provides models for language and speech. Vocalization rate is highly associated with later word use (Scherer et al., 2013). It is no surprise that early intervention programs for children with CLP included one or more of these behaviors as goals.

ASSESSMENT OF SPEECH AND LANGUAGE DEVELOPMENT

A thorough assessment of both speech and language performance is essential for intervention planning. Routine cleft palate team follow-up provides a screening of performance in order to recommended intervention, if appropriate. Additional assessment is necessary to determine intervention goals. Assessment of speech and language skills is challenging for young children. Guiding principles for assessment of children under 3 years of age, specified by the American Speech-Language-Hearing Association (ASHA), indicate that the assessment should (a) be an ongoing process, (b) include direct observation of child behaviors, (c) include parents, and (d) provide guidance for treatment decisions (ASHA, 2008).

Assessment methods for young children include a range of standardized tests, normative guidelines, and informal assessment procedures. Each has a role in the assessment process. Standardized tests provide a normative comparison for eligibility purposes; however, they fall short of providing sufficient information for intervention planning. The most helpful measures for intervention planning are those that capture communication in naturalistic settings.

Language and speech assessment is important for young children with CLP because speech sounds are taught in the context of whole words (Scherer & D'Antonio, 1995; Scherer et al., 2013; Scherer, Williams, & Proctor-Williams, 2008). For children who are not talking, assessment is best conducted from a sample of vocalization and should focus on measures of

- vocalization diversity (number of different consonant sounds used);
- vocalization complexity (syllable shapes, e.g., Consonant–Vowel (CV), VC, CVC, etc.);
- developmental stage of vocalization (canonical [e.g., mama] or variegated forms [e.g., maba]);
- vocalization rate (number of vocalizations per minute); and
- use of communicative gesture.

In keeping with the guiding principles of assessment, parent questionnaires are an important source of children's language use. The MacArthur-Bates Communication Inventories (CDI: Fenson et al., 2008; http://mb-cdi.stanford.edu/cdi-welcome.htm) is a reliable measure of the child's word and phrase comprehension, gesture, and words provided by the parents. The CDI is also available in many languages other than English. This measure has proved instrumental in determining prelinguistic goals for intervention and to monitor progress over time (Scherer, 1999; Scherer & D'Antonio, 1995; Scherer, D'Antonio, & McGahey, 2008; Scherer et al., 2008; Synder & Scherer, 2004). By 12 months of age, most nonsyndromic children with CLP in the United States have had their palates repaired. However, some children with associated syndromes or other conditions may not have had their palates repaired. If this were the case, then the focus of early intervention would be on language comprehension and vocalization rate and less on vocalization complexity or diversity.

Assessment of the velopharyngeal mechanism will be addressed over time as the child's consonant inventory and sentence length increases. Nasal resonance and audible nasal emission may be observed even after surgery but will not be addressed directly until the child's speech and language skills and behavioral compliance are adequate for a complete assessment. The child must be able to attempt oral and nasal consonants within a clinical setting when requested. (Chapter 8 describes some elicitation procedures that might be successful with a younger child who is saying words.) Intervention will facilitate change in the speech sound system, and as that change happens, resonance could change as well given that the child has the physiologic capability for adequate velopharyngeal function (Peterson-Falzone, Trost-Cardamone, Karnell, & Hardin-Jones, 2006). Early intervention has the potential then to monitor resonance that may need to be assessed further as the child's speech and language develops.

For children who have begun to use words, an assessment should include both a language and speech sample and parent questionnaire regarding early vocabulary and sentence complexity (Scherer, Frey, & Kaiser, 2014). For the language sample, the parents can collect a video or audio sample of the child with some instructions about how to collect the sample. A 10- to 15-minute sample is adequate and can be recorded by the parents when the child is typically vocal. A parent measure of early vocabulary and sentence complexity is also an important component of the assessment of young children. The MacArthur-Bates Communicative Development Inventories (CDI) Words and Sentences provides a parent report measure of vocabulary and sentence complexity for children from 16 to 36 months of age. The measures that are most important for intervention planning and tracking progress include the

- vocabulary size from the CDI;
- total number of words, from the language sample;
- number of different words from the language sample; and
- mean length of utterance (MLU) from the language sample for both *child and parent.*

If the language sample is transcribed in SALT (Systematic Analysis of Language Transcripts, 2012), measures for parent and child are analyzed as well as other measures related to intelligibility, talking rate, responsivity, and sentence types can be analyzed. The language sample can also be used to collect a spontaneous speech sample that can be compared to the single word speech sample described below.

The speech sample should include an object naming activity with toys representing early acquired sounds in initial and final word position that can be used to collect word level speech sound production information (Scherer, Williams, Stoel-Gammon, & Kaiser, 2012). The Profiles of Early Expressive Phonology (PEEPS) (Williams & Stoel-Gammon, 2014) is a test that is being developed for children 18 to 36 months of age. Table 7–1 includes a list of words from the PEEPS.

Table 7–1. PEEPS Word Lists 1 and 2

List 1	List 2
baby	ball
bed	balloon
bib	banana
cup	cheese
dog	cookie
car	cow
ear	doll
eye	duck
finger	fish
foot	go
hand	hair
hat	juice
light	kitty
mouth	moo
nose	mouse
peekaboo	pig
rock	puppy
shoe	quack
sock	truck
toe	woof
tummy	

The measures that are collected from the single word naming activity are

- consonant inventory (sounds used at least once during the sample in any position, with or without nasality);
- Percent Consonants Correct (PCC) (Shriberg et al., 1997);
- percent omissions and substitutions for initial and medial/final word position; and
- percent of compensatory articulation errors.

If the child has more than 15 words on the PEEPS, then PCC for manner categories may be computed. The nasal, stop, and fricative categories change the most for young children with CLP, so those are a higher priority for monitoring progress.

EARLY SPEECH AND LANGUAGE INTERVENTION

The purpose of early intervention for speech and language development is to provide services for families and children who are at risk for or who show early delays in communication, play, feeding or swallowing, and early literacy. For children with CLP, early intervention may include activities to reduce the impact of the cleft on later speech and language development and to identify deficits in speech and language development that require evaluation and referral. If recommended, intervention may take many forms from direct weekly intervention with a speech-language pathologist to monitoring on a less regular basis. Often, parent training is a major component of the intervention to maximize child progress.

Goals for early intervention may be different before and after palate repair. Prior to palate repair, intervention is more focused on promoting communicative interaction and vocalizations, but keeping in mind that some sounds may be difficult for babies with cleft palate to produce at this time. Following surgery, intervention expectations change to improving speech intelligibility and language use. Goals will then focus on stimulating production of pressure consonants (p, b, t, d, etc.), expanding vocabulary, and eventually the grammatical forms if speech and language delays persist.

Determining Goals for Intervention

Young children acquire speech and language skills simultaneously within contexts that support their interaction and activity (Kaiser, 1993). Given that assumption, goals for early intervention must take into consideration both speech and language assessment information and then integrate those into a single set of goals. This is different from intervention for children older than 3 years when speech and language goals may be addressed separately (Scherer & Kaiser, 2007). Additionally, speech and language development for infants and toddlers occurs within meaningful contexts. So, drill-based activities are not appropriate. Rather, activities that are functional and promote engagement with the child must serve as the intervention platform.

Determining Consonant Inventory

Using the language and speech assessment to develop intervention goals, it is important to identify a list of sounds that

the child uses and in what word position and syllable form (e.g., CV, CVC). These sounds are considered in the child's sound inventory even though there may be limited exemplars from diagnostic information initially. Stoel-Gammon and Otomo (1986) and Chapman, Hardin-Jones, and Halter (2003) have suggested that we separate glide and glottal consonants (i.e., w, j, h, glottal stop) from other oral consonants or true consonants. These true consonants (nasal, stop, fricative, affricate, and liquids), with the exception of nasals, are the sounds that are often slow to develop in children with CLP and are the focus of intervention goals. In addition to noting all the consonants in the child's sound inventory, it is important to identify true consonants already in the child's sound inventory. Prognostically, the appearance of true consonants is positive. In most cases, the sound categories that will comprise the goals will come from the high-pressure sound categories of stops and fricatives. These are the sound classes that children are acquiring during the toddler and preschool period.

Integrating Speech and Vocabulary Goals

The second step in goal selection is then to integrate the sound class goals with vocabulary. The CDI inventory can be helpful in identifying a list of possible target words for intervention that include the sound classes for intervention. It is suggested that approximately 20 words be selected as target words for beginning intervention. However, it is important to keep in mind that the clinician must be flexible in using a variety of words with the target sound classes in them. The goal in early intervention is to expose the child to a variety of words with stop consonant sounds, for example, and not to "teach" or target only one or two sounds. After the child has expanded their consonant inventory, intervention can focus on more traditional phonologic or articulatory goals. The target word list is helpful when training parents but should not be used as the exclusive list of words used to facilitate the goals.

Intervention Model for Young Children with CLP

Figure 7–1 displays a model of the early intervention for children with CLP (Scherer & Kaiser, 2010). In this model, the target goals of intervention are to increase consonant inventory and vocab-ulary simultaneously with the intervention outcome of improved intelligibility. However, in order to implement these intervention goals, the child must be attempting to communicate so that we can provide feedback to expand and modify their attempts. Early interventions must provide some strategies to promote and maintain the child's communicative engagement. Most interventions use some form of responsive interaction and environmental arrangement to facilitate the child's communicative attempts. Responsive interaction includes strategies to follow the child's lead by responding to the child's nonverbal or verbal communicative intent. Environmental arrangement assists to increase communicative attempts through manipulating the physical environment, activities, routines, and

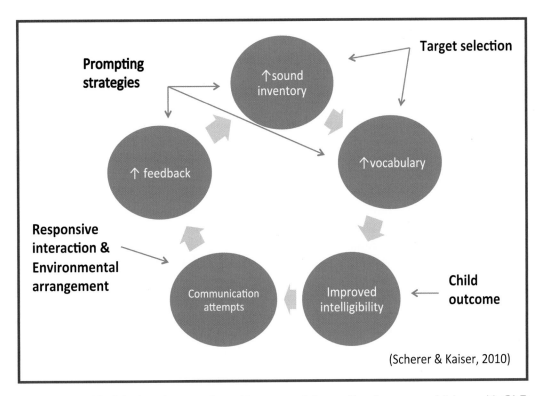

(Scherer & Kaiser, 2010)

Figure 7–1. Model of early speech and language intervention for young children with CLP.

behavioral support, and creating opportunities for the child to respond within the intervention. Once the child is engaged in an activity, strategies to facilitate speech and language can then be used to model both speech and language and to provide corrective and supportive feedback.

Intervention Approaches

There are limited data on intervention outcomes for children with CLP, especially in the birth to 3-year period. Bessell and colleagues (2013) completed a systematic review of speech-language interventions for children with CLP. Seventeen studies were examined with only three reporting data for children less than 3 years of age. Overall, the authors concluded that most studies found positive benefits of intervention; however, small participant numbers and methodological weaknesses limited any conclusive interpretations. Although data are limited presently, there are approaches that have data supporting their use for children with CLP and have additional data supporting their use with other populations of children with speech and language impairments (Girolametto, 1988; Girolametto, Greenberg, & Manolson, 1986; Girolametto, Pearce, & Weitzman, 1996, 1997; Scherer & Kaiser, 2010. Two major approaches that have been applied to children with CLP are Focused Stimulation (e.g., Hanen) and Enhanced Milieu Teaching (e.g., Enhanced Milieu Teaching with Phonological Emphasis).

In studies of early intervention for children with CLP, researchers are currently exploring the use of naturalistic models of intervention that have been successful with noncleft children who have speech and language impairments (Girolametto, 1988; Girolametto et al., 1996,

1997). Naturalistic intervention models use everyday interaction to facilitate language and speech that is functional for the child. Models exist on a continuum from those that are like everyday interactions, such as Floor Time (Greenspan & Wieder, 1997) to those that are hybrid models and combine prompting language with natural conversational contingencies, such as Enhanced Milieu Training (EMT) (Kaiser, Hancock, & Hester, 1998), EMT with Phonological Emphasis (EMT/PE) (Scherer & Kaiser, 2010), and Focused Stimulation (FS) (Girolametto, 1988; Girolametto et al., 1996, 1997). Presently, the impact of the hybrid models of early language intervention has been examined with young children with CLP in two models: FS and EMT/PE. The EMT/PE model is a naturalistic intervention that applies behavioral principles to prompt and support functional language use in routine daily activities (Kaiser, 1993; Kaiser et al., 1996). The FS model is a naturalistic intervention that emphasizes modeling and responsive interaction with use of modeling and little direct prompting of the child's language production (Baxendale & Hesketh, 2003; Girolametto et al., 1986, 1996, 1997, 1998). The two hybrid models are described in Table 7–2. The models share some fundamental characteristics:

- Each assumes that language is learned in meaningful communicative interaction.
- Each is designed to be used in everyday activities to teach language that is functional to the child.
- Each uses environmental arrangement to enhance opportunities for facilitating language.
- Each uses prompting to facilitate language use.

Table 7–2. Key Components of Focused Stimulation (FS), Enhanced Milieu Teaching (EMT), and Enhanced Milieu Teaching With Phonological Emphasis (EMT/PE)

Approach	Key Components
Enhanced Milieu Training (EMT)	Responsive interaction: Responding to child's communication
Enhanced Milieu Training With Phonological Emphasis (EMT/PE)	Arranging the environment to promote engagement
	Modeling: Words with target sounds
	Questions: Asking questions to initiate interaction (e.g., Do you want the truck or the car?)
	Time delay: Waiting a few seconds before initiating
	Expansion: Adding lexical or syntactic complexity to child's sentences
	Incidental teaching: Using all strategies
	Speech recasting: Repeating child's incorrect production emphasizing the correct target sound
Focused Stimulation	Follow child's lead
	Facilitate conversation through games and books
	Use intensive modeling and expansion
	Interact responsively

■ Each uses conversational partners to promote learning of vocabulary and word combinations.

Although the models share many attributes, they differ in the density and type of prompting used to facilitate language. FS uses a high density of modeling, while EMT/PE uses modeling as one of a number of prompting strategies, resulting in low density of modeling. EMT/PE is the only approach that has a specific strategy to facilitate speech (i.e., speech recasting).

Of the studies examining early intervention of children with CLP younger than 3 years, Scherer (1999) reported that a vocabulary intervention conducted by clinicians could improve both vocabulary and speech sound acquisition simultaneously. The intervention used an EMT model to facilitate vocabulary growth. In a subsequent randomized control study (Scherer, Kaiser, Frye, & Roberts, in preparation), EMT/PE was used to facilitate vocabulary and speech sound production in 15- to 36-month-old children with CLP. The children in the EMT/PE group had significantly greater improvement in speech accuracy and production of stop consonants and reduction in substitution errors during the intervention than the control group.

Parent Training

The effects of parent-implemented speech and language intervention on the development of noncleft children with delays have been known for some time (Brown,

2012; Kaiser & Roberts, 2013; Kaiser et al., 1996; Roberts & Kaiser, 2011, 2012). Roberts and Kaiser (2011) conducted a meta-analysis of published studies of parent-implemented language intervention and found support for the effectiveness of parent-implemented intervention in facilitating language development in children with language impairments. However, the composition of the parent training varied widely, and many studies did not assess treatment fidelity for the parents. The most effective approach was a combination of parent-implemented and clinician-implemented intervention. There are several variables that could impact the effectiveness of parent training: the parent's education level, the child's developmental level, and behavior. The choice of approach to train parents may differ based on these variables and cost of the training.

Early intervention has been a recent focus for children with CLP, and as such, parent training is often included in some form. The data on the intervention effects of a combined clinician and parent-implemented therapy have been well established for young children with communication impairments (Kaiser & Roberts, 2013; Roberts & Kaiser, 2011). However, the type and intensity of the training vary widely and impact the relative effectiveness of the parent-implemented component (Kaiser & Roberts, 2013). Parent training has often been provided indirectly through observation of clinician-child interaction or through provision of handouts describing therapy goals and therapeutic techniques without examining the parents' implementation of the techniques. Parents of children with CLP are given handouts on early speech and language development and feeding as part of their team visits. The literature suggests that more active engagement

with parents to provide strategies for promoting early speech and language development is warranted (Scherer et al., 2008). These strategies include demonstrating or showing video examples of different techniques or strategies to facilitate speech and language or reduce use of compensatory articulation, clinician demonstration of techniques on their child, provision of training materials to use in the home. An example of the types of strategies that have been effective in parent implemented interventions include

- Modeling: Adults increase the frequency of target word use in interactions with their child. The target words are selected based on phonologic and lexical characteristics determined in consultation with the child's speech-language pathologist. This is a strategy that is highly effective in increasing the likelihood that the child will attempt the target words. However, some children may need more direct methods to facilitate word attempts. In this case, parents can model the word within a request to imitate, for example, Adult: Say "ball." Child: Ball. This more direct method can be dropped once the child begins to spontaneously imitate target words.
- Expansions: Adults expand the lexical or syntactic complexity of their child's utterances, for example, Child: Ball. Adult: Throw the ball. Child: Throw ball. Expansions provide an opportunity for the child to practice sound production in contexts above single words. It is not uncommon for children to produce new sounds in single words but not in longer

sentences. Expansions provide those opportunities to practice in longer contexts.

■ Use of requests: Adults can use requests to gain a response from their child. Choice requests (e.g., Do you want the car or the truck?) are particularly effective in eliciting a response from the child. Requests provide a way for adults to start a conversation, but they should be used sparingly so as not to monopolize the conversation.

■ Balance turns: Adults respond to all verbal or nonverbal communicative attempts from their child. Adults are trained to respond and map language onto their child's actions or vocalizations. Some parents need assistance identifying nonverbal communicative attempts or interpreting early vocalizations.

■ Wait: Many of the strategies given parents serve to elicit responses from their child, but the goal for any intervention is to transition the child from a responsive contributor to an initiator in conversation. One strategy that is effective is to have the adult wait a few seconds before talking during an activity with their child. This gives the child an opportunity to contribute first. Then the adult can follow the child's lead. Another way to use the "wait" strategy is within games or routines. The adult can "wait" to take their turn to give the child a chance to take the turn.

■ Speech recasting: Adults can emphasize a sound in a word that the child has produced incorrectly (e.g., Child: "no," Adult: Oh that's your toe). This strategy gives the child corrective feedback for sound

production at the time that is meaningful to them.

Some parent training programs have used a coaching model for parents that has been positively associated with better treatment fidelity (Scherer et al., 2008). The coaching model begins with a description of an individual language facilitation strategy through handouts, scripts, video examples, or role-play, then the clinician demonstrates the techniques with the child and the parent takes over, and the clinician coaches the parent by giving short positive feedback on activities and use of techniques. The clinician can provide simple suggestions when the parent is not using the strategy correctly to promote success. In a recent study in which parents were trained through coaching to implement an EMT/PE approach, children made vocabulary and gains in their overall speech accuracy and specifically in the stop consonant class of sounds which was a focus of the intervention (Scherer et al., 2014). The parents were able to achieve fidelity with the training program using coaching.

A popular model of parent training is a group parent training session such as the Hanen Early Language Parent Program (Girolametto et al., 1986). The Hanen program was used in the Scherer et al. (2008) study and demonstrated positive improvements in the children with CLP in language and speech production. Scherer et al. (2008) focused on expanding vocabulary development and did not specifically train parents to facilitate words with specific sounds. This study demonstrated that parents can be trained in the group model; however, home visits were included with the group training to support individualization of the parent training.

CHAPTER SUMMARY

Young children with CLP demonstrate early vocabulary and speech delays that persist even after palate repair. Speech and language performance should be monitored routinely in the first 3 years of life as part of the child's cleft palate team. Given the high risk of early speech and vocabulary delays, parent training in early speech and language facilitation techniques can serve as a preventive treatment even before the child's palate is repaired. After repair, careful assessment of speech and language performance is recommended, and referral for early intervention if needed. Evidence-based early intervention approaches for children with CLP include naturalistic language and speech intervention such as FS, EMT, and EMT/PE. Parent training using a parent plus clinician intervention model with coaching results in the greatest gains in child outcome measures, but other less intense methods may have application in circumstances where the family has limited access to professionals. Further study of adaptions of these approaches in terms of dosage, maintenance of intervention gains, and social validity are still needed.

REFERENCES

American Speech-Language-Hearing Association. (2008). *Core knowledge and skills in early intervention speech-language pathology practice* [Knowledge and skills]. Available from http://www.asha.org/policy.

Baxendale, J., & Hesketh, A. (2003). Comparison of the effectiveness of the Hanen Early Parent Programme and traditional clinic therapy. *International Journal of Language and Communication Disorders, 38*(4), 397–415.

Bessell, A., Dip, C., Sell, D., Whiting, P., Roulstone, S., Albery, L., . . . Ness, A. (2013). Speech and language therapy interventions for children with cleft palate: A systematic review. *Cleft Palate-Craniofacial Journal, 50*(1), e1–e17.

Broen, P. A., Devers, M. C., Doyle, S. S., Prouty, J., & Moller, K. T. (1998). Acquisition of linguistic and cognitive skills by children with cleft palate. *Journal of Speech-Language Hearing Research, 41*, 676–678.

Brown, J. (2012). Exploring coaching strategies in a parent-implemented intervention for toddlers (Order No. 3551114). Available from ProQuest Dissertations & Theses Global (1287780373). Retrieved from http://login.ezpraxy1lib.asu.edu/login?url=http://search.proquest.com/docview/1287780373?Accounted=4485

Chapman, K. (1991). Vocalizations in toddlers with cleft palate. *Cleft Palate-Craniofacial Journal, 28*(2), 172–178.

Chapman, K. (2004). Is presurgery and early postsurgery performance related to speech and language outcomes at 3 years of age for children with cleft palate? *Clinical Linguistics and Phonetics, 18*(4–5), 239–377.

Chapman, K., Hardin-Jones, M., & Halter, K. A. (2003). Relationship between early speech and later speech and language performance for children with cleft lip and palate. *Clinical Linguistics and Phonetics, 17*(3), 173–197.

Chapman, K., Hardin-Jones, M., Schulte, J., & Halter K. A. (2001). Vocal development of 9-month-old babies with cleft palate. *Journal of Speech Language Hearing Research, 44*, 1268–1373.

Estrem, T., & Broen, P. A. (1989). Early speech production of children with cleft palate. *Journal of Speech and Hearing Research, 39*, 12–23.

Fenson, L., Marchman, V., Thal, D., Dale, P., Reznick, J. S., & Bates, E. (2008). *MacArthur-Bates Communicative Development Inventories* (2nd ed.). Baltimore, MD: Brookes.

Girolametto, L. (1988). Improving the social-conversational skills of developmentally delayed children: An intervention study. *Journal of Speech and Hearing Disorders, 53*, 156–167.

Girolametto, L., Greenberg, J., & Manolson, H. A. (1986). Developing dialogue skills: The Hanen Early Language Parent Program. *Seminars in Speech Language, 7*(4), 367–382.

Girolametto, L., Pearce, P., & Weitzman, E. (1996). Interactive focused stimulation for toddlers with expressive language delay. *Journal of Speech and Language Research, 39*(6), 1274–1284.

Girolametto, L., Pearce, P., & Weitzman, E. (1997). The effects of intervention on the phonology of Late Talkers. *Journal of Speech and Hearing Research, 40*(2), 338–348.

Greenspan, S. I., & Wieder, S. (1997). An integrated developmental approach to interventions for young children with severe difficulties in relating and communicating. *ZERO TO THREE: National Center for Infants, Toddlers, and Families, 17*(5), 5–18.

Hardin-Jones, M., & Chapman, K. (2014). Early lexical characteristics of toddlers with cleft lip and palate. *Cleft Palate-Craniofacial Journal, 6*(51), 622–631.

Hardin-Jones, M., Chapman, M., & Schulte, J. (2003). The impact of cleft type on early vocal development in babies with cleft palate. *Cleft Palate-Craniofacial Journal, 40*(5), 453–459.

Jones, C. E., Chapman, K., & Hardin-Jones, M. A. (2003). Speech development of children with cleft palate before and after palatal surgery. *Cleft Palate-Craniofacial Journal, 40*(1), 19–37.

Kaiser, A. (1993). Parent-implemented language intervention: An environmental system perspective. In A. P. Kaiser & D. B. Gray (Eds.*), Enhancing children's communication: Research foundations for intervention* (pp. 63–84). Baltimore, MD: Brookes.

Kaiser, A., Hancock, T., & Hester, P. (1998). Parents as cointerventionists: Research on application of naturalistic language teaching procedures. *Infants and Young Children, 10*, 46–55.

Kaiser, A., Hemmeter, M., Ostrosky, M., Fisher, R., Yoder, P., & Keefer, M. (1996). The effects of teaching parents to use responsive interaction strategies. *Topics in Early Childhood Special Education, 16*(3), 375–406.

Kaiser, A., & Roberts, M. (2013). Parent-implemented enhanced milieu teaching with preschool children who have intellectual disabilities. *Journal of Speech, Language, and Hearing Research, 56*(1), 295–309.

Peterson-Falzone, S., Trost-Cardamone, J., Karnell, M., & Hardin-Jones, M. (2006). *A clinician's guide to treating cleft palate speech.* Cambridge, MA: Mosby.

Roberts, M., & Kaiser, A. (2011). The effectiveness of parent-implemented interventions: A meta-analysis. *American Journal of Speech-Language Pathology, 20*(3), 180–199.

Roberts, M., & Kaiser, A. (2012). Assessing the effects of a parent-implemented language intervention for children with language impairments using empirical benchmarks: A pilot study. *Journal of Speech, Language. amd Hearing Research, 55*(6), 1655–1670.

Scherer, N. J. (1999). The speech and language status of toddlers with cleft lip and/or palate following early vocabulary intervention. *American Journal of Speech-Language Pathology, 8*, 31-40.

Scherer, N. J., Boyce, S., & Martin, G. (2013). Pre-linguistic children with cleft palate: Growth of gesture, vocalization, and word use. *International Journal of Speech-Language Pathology*, 15(6), 586–592. doi:10.3109/1754 9507.2013.794475

Scherer, N. J., & D'Antonio, L. (1995). Use of a parent questionnaire for screening language in children with cleft lip/palate. *Cleft Palate-Craniofacial Journal, 32*, 7–14.

Scherer, N. J., D'Antonio, L., & Kalbfliesch, J. (1999). Early speech and language development in children with velocardiofacial syndrome, *American Journal of Medical Genetics, 88*(6), 714–723.

Scherer, N. J., D'Antonio, L., & McGahey, H. (2008). Early intervention for children with cleft palate. *Cleft Palate-Craniofacial Journal, 45*(1), 18–31.

Scherer, N. J., Frey, J., & Kaiser, A. (2014). *Competence-performance gaps in young children with cleft palate: Evidence from assessment.* Presentation at the 15th International Clinical Phonetics and Linguistics Conference, Stockholm, Sweden.

Scherer, N. J., & Kaiser, A. (2007). Early intervention in children with cleft palate. *Infants and Young Children, 20*, 355–366.

Scherer, N. J., & Kaiser, A. (2010). Enhanced milieu teaching/phonological emphasis: Application for children with cleft lip and palate. In L. Williams & R. McCauley (Eds.), *Speech sound disorders in children*. Baltimore, MD: Brookes.

Scherer, N. J., Kaiser, A., Frey J., & Roberts, M. (in preparation). A pilot study of the efficacy of an early speech intervention on the speech sound development of young children with cleft palate. Manuscript submitted for publication.

Scherer, N. J., Williams, A. L., & Proctor-Williams, K. (2008). Early and later vocalization skills in children with and without cleft palate. *International Journal of Pediatric Otorhinolaryngology, 72*, 827–840.

Scherer, N. J., Williams, A. L., Stoel-Gammon, C., & Kaiser, A. (2012). Assessment of single word production for children under three years of age: Comparison of children with and without cleft palate. *International Journal of Otolaryngology, Cleft–VPI Special Issue,* Article ID 724214. doi:10.1155/2012/724214

Shriberg, L. D., Austin, D., Lewis, B. A., McSweeny, J. L., & Wilson, D. L. (1997). The percentage of consonants correct metric: Extensions and reliability data. *Journal of Speech, Language, and Hearing Research, 40*, 708–722.

Snyder, L., & Scherer, N. J. (2004). The development of symbolic play and language development in toddlers with cleft palate. *American Journal of Speech-Language Pathology, 13*, 66–80.

Stoel-Gammon, C., & Otomo, M. (1986). Babbling development of hearing-impaired and normally-hearing subjects. *Journal of Speech and Hearing Disorders, 51*(1), 33–45.

Systematic Analysis of Language Transcripts. (2012). Retrieved from http://saltsoftware .com/

Willadsen, E. (2013). Lexical selectivity in Danish toddlers with cleft palate, *Cleft Palate-Craniofacial Journal, 50*, 456–465. doi:http://dx.doi.org/10.1597/11-022

Williams, A. L., & Stoel-Gammon, C. (2014). Profiles of early expressive phonology. Manuscript in preparation.

PART III

Early to Middle School Age

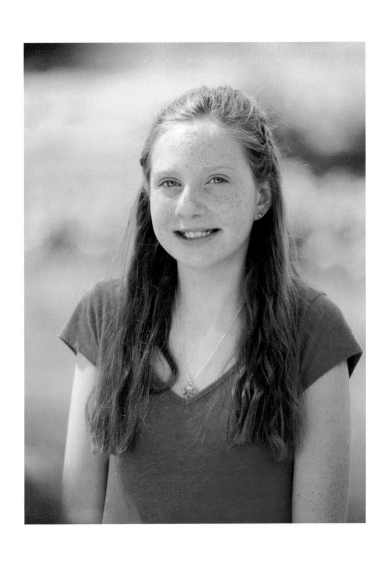

Normal speech is the goal for the child born with cleft lip and palate by the time he or she enters school. In this section, we begin by describing the speech and resonance characteristics that may impact this goal. To be sure, hypernasality and various types of audible nasal air emission are the most frequent perceptual symptoms that result from velopharyngeal inadequacy. In Chapter 8, we emphasize the physiologic and acoustic-perceptual characteristics of hypernasal resonance and audible nasal air emission. We also describe the articulation, voice, fluency, and intelligibility characteristics of children with repaired cleft palate. Regarding articulation, we present evidence that questions the long-held assumption that some common misarticulations such as mid-dorsum palatal stops and posterior nasal fricatives are compensatory to velopharyngeal inadequacy. Rather, the evidence suggests that other structural and hearing anomalies may contribute to the development of these articulations.

In Chapter 9, we describe perceptual and instrumental techniques to assess resonance, nasal air emission, and velopharyngeal function. We draw on our combined clinical experience to focus on practical procedures. Although perceptual assessment is the gold standard, we stress that comprehensive assessment of the child must include instrumental measures. We describe a novel use of the Nasometer—an instrument available to many clinicians—to differentially identify passive (obligatory) nasal air emission from active (learned) nasal air emission that is part of the articulation of nasal fricatives.

In Chapter 10, Dennis Ruscello provides a comprehensive protocol for treating the child with articulation disorders in the school setting. He describes models for collaboration between the school-based clinician and the craniofacial team. He stresses that most children will need coordinated services and that communication between school and team personnel is essential. Ruscello further advocates the use of phonetic teaching for misarticulations such as compensatory errors that are not stimulable by perceptual techniques. He discusses sequencing of target sounds and working with the older, adolescent child in the school setting.

In Chapter 11, we describe secondary management of velopharyngeal inadequacy in the school-aged child. Although physical management such as additional palatal surgery or prosthetic speech appliances is usually the standard, we review some behavioral management options that may be considered in some cases.

Finally, in Chapter 12, Joseph Napoli describes the orthodontic preparation and surgical management of the older school-aged child relative to alveolar cleft repair. Alveolar bone grafting is usually the final surgery required for most children with complete cleft lip and palate to close the cleft defect. Although it is primarily intended to restore bony continuity of the upper gum ridge to support eruption of permanent teeth, there are multiple other benefits. These include elimination of nasal drainage into the oral cavity, elimination of reflux of foods and liquids into the nasal cavity, and improved aesthetic contour of the upper lip. Possible speech benefits include the elimination of obligatory nasal air escape from anterior oronasal fistulae and, if maxillary expansion was done, normalization of backed articulatory placement for lingual-alveolar sounds either spontaneously or through follow-up speech therapy.

8

Speech and Resonance Characteristics

INTRODUCTION

The young child with repaired cleft palate can be a diagnostic challenge for clinicians, even experienced ones. The child may present with speech, resonance, and nasal air emission characteristics determined by many conditions other than the cleft. These include but are not limited to phonological disorders, sensorineural hearing loss, dysarthria, apraxia, or some combination of conditions. In essence, the child born with a palatal cleft is not immune from other developmental and organic disorders.

Some children with palatal clefts exhibit speech symptoms such as hypernasality and audible nasal air emission that are the direct result of an inadequate velopharyngeal mechanism. These symptoms are considered *obligatory*. Some of these children may learn *compensatory* articulations that circumvent the velopharyngeal valve. Others may exhibit articulation errors or distortions that are related to anterior maxillary arch or dental anomalies. Still others may exhibit phonetic or phonological errors that are

unrelated to their cleft condition. Finally, there are some children with clefts who do not exhibit speech symptoms or articulation errors at all.

The task of the speech-language pathologist (SLP) relative to the young child with repaired cleft palate is two-fold. First, the SLP must carefully assess the child relative to multiple speech characteristics including resonance, nasal air emission, articulation, phonation, fluency, and intelligibility. Second, the SLP must make appropriate diagnostic and management decisions based on sound clinical judgment using both perceptual and instrumental findings. The objective of this chapter is to describe the speech characteristics of children with repaired cleft palate. Perceptual and instrumental assessment procedures are covered in Chapter 9.

RESONANCE CHARACTERISTICS

Hypernasal resonance is perhaps the most defining feature of children with repaired cleft palate who have velopharyngeal inadequacy (VPI). Therefore, it is critical that clinicians have a clear understanding of the nature of normal resonance and clinical procedures to identify and assess hypernasal resonance. Resonance is a complex acoustic-perceptual phenomenon. Resonance occurs when a vibrating sound source excites an air-filled cavity. In human speakers, the vibrating sound source is the vocal folds and the air-filled cavities include the pharynx, oral cavity, and nasal passages. Each individual has a unique resonance that is determined by the frequency of vocal-fold vibration and the physical dimensions—length, width (or cross-sectional area), and volume—of the resonating cavities. Because voicing is required, resonance occurs only on vowels or voiced consonants, not voiceless consonants. For an individual without structural anomalies and normal velopharyngeal closure, resonance during production of vowels and voiced oral consonants occurs primarily in the pharyngeal and oral cavities. During production of nasal consonants and nasalized vowels when the velum is lowered, the nasal cavity becomes an additional resonator.

Hypernasality is excessive resonance of the nasal cavity during production of vowels and voiced oral consonants. Conversely, *hyponasality* involves reduced resonance of the nasal cavity during production of nasal consonants and vowels adjacent to nasal consonants. Individuals with repaired cleft lip and palate may exhibit both hypernasality and hyponasality. Hyponasal resonance may occur due to posterior anomalies such as enlarged tonsils, enlarged adenoids, choanal atresia, and a shallow nasopharynx. Hyponasal resonance may also occur due to anterior anomalies such as a collapsed nasal valve or hypertrophic (enlarged) turbinates.

Cul-de-sac resonance is a distinctive type of resonance that has been described differently by various authors. We consider cul-de-sac as the lack of normal oral resonance that often results in a muffled, nasopharyngeal quality. Kummer (2014) calls this pharyngeal cul-de-sac and attributes the quality to enlarged tonsils that impede efficient oral resonance. Some children with syndromes such as Treacher Collins may exhibit cul-de-sac resonance due to a small and retracted mandible (Vallino, Peterson-Falzone, & Napoli, 2006). Still other authors consider cul-de-sac a variant of hyponasal resonance that, as noted above, is caused by anterior obstruction of the nasal cavity (Peterson-Falzone, Hardin-Jones, & Karnell, 2001). Peterson-Falzone et al. (2001) note that this type of resonance can be simulated by repeating the syllable "mi" normally and then with the nostrils pinched closed. Finally, it should be reemphasized that there is little consensus among clinicians regarding the term *cul-de-sac* and little, if any, objective acoustic-perceptual research on this type of resonance.

It is important to note that although hypernasality primarily occurs due to an open velopharyngeal port and direct acoustic coupling of the oral and nasal cavities, some nasal resonance can also occur in the presence of complete velopharyngeal closure (Bundy & Zajac, 2006; Gildersleeve-Neumann & Dalston, 2001). In such a situation, the nasal air mass is excited indirectly (or sympathetically) by velar tissue vibration against the posterior pharyngeal wall during closure (Moll, 1960). This phenomenon is responsible to some extent for the unique resonance of an individual, in addition to other factors such as the relative size and shape of the resonating cavities.

Acoustic Characteristics of Hypernasality

Acoustic analysis has long been used in an attempt to identify correlates of hypernasality. Because nasality can be reliably perceived by a listener, clinicians and researchers have assumed that some invariant feature or set of features must be present in the acoustic signal. As pointed out by Baken and Orlikoff (2000), this assumption implies that the nasal cavity acts as a fixed resonator that simply adds some component to the acoustic signal. Curtis (1968), however, suggested that the acoustics associated with perceived nasality are dependent on complex interactions with the oral and pharyngeal resonators that vary across speakers and specific vowels. As summarized by Baken and Orlikoff (2000), "coupling of the nasal cavity to the rest of the system does not add an invariant resonator, but rather it just changes the overall nature of a complex acoustic system" (p. 462).

Schwartz (1968) identified four common spectral changes that occur as a function of nasalization: (a) reduction in intensity of the first formant, (b) presence of antiresonances, (c) presence of extra resonances or formants, and (d) shift in frequency of formants. Schwartz noted that a reduction in intensity of the first formant was the most frequently reported spectral change across studies and attributed this to acoustic damping by the nasal cavity. Although not identified by Schwartz, an increase in the bandwidth of formants is also a commonly recognized correlate of nasalization (Bloomer & Peterson, 1955; Dickson, 1962; House & Stevens, 1956). The increase in formant bandwidth is also due to excessive damping by the nasopha-ryngeal cavity (see discussion of Dwyer, Robb, O'Beirne, & Gilbert, 2009, later in the chapter).

Some acoustic and spectral changes in the vowel /i/ due to nasalization are illustrated in Figure 8–1. The speaker was an adult male without palatal anomalies who first produced the vowel normally and then with the velum voluntarily lowered to simulate hypernasality. The speaker was recorded using a high-quality, head-mounted condenser microphone to maintain a constant mouth-to-microphone distance. The speaker also monitored his electroglottographic (EGG) activity in an attempt to maintain the same vocal effort level during production of the nasalized vowel. EGG is a noninvasive technique that monitors impedance changes of the vibrating vocal folds (see Baken & Orlikoff, 2000). Figure 8–1A displays the microphone signal (top), the EGG signal (middle), and the root-mean-square (RMS) intensity level of the EGG signal (bottom). As indicated by the RMS of the EGG signal, the speaker produced both vowels at approximately the same effort level. Nevertheless, the nasalized production was reduced in overall acoustic amplitude as reflected by the envelope of the microphone signal, due to damping by the nasal cavity. Figure 8–1B shows spectral changes in the vowel due to nasalization as determined by linear predictive coding (LPC) analysis. The primary spectral change that occurred during nasalization was reduction in the amplitude of all formants (F1, F2, and F3 are labeled in the figure). Additional spectral changes included (a) an upward shift in frequency of F1 and F2, (b) the presence of an extra resonance at approximately 3.5 kHz, and (c) reduced intensity or an antiresonance at approximately 5.5 kHz.

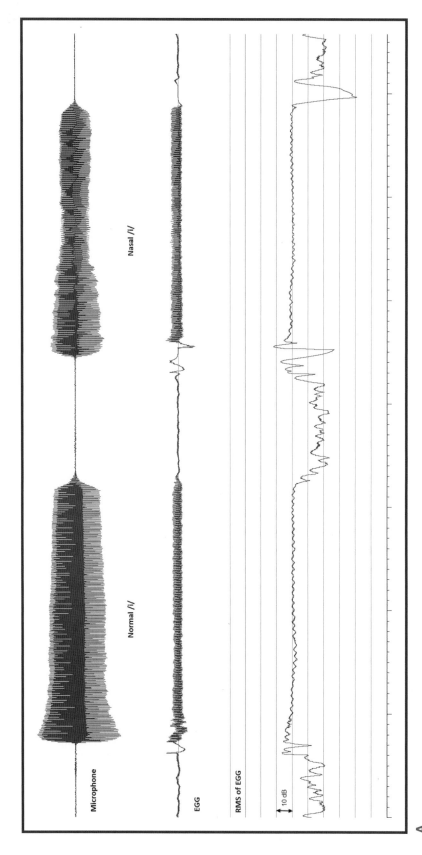

Figure 8–1. A. Microphone signal (*top*), electroglottographic (EGG) signal (*middle*), and RMS amplitude of EGG (*bottom*) of normal and nasalized /i/. Vocal effort was the same for both productions as indicated by the RMS amplitude of the EGG; the nasalized vowel, however, was reduced in acoustic amplitude as reflected by the microphone signal. *continues*

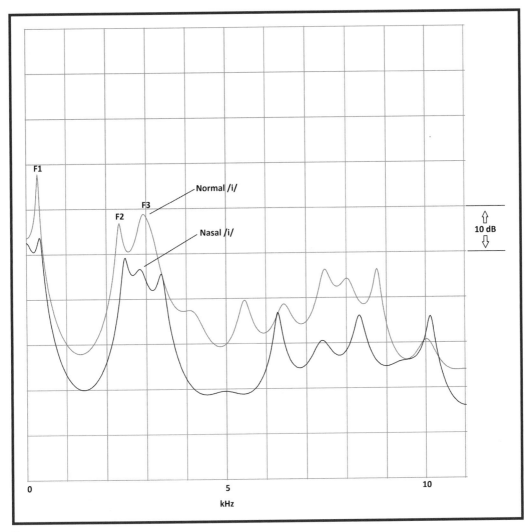

B

Figure 8–1. *continued* **B.** Spectra of the normal and nasalized vowels shown in **A** using linear predictive coding. See text for description.

These changes are consistent with those typically reported in the literature for nasalized vowels (e.g., Schwartz, 1968).

Factors Affecting Hypernasality

Many factors may affect the perception of nasality including phonetic context, vocal quality (i.e., loudness, pitch, breathi-ness, and hoarseness), and speaking rate. Among speakers without cleft palate, low vowels are typically perceived as more nasal than high vowels (Carney & Sherman, 1971; Lintz & Sherman, 1961). The converse, however, has been reported for speakers with cleft palate in that high vowels are perceived as more nasal than low vowels (Carney & Sherman, 1971; Hess, 1959; Spriesterbach & Powers, 1959).

Although the reason for this discrepancy is not exactly clear, it should be noted that Gildersleeve-Neumann and Dalston (2001) reported that sympathetic vibration of the nasal cavity was greatest on high vowels in speakers without cleft palate. High vowels, therefore, may be more susceptible to sympathetic transfer of nasal acoustic energy in speakers with surgically repaired cleft palate. This may occur due to altered tissue biomechanics.

Phonetic assimilation also affects perceived nasality. A given speaker is likely to sound more nasal when the phonetic context includes nasal consonants due to anticipatory and carryover effects to adjacent vowels and voiced consonants. Relative to carryover nasalization, there is some evidence that speakers with repaired cleft palate take longer to achieve velopharyngeal closure in a nasal-plosive sequence (Dotevall, Ejnell, & Blake, 2001). If so, then carryover nasality on vowels also may be greater.

Vocal characteristics such as loudness and quality may affect the perception of nasality. Some children with repaired cleft palate tend to habitually speak with reduced loudness. McWilliams, Morris, and Shelton (1990) referred to this as "soft voice syndrome" and suggested that children may reduce loudness in an attempt to reduce nasality or other obligatory symptoms of VPI. Vocal dysfunction such as hoarseness or breathiness may also make it difficult to assess resonance. It has been our clinical experience that speakers with suspected VPI who exhibit moderate to severe hoarseness are especially difficult to judge relative to resonance. This most likely occurs due to reduced signal-to-noise ratio that eliminates or alters spectral clues in the acoustic signal.

Vocal pitch of an individual might also affect judgments of resonance. Young children with relatively high fundamental frequencies, for example, may be perceived as more nasal than older children. In one of our clinics, an experienced surgeon commented that he was baffled by the hypernasality of a 5-year-old girl with repaired cleft palate as she appeared to demonstrate complete velopharyngeal closure during phonation on oral examination. To be sure, both pressure-flow measures and nasometry (reviewed in the next chapter) were well within normal limits. The girl's pitch, however, was high for her age and that may have contributed to the perception of nasality.

Although the effect of vocal pitch has been relatively neglected in the literature on resonance, two recent studies should be noted. Mandulak and Zajac (2009) determined acoustic nasalance of men and women without cleft palate who sustained vowels at targeted sound pressure levels and fundamental frequency ranges. They reported increased nasalance for men during production of the vowel /a/ when a higher than normal fundamental frequency was targeted. Zajac et al. (2015) had adult listeners use direct magnitude estimation (DME) (described in Chapter 9) to determine hypernasality of 23 children with repaired cleft palate at 6, 7, and 8 years of age. They reported that DME ratings of hypernasality decreased by 20% from the youngest to the oldest age. Although fundamental frequency of the children also decreased slightly with age, it did not account for the change in nasality. Other unknown factors, therefore, apparently contributed to the finding of reduced nasality as function of increased age.

Speaking rate may also affect the perception of nasality. Jones, Folkins, and

Morris (1990) manipulated speech production time in children with cleft palate and hypernasality. Although overall effects were not statistically significant, they reported that some children with cleft palate were judged to be less hypernasal when speaking time was decreased (i.e., when speaking rate was increased). One possible reason for this finding might be that listeners simply had less time to judge the extent of nasality. Dwyer et al. (2009) reported decreased nasality as a function of increased speaking rate in adults with hearing impairment who were hypernasal. They reported that listeners' judgments of nasality were significantly reduced when the speakers doubled their speaking rate. Dwyer et al. also reported that reduced judgments of nasality were associated with a reduction (narrowing) of formant bandwidths of vowels via acoustic analysis. As noted previously, wide or broad bandwidths of vowels are often reported as an acoustic characteristic of hypernasality. Dwyer et al. speculated that increased speaking rate might increase tension of the vocal tract walls that in turn reduce acoustic damping and bandwidth.

It should be noted that the above findings relative to speaking rate, albeit limited, do not support some common clinical beliefs. Some clinicians, for example, believe that hypernasality will be reduced at slower speaking rates as this will facilitate greater movement of the velum (i.e., eliminate articulatory undershoot). Given the complexity of hypernasality relative to the many factors that might affect it, clinicians should be cognizant that different approaches to reduce nasality may work for different speakers. To be sure, clinicians should use stimulability testing and attempt to modify various parameters of speech in different ways to determine the effects on perceived resonance.

NASAL AIR EMISSION

Following hypernasal resonance, nasal air emission is the second most defining feature of children with repaired cleft palate and VPI. Many graduate students mistakenly consider nasal air emission to be synonymous with hypernasality. Even though hypernasality and nasal air emission can certainly co-occur in a speaker, these are distinct perceptual symptoms that occur on different speech segments for different physiological reasons (Table 8–1). Whereas hypernasality is a resonance phenomenon that occurs on vowels and voiced consonants, nasal air emission is an aerodynamic event that occurs primarily on obstruent consonants, especially voiceless consonants. Actually, hypernasality can be associated with relatively little nasal airflow. This occurs because during production of a vowel the oral cavity is open and typically has much less impedance to airflow than the nasal cavity. The aerodynamics of hypernasality and nasal air emission can be easily demonstrated using devices such as the See-Scape (see Chapter 9, Figure 9–5). During production of nasalized stop consonants such as /p/, the float of the See-Scape rises excessively. Conversely, during production of a prolonged nasalized vowel such as /i/ or /a/, there is little movement of the float.

In the absence of neuromotor dysfunction, oronasal fistula, or articulatory mislearning (see section on articulation in this chapter), nasal escape of air during production of oral pressure consonants occurs as a direct consequence of VPI (i.e.,

Table 8–1. Distinguishing Characteristics of Hypernasality and Nasal Air Emission

Hypernasality	Nasal Air Emission
Resonance phenomenon	Aerodynamic phenomenon
Occurs on vowels and voiced consonants	Occurs on obstruent consonants, especially voiceless
Associated with little nasal airflow	Nasal emission (NE) can be visible only, audible, or turbulent • Visible NE—detected by mirror • Audible NE—turbulence created at anterior nasal valve • Turbulent NE—turbulence created at VP port (often with tissue flutter)

an obligatory symptom). There is robust evidence to show that velopharyngeal closure is essentially airtight during production of oral pressure consonants across the lifespan of individuals without structural anomalies (see Zajac, 2015b, for a review). In the presence of an unrepaired cleft of the palate, there will always be some degree of nasal air escape during production of oral pressure consonants if the nasal airway is unobstructed. Likewise, even following surgical repair of a palatal cleft, nasal air emission may occur. Zajac (2003) used the pressure-flow method to study 176 individuals with repaired cleft palate and 223 individuals without cleft palate aged 5 to 51 years. Zajac reported that 54 (31%) of the speakers with cleft palate exhibited nasal airflow during production of the /p/ segment of the syllable /pi/ that exceeded 20 mL/s compared to 3 (1%) of the speakers without cleft palate. Zajac used a 20 mL/s nasal air flow criterion to safeguard against including speakers who may have exhibited small rates of nasal airflow that were due to normal movement of a closed velum (i.e., velar bounce, see below and Chapter 9). It must

be noted that not all of the speakers with cleft palate who exhibited nasal airflow also presented with perceptual symptoms of audible nasal air escape. This point is discussed next.

Types of Nasal Air Emission

Nasal air emission can occur across a continuum from inaudible (visible only) to audible. There have been many different, and confusing, terms used to describe obligatory nasal air emission. Some of the terms found in the literature include audible nasal air emission, turbulent nasal air emission, nasal rustle, and passive nasal fricatives. Nasal emission typically occurs during production of obstruent consonants—stops, fricatives, and affricates—that require relatively high levels of oral air pressure, especially voiceless obstruents. Peterson-Falzone et al. (2010) describe the continuum of nasal air emission as visible only (i.e., detected by mirror testing) to audible to turbulent. Audible nasal air emission can be simulated by forcefully exhaling through the nose. In this situation, air becomes turbulent as it passes through the smallest cross-sectional area of the nose, typically the anterior nasal valve (Proctor, 1982). Peterson-Falzone et al. (2010) describe nasal "turbulence" as the sound of extra noises that occur when "marked intranasal or velopharyngeal resistance to air flow is present" (p. 223). Specifically, they state that the extra noises occur due to vibration of soft tissue or displacement of mucous that pools in the constriction. Nasal turbulence has been called "nasal rustle" by Kummer and colleagues. They attribute the noise of "nasal rustle" to bubbling of secretions in a small velopharyngeal port (Kummer, Briggs, & Lee, 2003; Kummer, Curtis, Wiggs, Lee, & Strife, 1992). Regardless of the specific terms used, the important point is that extra noises are generated in addition to turbulence as air is forced through a small velopharyngeal port. Peterson-Falzone et al. (2010) consider nasal turbulence to be perceptually more severe than audible nasal air emission due to the loud and distracting nature of the extra noise.

Although displacement (or bubbling) of mucus can undoubtedly cause some noise, the perceptually prominent extra noise associated with nasal turbulence is most likely due to vibration (or flutter) of tissue at the velopharyngeal port (Zajac & Preisser, 2015). Trost (1981) used video radiography to identify velar flutter as a component of the posterior nasal fricative. Whereas posterior nasal fricatives are active (or learned) alternative articulations for oral fricatives (see section on articulation later in the chapter), a similar or even identical sound can occur during production of high-pressure consonants as a passive (or obligatory) consequence to incomplete velopharyngeal closure (Peterson-Falzone, Trost-Cardamone, Kar-

nell, & Hardin-Jones, 2006). As illustrated in Figure 8–2, passive tissue flutter may occur when the velum is closely approximated to the posterior pharyngeal wall (or adenoids), and oral air pressure is high enough to set the marginal edges of the velum into vibration. This event is similar to vocal fold vibration that occurs due to known aerodynamic-myoelastic forces.

Factors Affecting Nasal Air Emission

The occurrence of nasal air emission may be influenced by several factors. Zajac and Preisser (2015) investigated the effects of age and phonetic context on the occurrence of turbulent nasal air emission. They studied 30 children with repaired cleft palate who exhibited nasal turbulence with either consistent or inconsistent velar flutter. The children were recorded using the oral and nasal microphones of the Nasometer while producing consonant-vowel (CV) syllables that contrasted plosives and fricatives (/p/–/t/ versus /f/–/s/) with high and mid-low vowels (/i/ versus /ʌ/). The consonants were coded as either having flutter or not having flutter using a combination of auditory-perceptual and spectral analysis of the nasal audio signals (see Chapter 9). Zajac and Preisser found that although velar flutter tended to occur at approximately equal rates on plosives and fricatives (54% and 58%, respectively), it occurred significantly more often on consonants in syllables with high versus mid-low vowels (62% and 50%, respectively). Because high vowels are produced with greater velar height than low vowels (Moll, 1962; Moll & Shriner, 1967), these findings indicate that velar flutter is more likely to be triggered by relatively small velopharyngeal openings. Kummer and colleagues also

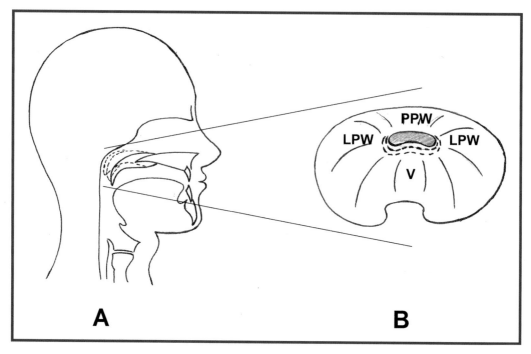

Figure 8–2. A. Lateral view illustrating passive velar tissue flutter during the stop phase of a bilabial plosive consonant. **B.** Superior view illustrating flutter of the marginal edges of the velum. (PPW, posterior pharyngeal wall; LPW, lateral pharyngeal wall; V, velum.)

reported small velopharyngeal openings in speakers who exhibited nasal rustle (Kummer, Briggs, & Lee, 2003; Kummer, Curtis, Wiggs, Lee, & Strife, 1992).

Age may also influence the occurrence, and perhaps the severity, of nasal air emission. In general, the occurrence of nasal emission is determined by the magnitude of oral air pressure that drives nasal airflow, the size of the velopharyngeal port, and the size of the nasal passages. Audible nasal air emission that is generated at the anterior nasal valve, for example, is likely to occur if the speaker uses high oral air pressure, has a large velopharyngeal gap, and has a small nasal valve area. Likewise, turbulent nasal air emission that is generated at the velopharyngeal port is likely to occur if the speaker uses high oral air pressure but has

a small velopharyngeal opening. Because younger children have smaller nasopharyngeal dimensions (Vorperian et al., 2009) and use greater oral air pressure during production of stop consonants (Searl & Knollhoff, 2013; Zajac, 2000), they may be more susceptible than older children to produce either audible or turbulent nasal air emission. Zajac and Preisser (2015), however, found no statistically significant relationship between age and frequency of occurrence of nasal turbulence with flutter in children with repaired cleft palate. One possible reason for this negative finding might have been preferred loudness levels of the children. All of the children studied by Zajac and Preisser produced CV syllables at self-determined loudness levels. It is possible that some of the children may have exhibited "soft voice syndrome" as suggested by McWilliams et al. (1990). If so, then the occurrence of nasal turbulence and flutter may have been reduced for some children.

Weak Oral Air Pressure

Weak or reduced oral air pressure during production of obstruent consonants is associated with severe VPI. It is discussed here, rather than in the section on articulation, as it is an obligatory symptom directly related to nasal air emission. When a relatively large velopharyngeal gap is present, oral air pressure during the stop phase of a plosive will bleed into the nose resulting in audible nasal air emission and reduced oral air pressure. This loss of aerodynamic energy can alter the acoustics of the oral release burst and reduce intelligibility. Weak oral air pressure, therefore, usually occurs in conjunction with audible nasal air emission, but not nasal turbulence. As discussed previously, nasal turbulence with or without flutter is triggered by a relatively small velopharyngeal gap and relatively high oral air pressure.

Nasal Grimace

A nasal grimace sometimes accompanies audible nasal air emission in children with severe VPI. The grimace is characterized by constriction of the nares, most likely due to contraction of the transverse part of the nasalis muscle. The nasalis is a paired muscle that arises from the surface of the maxilla and inserts into the midline of the nose (Dickson & Maue-Dickson, 1982). The cause of a nasal grimace is somewhat controversial. Kummer (2014) considers the nasal grimace a type of obligatory

distortion that occurs due to "overflow muscle reaction" in an attempt to achieve velopharyngeal closure. Warren (1986), however, believes that a nasal grimace occurs as a compensatory attempt to regulate vocal tract air pressure in the presence of a defective velopharyngeal valve. At times, a nasal grimace also occurs as part of the articulation of anterior nasal fricatives. As discussed below, the nasal grimace may function to increase turbulence when produced with an anterior nasal fricative.

ARTICULATION CHARACTERISTICS

Hypernasality and nasal air emission are *obligatory* symptoms of velopharyngeal dysfunction. Children who have incomplete velopharyngeal closure will exhibit some degree of hypernasality and nasal air emission depending on the size of the velopharyngeal gap and speech production factors (e.g., respiratory effort level). Some children with repaired cleft palate or VPI also exhibit articulation errors that are considered *compensatory* in nature. This means that the child has actively learned some type of maladaptive articulation in response to a structural defect, either VPI or anterior structural anomalies. Some compensatory articulations are clearly in response to VPI in that articulatory constriction is below the velopharyngeal valve. Warren (1986) considers "gross" misarticulations such as glottal stops and pharyngeal fricatives (described later in this section) as attempts by the child to fulfill the respiratory and aerodynamic demands of speech by bypassing a defective velopharyngeal mechanism, even at the expense of intelligibility. Trost (1981) described several additional maladaptive articulations that were associated with the speech of children with cleft palate. Some of these articulations, such as the pharyngeal stop, are clearly compensatory to a defective velopharyngeal mechanism. Others, however, such as the mid-dorsum palatal stop are problematic in that articulation occurs in the oral cavity and does not circumvent the velopharyngeal mechanism. There is a growing body of clinical research (described later in the chapter) to suggest that some of these maladaptive articulations may be compensatory to anterior structural defects such as collapsed or narrow maxillary arches.

Children with repaired cleft lip and palate are also susceptible to obligatory articulation distortions due to skeletal malocclusion and dental anomalies. Children with palatal clefts are at risk for maxillofacial growth restrictions that predispose them to skeletal Class III malocclusion (see Chapter 13). When severe, Class III malocclusion can significantly distort sibilants and affricates, causing various types of lisp. Missing, misshaped, rotated, extra, or ectopic teeth can also contribute to obligatory distortion of sibilants and affricates.

Compensatory Articulations

Articulations that are clearly compensatory to velopharyngeal inadequacy are glottal stops, pharyngeal stops, pharyngeal fricatives, and pharyngeal affricates. These articulations modify the airstream well below the velopharyngeal valve.

Glottal Stops

Glottal stops are produced by a rapid and forceful adduction of the vocal folds that momentarily stops all expiratory airflow

at the level of the glottis. Linguists have typically described glottal stops as voiceless in that no vocal fold vibration occurs. Glottal stops are produced as allophones of /t/ in many American English dialects. Some examples are productions of words such as "button" and "kitten" where the voiceless alveolar stop (or flap) is replaced by a glottal gesture. In children with VPI, glottal stops are produced in place of oral stops, with some children also replacing sibilants such as /s/ with glottal stops. Glottal stops may also be co-produced with oral stops by some children. Typically, this occurs during production of bilabial stops. It is not clear if these co-productions develop spontaneously or if they occur as a result of ineffective speech therapy.

Henningsson and Isberg (1986) observed limited velopharyngeal movement, especially lateral pharyngeal wall motion, in speakers who produced gross compensatory articulations such as glottal stops. When those speakers produced oral stops, "moderate-to-good" velopharyngeal movements were observed. As discussed in Chapter 9, these findings have significant implications for the instrumental assessment of velopharyngeal function in children who produce pervasive glottal stop substitutions.

Pharyngeal Stops and Fricatives

Pharyngeal stops are produced by complete retraction of the root of the tongue against the posterior pharyngeal wall to stop expiratory airflow. Trost (1981) noted that these articulations are typically substituted for /k/ and /g/. To understand how a pharyngeal stop is made, first produce /k/ then quickly lower the jaw and drop the base of the tongue against the pharynx. Figure 8–3 illustrates tongue

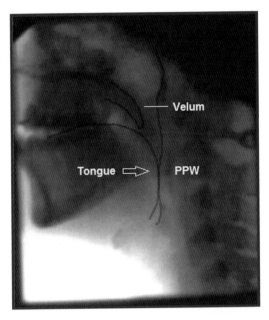

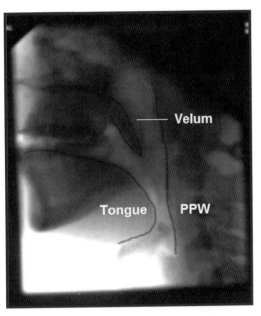

Figure 8–3. Lateral view fluoroscopy showing positions of the tongue, velum, and posterior pharyngeal wall (PPW) during production of a pharyngeal stop.

Figure 8–4. Lateral view fluoroscopy showing positions of the tongue, velum, and posterior pharyngeal wall (PPW) during production of a pharyngeal fricative.

retraction during production of a pharyngeal stop by an adult speaker with repaired cleft lip and palate. Of Interest, this speaker produced pharyngeal stops as replacements for /t/.

Pharyngeal fricatives are also produced by retracting the root of the tongue to the posterior pharyngeal wall but not completely as for a stop. Pharyngeal fricatives are typically substituted for /s/. Prolonging the release of a pharyngeal stop will simulate the acoustics of a pharyngeal fricative, resulting in a low-frequency, turbulent sound. Clinicians should not confuse pharyngeal fricatives with posterior nasal fricatives that are described later in this chapter. Figure 8–4 illustrates tongue retraction during production of a pharyngeal fricative. The speaker is the same as in Figure 8–3.

Pharyngeal Affricates

Pharyngeal affricates, similar to oral affricates, are a combination of a stop followed by a fricative. A pharyngeal affricate, however, is produced with a glottal stop followed by a pharyngeal fricative. These articulations are typically substituted for velar stops.

SLPs must remember that not all children with VPI will develop gross compensatory articulations. But, when present, many clinicians consider these articulations as a sure sign of VPI, especially in a young child. This is likely because compensatory errors typically inhibit the need for velopharyngeal closure and increase the perception of hypernasality. Clinicians must be cognizant, however, that compensatory articulations may have been acquired prior to palate surgery and are retained errors. In addition, some compensatory articulations occur for other reasons. Children with moderate to severe hearing loss, for example, often develop glottal stop articulations (Lach, Ling, Ling, & Ship, 1970; Smith, 1975; Stoel-Gammon, 1982).

Other Maladaptive Articulations

Children with repaired cleft palate also produce maladaptive articulations such as mid-dorsum palatal stops and posterior nasal fricatives. Other textbooks and sources (e.g., the Core Curriculum developed by the American Cleft Palate-Craniofacial Association) consider these articulations as compensatory to VPI. As noted previously, articulations produced in the oral cavity anterior to the velopharyngeal valve are problematic to describe as compensatory to VPI. For this reason and others discussed below, we describe these articulations as separate from "gross" compensatory articulations.

Mid-Dorsum Palatal Stops

Trost (1981) described the *mid-dorsum palatal stop* as a hybrid articulation between alveolar and velar stops. Whereas alveolar stops are produced with the tongue tip contacting the alveolar ridge and velar stops are produced with the back of the tongue contacting the velum, mid-dorsum palatal stops are produced with the tongue tip down and the middle of the tongue contacting the hard palate, a placement between alveolar and velar stops. Although Trost stated that these productions replace both alveolar and velar stops, recent research suggests that /t/

and /d/ are primarily affected (Gibbon, Ellis, & Crampin, 2004; Zajac, Cevidanes, Shah, & Haley, 2012). Gibbon et al. (2004) noted that a large percentage of children with cleft palate used simultaneous alveolar-velar double articulations when targeting alveolar stops. This was determined by electropalatography, a technique that uses multiple contact electrodes embedded in an artificial palate. Some studies suggest that mid-dorsum palatal stops may be one of the most frequently used maladaptive articulations. Chapman and Hardin (1992), for example, reported that half of 10 toddlers with cleft palate exhibited mid-dorsum palatal stops.

The perception of mid-dorsum palatal stops is difficult for many English-speaking clinicians. Santelmann, Sussman, and Chapman (1999) demonstrated that both trained and untrained listeners could not reliably identify mid-dorsum palatal stops as different from /t/ and /k/. This is due to the fact that mid-dorsum palatal stops are not phonemic in English. Listeners, therefore, typically perceive it as either an alveolar or velar stop.

The reason why children with palatal clefts use mid-dorsum palatal stops is not entirely clear. As noted above, Trost (1981) and others typically consider it as a compensatory articulation due to VPI. Other researchers, however, have suggested that anterior structural anomalies may be the precipitating cause. Okazaki, Kato, and Onizuka (1991) determined maxillary arch width, length, and height in three groups of Japanese-speaking children. The first group (*n* = 30) had repaired cleft lip and palate (CLP) and exhibited palatalized articulation. The second group (*n* = 30) had repaired CLP but without palatalized articulation. The third group (*n* = 30) did not have CLP and had normal articulation. Palatalized articulation was defined as the backing of dental and alveolar tongue-tip sounds to the mid-palate with broad and central tongue contact, a description quite similar to mid-dorsum palatal stops. Okazaki et al. reported that the maxillary arches of children who exhibited palatalized articulations were significantly narrow, short, and shallow compared with those of the other groups of children.

Zajac et al. (2012) studied five children with repaired CLP who produced mid-dorsum palatal stops for alveolar stops, six children with repaired CLP who did not produce mid-dorsum palatal stops, and eight typically developing children with normal articulation. All were native-English speakers. Mid-dorsum palatal stops were identified clinically and confirmed by listeners via a forced-choice identification task. The listeners identified both alveolar and velar stops of the latter two groups with 91% to 100% accuracy, but they were only 50% accurate in identifying alveolar stops of the children clinically judged to produce mid-dorsum palatal stops. Zajac et al. also reported that these children had the narrowest maxillary arch width at the canine teeth relative to arch width at the molar teeth as determined from dental casts. Zajac et al. concluded that mid-dorsum palatal stops might occur in children with repaired CLP in response to reduced anterior oral cavity space due to restricted (or collapsed) maxillary arches.

Eshghi, Zajac, Bijankhan, and Shirazi (2013) studied 11 Persian-speaking children with repaired CLP who were undergoing orthodontic treatment for maxillary collapse (see Chapter 12). Four of the 11 children were clinically judged to produce mid-dorsum palatal stops for

the alveolar /t/. It should be noted that in Persian, /t/ is typically produced with dento-alveolar tongue contact. Eshghi et al. determined the first spectral moment during the release of /t/ and /k/ of the 11 children with CLP and 20 additional Persian-speaking children without CLP. The first spectral moment is the mean frequency as computed from Fast Fourier transforms. Eshghi et al. reported that the frequency of the first spectral moment for /t/ and the difference in frequency between /t/ and /k/ were significantly reduced for the children with CLP. These findings are consistent with backed articulation of /t/ by the children with CLP, suggesting that maxillary collapse was a factor in the findings.

Some clinicians have suggested that anterior oronasal fistulas or Class III malocclusion might contribute to the occurrence of mid-dorsum palatal stops (Golding-Kushner, 1995; Kummer, 2008). None of the children studied by either Okazaki et al. (1991) or Zajac et al. (2012), however, had oronasal fistulas at the time of the respective studies. Both studies also controlled for type of skeletal occlusion. Although a child may use mid-dorsum palatal stops in the presence of an anterior oronasal fistula as a way to circumvent loss of oral air pressure, the impact of skeletal Class III malocclusion is less clear. Individuals without cleft palate who have Class III malocclusion, for example, typically exhibit dental or interdental distortion of consonants, not backed articulation (Vallino & Thompson, 1993).

Finally, it is possible that a child who uses mid-dorsum palatal stops for alveolar stops might also use palatal fricatives for alveolar fricatives. We have observed this pattern in some children with repaired CLP. Clinicians, therefore, should be aware of this possibility when evaluating young children with repaired CLP.

Nasal Fricatives

Nasal fricatives are unusual maladaptive articulations used by children both with *and* without palatal anomalies. Nasal fricatives are produced through the nose and are used to replace oral fricatives, affricates, and derived affricates (e.g., /tr/). Nasal fricatives vary in articulatory, aerodynamic, and acoustic-perceptual characteristics. Two generally distinct types have been described (Zajac, 2015a). *Anterior nasal fricatives* are produced without significant velopharyngeal constriction resulting in turbulent airflow generated at the anterior nasal valve of the nose. *Posterior nasal fricatives* are produced with velopharyngeal constriction that results in turbulent nasal airflow and, frequently, tissue vibration (flutter) at the velopharyngeal port. Recall that we previously described passive (obligatory) audible and turbulent nasal air emission as occurring at the anterior nasal valve and posterior velopharyngeal port, respectively. Anterior and posterior nasal fricatives, however, are "active" articulations in that the child occludes the oral cavity to direct all airflow through the nose (Harding & Grunwell, 1998). It is this oral airflow stopping gesture that differentiates nasal fricatives from passive audible and turbulent nasal air escape that may sound similar or even identical.

Anterior Nasal Fricatives. Anterior nasal fricatives are produced when the oral cavity is occluded and all airflow is forced through the nose. Turbulence and frication are created when airflow reaches the anterior nasal valve, the smallest cross-sectional area of the nose. Anterior nasal fricatives can be considered as voiceless nasal consonants produced with turbulent nasal airflow (Harding & Grunwell, 1998; Sell, Harding, & Grunwell, 1999). Oral stopping of airflow can occur at the three typical places of nasal consonant articulation—bilabial, alveolar, and velar—or at atypical locations such as the hard palate, similar to a mid-dorsum palatal stop.

As indicated above, anterior nasal fricatives may sound similar or even identical to audible nasal air emission that is obligatory to velopharyngeal inadequacy. As with obligatory nasal air emission, the child may also exhibit a nasal grimace during production of anterior nasal fricatives. Zajac, Mayo, Kataoka, and Kuo (1996) suggested that a nasal grimace would further constrict the nasal valve and enhance generation of aperiodic noise. A clinical procedure that may help differentiate active nasal fricatives from obligatory nasal air emission is to occlude the nostrils of the child while /s/ is prolonged. If the child has actively stopped oral airflow as part of a nasal fricative, then nasal airflow and frication will abruptly stop. A nasometric recording technique is described in Chapter 9 to identify the oral stop component and differentiate nasal fricatives from passive nasal air emission more reliably.

Posterior Nasal Fricatives. Posterior nasal fricatives are produced when the oral cavity is occluded, the velopharyngeal port is partially constricted, and all airflow is forced through the velopharyngeal port. In this situation, the relatively small velopharyngeal port is the source of turbulent nasal airflow and, often, tissue flutter. As previously illustrated in Figure 8–2, flutter is dependent on aerodynamic and biomechanical factors that cause the marginal edges of the velopharyngeal sphincter to vibrate. Similar to an anterior nasal fricative, clinicians may find it difficult to perceptually differentiate an active posterior nasal fricative from passive nasal turbulence.

Trost (1981) used radiographic imaging to describe some of the articulatory components of the posterior nasal fricative. Trost noted that while the velum approximated the posterior pharyngeal wall, it did not make contact. She also noted that the tongue elevated and contacted the velum in some patients. Peterson (1975) and Peterson-Falzone and Graham (1990) also noted a retracted tongue that appeared to contact the soft palate. Trost (1981) reported that the velum tended to flutter—seen as a blurring on the video—during production of the posterior nasal fricative. Even though some clinicians attribute the distinctive sound of the posterior nasal fricative to turbulent nasal airflow or bubbling of mucous, it is the flutter component that is most perceptually salient (Zajac, 2015a). Acoustic and spectral evidence of velar flutter as a component of the posterior nasal fricative is illustrated in Chapter 9.

The perceptual characteristics of posterior nasal fricatives tend to vary across children. In some children, turbulence is prominent. In others, velopharyngeal flutter is prominent. The flutter component also varies to the extent that it may be absent in some productions of the same syllable by the same speaker. When flutter is absent, a posterior nasal fricative may sound similar to an anterior nasal fricative. The variability in the occurrence and extent of flutter is likely dependent on multiple anatomical and speech production factors that include physical characteristics of the velum (e.g., length, thickness, presence of scarring) and magnitude of the driving respiratory air pressure. These same factors also determine the occurrence of flutter as a component of *obligatory* nasal turbulence previously described.

Posterior nasal fricatives are a hallmark of *phoneme-specific nasal emission* in children *without* cleft palate or other structural anomalies (Peterson, 1975; Peterson-Falzone & Graham, 1990). Peterson-Falzone and Graham made several important observations regarding children both with and without palatal anomalies who exhibited phoneme-specific nasal emission. First, the children used a wide range of phonological processes with gliding and stopping occurring most frequently overall. Second, there was no significant difference between the groups of children regarding overall number of phonological processes. Third, although Peterson and Graham were unable to adequately document early episodes of otitis media in the children, they nonetheless noted "suspicious" histories of middle ear disease in 64% of the children without palatal anomalies and 94% with palatal anomalies. The potential significance of early middle ear disease and conductive hearing loss regarding the use of nasal fricatives is discussed next.

Etiology of Nasal Fricatives. Children with repaired cleft who use nasal fricatives traditionally have been assumed to have inadequate velopharyngeal function. To be sure, if a child cannot achieve velopharyngeal closure during acquisition of early plosive consonants, then it is understandable that he or she may learn to replace later acquired oral fricatives with nasal fricatives. This line of reasoning, however, becomes tenuous when applied to the child without palatal anomalies who exhibits phoneme-specific nasal emission. In this case, the child acquires early stop consonants with complete velopharyngeal closure but, for some reason, acquires nasal fricatives as substitutes for oral fricatives. It is not clear why a young child learning the phonetics and phonology of his or her language would make an already complex motor behavior such as fricative production even more complicated.

A New Perspective on Nasal Fricatives. Zajac (2015a) presented a theoretical framework that appears to account for the acquisition of nasal fricatives by children both with and without palatal anomalies (Figure 8–5). The model assumes that nasal fricatives are a learned speech sound disorder that is caused by underlying conductive hearing loss in conjunction with various precipitating events that trigger turbulent nasal airflow. The precipitating events can be respiratory or speech related in nature. According to the model, a child with conductive hearing loss may benefit from enhanced bone-conducted auditory feedback—and perhaps vibratory-tactile feedback—during production of nasal fricatives. If the conductive hearing loss is chronic or occurs during critical learning periods, then the

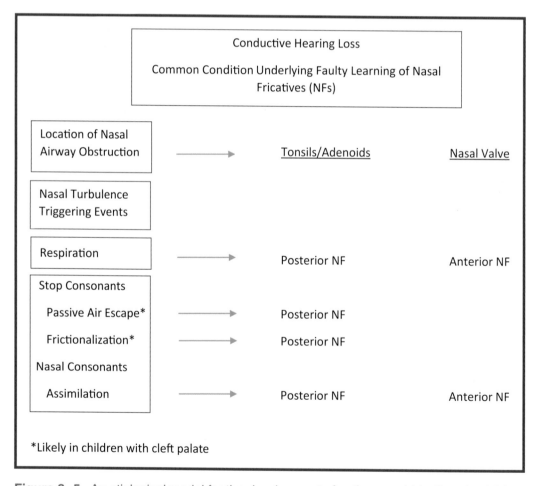

Figure 8–5. An etiological model for the development of active nasal fricatives in children with and without cleft palate. See text for description.

child may come to accept nasal frication as an auditory-perceptual model for the production of fricatives.

As indicated in Figure 8–5, respiratory events such as end-of-utterance expiration can create turbulence and audible frication in children who have either posterior or anterior nasal airway obstruction. Both of these conditions are more common in children with repaired cleft palate (Abdel-Aziz, 2012). The model also assumes that various speech events can trigger turbulent nasal airflow. Some speech events are more common in children with cleft palate, such as passive nasal air escape during production of obstruent consonants. Children without cleft palate, however, might also experience passive nasal air escape during obstruent consonants due to large and obstructing tonsils or large and irregular adenoids (Figure 8–6). Finally, assimilatory processes that simplify word production such as consonant harmony also might trigger nasal turbulence in children

either with or without palatal anomalies. Young children, for example, commonly experiment with fricative production. Some parents report that their children go through a period of producing nasal fricatives for oral targets only in words such as "snip." One parent, who was also an SLP, noted that this behavior coincided with a period of chronic otitis media in her toddler. She further reported that her child's use of nasal fricatives ended about the time that the otitis media resolved.

Zajac (2015a) provided some evidence in support of the model. He reported the longitudinal observation of a young child with repaired bilateral cleft lip and palate who was participating in a research study. The mother reported that the child experienced congestion and difficulty breathing through the nose since birth. As part of the child's participation in the study, nasal ram pressure (NRP) data (see Chapter 9) during respiration and speech were obtained every 2 months beginning at 14 months of age. The child's production

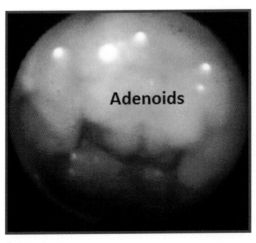 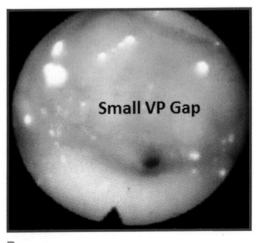

A   B

Figure 8–6. A. Nasoendoscopy image showing large and irregular adenoids of a child at rest. **B.** Same child during attempted velopharyngeal closure during speech. Note the small circular gap that remains during speech.

of stop consonants at 16 months of age was characterized by incomplete velopharyngeal closure as determined by positive NRP occurring during production of stop consonants. At 18 months of age, the child began producing anterior nasal fricatives for oral fricatives in word final position, often with an accompanying nasal grimace. This child also exhibited frication-like noise as part of end-of-utterance exhalation that was perceptually similar to the anterior nasal fricatives. At 24 months of age, while incomplete velopharyngeal closure persisted for stop consonants, the child was no longer producing anterior nasal fricatives. It must be noted that tympanometry performed at the study visits indicated middle ear dysfunction in at least one ear. An audiologic assessment at 24 months of age, however, indicated hearing was within normal limits.

Zajac and Vallino (2015) provided additional evidence in support of the model. They studied eight children who produced posterior nasal fricatives and four who produced anterior nasal fricatives as substitutions for /s/. All of the children had either repaired cleft palate or unrepaired submucous cleft palate. Oral-nasal audio recordings and spectral analysis were used to confirm the presence and type of nasal fricatives (see Chapter 9). The pressure-flow method was used to determine the volume rate of nasal airflow during production of the nasal fricatives. Velopharyngeal port size was also estimated during production of /pi/ syllables. Zajac and Vallino reported a median rate of nasal airflow for the children who produced posterior nasal fricatives of 174 mL/s compared to 365 mL/s for the children who produced anterior nasal fricatives. This finding is consistent with a relatively small velopharyngeal port limiting airflow during production of posterior nasal fricatives. Of greater significance, however, seven of eight children who produced posterior nasal fricatives had adequate velopharyngeal closure as reflected by areas under 5 mm^2 during production of /pi/. These findings are obviously not consistent with the assumption that posterior nasal fricatives are compensatory to velopharyngeal inadequacy, at least gross inadequacy.

Admittedly, the above findings in support of the model are limited. Nonetheless, the findings are consistent with the main tenets of the model in that (a) nasal fricatives are considered to be a speech sound disorder that are acquired as a consequence of early chronic conductive hearing loss, not as compensation to velopharyngeal inadequacy, and (b) nasal fricatives may spontaneously resolve in some children if adequate hearing is restored.

Nasal Substitutions

As described in the previous chapter, the phonetic inventory of infants with cleft palate prior to surgery may be limited to nasal consonants, vowels, and nonobstruent oral consonants (e.g., /h/, /w/, /j/). Even following palate repair, some toddlers persist in using nasal substitutions for oral consonants (e.g., "my" for "bye"). The use of nasal substitutions by toddlers with repaired cleft palate, or unrepaired submucous cleft palate, is considered a red flag for velopharyngeal inadequacy by many SLPs. Recent evidence, however, suggests that this may not necessarily be the case. Hardin-Jones and Chapman (2015) studied 34 toddlers with repaired cleft palate and 20 noncleft toddlers longitudinally from 6 to 39 months of age. They reported that 76% and 40% of toddlers with and without palatal clefts, respectively, used nasal substitutions as part of their phonetic inventories. Hardin-Jones and Chapman further reported that use of nasal substitutions resolved in 62% of the toddlers with clefts by 39 months of age. In other words, only 38% of the toddlers with clefts who used nasal substitutions were eventually diagnosed with VPI. Hardin-Jones and Chapman cautioned that the presence of nasal substitutions following palate repair is not always an early sign of VPI and that speech therapy is needed to expand the child's consonant inventory in order to make an appropriate diagnosis.

Obligatory Oral Distortions

Children with repaired cleft lip and palate are likely to experience multiple dental and occlusal anomalies that might distort articulation. Occlusion is often classified as dental or skeletal. Dental occlusion refers to the natural fitting together of the upper and lower teeth when the jaws are closed, whereas skeletal occlusion refers to the relationship between the maxilla and mandible to each other. Malocclusion, therefore, is the abnormal relationship of the teeth (dental), jaws (skeletal), or a combination of both (dentoskeletal).

Dental Malocclusion

The standard and most widely used system for classifying dental malocclusion is that described by Angle (1899). The point of orientation is the relationship between the first permanent mandibular and maxillary molars. In a normal dental occlusion (Class I), the mesiobuccal cusp of the maxillary first molar rests in the buccal groove of the mandibular molar when the jaws are closed (Figure 8–7A). Mesiobuccal

refers to the first or front cusp along the cheek side of the tooth. Angle classified deviations from the normal relationship as Class II and Class III malocclusions. In Class II malocclusion (Figure 8–7B), the upper molar is anterior to the lower molar, whereas in Class III malocclusion (Figure 8–7C), the upper molar is posterior to the lower molar.

Dental malocclusions can also be classified according to the incisor relationship. An open bite occurs when the maxillary and mandibular incisors do not make contact (see Chapter 13, Figure 13–4). A deep bite is present when the maxillary incisors overlap the mandibular incisors by more than one half. An open-bite malocclusion frequently affects the production of sibilants, and often affricates, as the tongue protrudes through the opening between the teeth.

Skeletal Malocclusion

Skeletal malocclusion applies to the relationships between the upper and lower jaws caused by discrepancy in size, shape, or position of one or both jaws. The jaws simply do not match. Skeletal relationships have three classifications similar to Angle (1899). They are referred to as Class I, Class II (retrognathic), and Class III (prognathic) skeletal malocclusion. It is also possible for an open bite to be present with these conditions.

Children with a cleft or craniofacial condition are likely to have dental or skeletal anomalies that can affect speech, eating, and facial appearance. Dental anomalies include missing or extra teeth, often in the cleft site. At times, teeth may erupt in abnormal locations, called *ectopic eruption*. Ectopic teeth often erupt in the middle of the hard palate, affecting articulation of tongue-tip alveolar sounds (Figure 8–8).

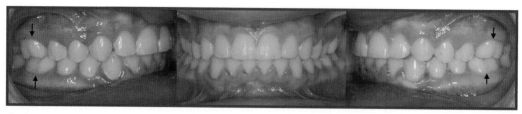

A

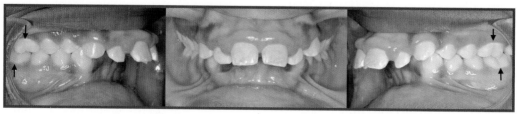

B

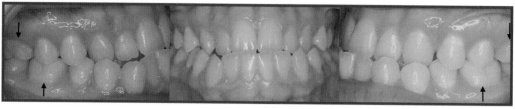

C

Figure 8–7. A. Angle Class I occlusion. **B.** Angle Class II malocclusion. **C.** Angle Class III malocclusion. (Courtesy of the Department of Orthodontics, University of North Carolina at Chapel Hill.)

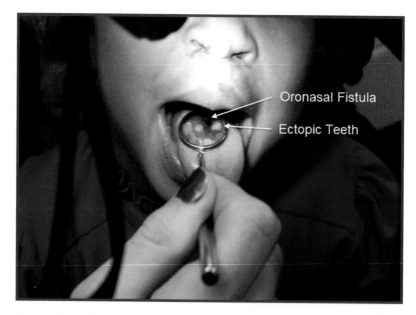

Figure 8–8. Ectopic teeth and oronasal fistula in a child with repaired bilateral cleft lip and palate.

Children with repaired cleft lip and palate are likely to develop Class III malocclusion and crossbite. Crossbite means that the upper anterior and posterior teeth are closer to the tongue than the lower teeth (Figure 8–9). Children with cleft palate and Class III malocclusion usually have anterior crossbite. If the maxillary arch is constricted or collapsed, also common in children with cleft palate, then a posterior crossbite may develop. Anterior and posterior crossbites may affect articulation of sibilants such as /s/. A protruding premaxilla or oronasal fistula, common with bilateral cleft lip and palate, also may be present. All of these dental-occlusal anomalies may distort speech.

Dental and Interdental Distortions

Production of the sibilant /s/ requires precise channeling of the airstream to produce

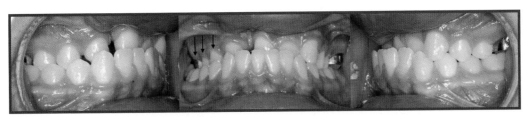

A

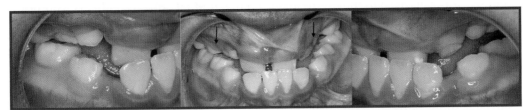

B

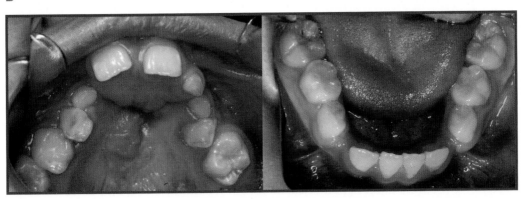

C

Figure 8–9. A. Class III malocclusion with anterior and unilateral posterior crossbites. Arrows indicate posterior crossbite. **B.** Class III malocclusion with anterior and bilateral posterior crossbites. Arrows indicate posterior crossbites. **C.** Constricted maxillary arch, protruding premaxilla, and oronasal fistula (*left image*). Patient had repaired bilateral cleft lip and palate. (Courtesy of the Department of Orthodontics, University of North Carolina at Chapel Hill.)

turbulence and aperiodic noise. The tongue is primarily responsible for this by forming a constriction (groove) along its length. This constriction will increase the velocity of the airstream and produce turbulence when the air exits the constriction. The teeth are also important in that they provide an obstacle to the escaping jet of air that creates additional turbulence (Hixon, Weismer, & Hoit, 2008). Hixon et al. note that fricatives produced with teeth as an obstacle (e.g., /s/) are greater in intensity than those produced without teeth as an obstacle (e.g., /f/). Teeth that are missing, misshaped, or rotated may result in distortion and reduction of fricative intensity. Likewise, a forward tongue posture as the result of a Class III malocclusion may also cause distortions. When the tip of the tongue is behind the lower incisors but distal to the upper incisors, common in Class III malocclusion, distortion, and reduction in intensity of frication is likely. This is called a *dental distortion* or dental lisp. When the tip of the tongue protrudes beyond the lower incisors, a more significant distortion can occur. This is called an *interdental distortion* or interdental lisp.

Lateral Distortions

During production of alveolar stops and fricatives, the sides of the tongue elevate to seal against the maxillary teeth, called lateral bracing (Fletcher, 1992; Lee, Gibbon, & Oebels, 2015). Children with repaired cleft lip and palate who have posterior crossbites, lateral open bites, or missing maxillary teeth may not be able to effectively seal one or both sides of the tongue during fricative production. The escape of airflow from the side(s) of the tongue during /s/ production is called a *lateral distortion* or lateral lisp. A child with unilateral posterior crossbite may shift the mandible to the affected side during /s/ production. Although the reason for this jaw movement is not clear, it may increase lateral bracing of the tongue to prevent air escape, or it may better position lower central teeth into the airstream to increase turbulence.

It must be stated that not all children with dental-occlusal anomalies, even severe, will exhibit speech distortions. Peterson-Falzone (1990) indicated that dental-occlusal anomalies are most likely to affect speech when combinations of conditions are present, conditions are present during early speech acquisition, and the anomaly alters the tongue-tip incisor spatial relationship. At times, we see children with significant posterior crossbites, multiple missing teeth, or Class III malocclusions whose speech is minimally, if at all, affected. This is testimony to the adaptability of the child in overcoming structural anomalies. Many children with these anomalies, however, will exhibit speech distortions. Some will have endured years of speech therapy with limited results. We are typically reluctant to recommend continued speech therapy for a young child who exhibits only obligatory distortions of a few phonemes and when prior speech therapy has not been successful. As discussed in later chapters, speech therapy to correct obligatory distortions may be most effective following surgical and orthodontic correction of the underlying structural conditions. Table 8–2 summarizes the articulation errors and distortions commonly encountered in children with repaired cleft lip and palate.

Phonation

Children with repaired cleft palate and VPI often exhibit perceptual voice disorders or laryngeal anomalies (D'Antonio, Muntz,

Table 8–2. Summary of Some Common Articulation Errors and Distortions Associated With Cleft Lip and Palate and Velopharyngeal Inadequacy (VPI)

Error/ Distortion	Articulatory Characteristics	Cause	Phonemes Affected
Glottal stop	Quick and forceful adduction of vocal folds	Compensatory for VPI	Stops and affricates, also fricatives
Pharyngeal stop	Tongue base contacts posterior pharyngeal wall	Compensatory for VPI	Velar stops, also alveolar stops
Pharyngeal fricative	Tongue base approximates pharyngeal wall	Compensatory for VPI	Alveolar fricatives
Mid-dorsum palatal stop	Middle of tongue contacts hard palate	A learned speech sound error likely due to anterior oral-nasal fistula or maxillary collapse*	Alveolar stops
Anterior nasal fricative	Oral stop with airflow directed through open VP port	A learned speech sound error that may be secondary to conductive hearing loss*	Alveolar fricatives
Posterior nasal fricative	Oral stop with airflow directed through a partially closed VP port; often with tissue flutter	A learned speech sound error that may be secondary to conductive hearing loss*	Sibilants and fricatives
Dental sibilants	Tongue tip contacts maxillary incisors	Class III dental malocclusion	Sibilants
Interdental sibilants	Tongue tip protrudes beyond maxillary incisors	Class III dental malocclusion, anterior open bite	Sibilants
Lateral sibilants	Lack of lateral tongue contact to maxillary teeth	Posterior crossbite, lateral open bite	Sibilants

Note. *Traditionally considered to be compensatory to VPI.

Providence, & Marsh, 1988; Marks, Barker, & Tardy, 1971; McWilliams, Bluestone, & Musgrave, 1969). McWilliams et al. (1969) performed laryngoscopic examinations on 32 children with cleft palate who also exhibited vocal hoarseness. They reported that 84% of the children had some type of vocal fold pathology, with 72% of the children having bilateral vocal fold nodules. The majority of the children also exhibited VPI to varying degrees. McWilliams et al. suggested that the children might have attempted to compensate with the laryngeal mechanism for inadequate velopharyngeal closure. Marks et al. (1971) estimated the occurrence of perceived vocal dysfunction in a sample of 102 speakers, including children, diagnosed with palatal anomalies. Marks et al. reported that 34% of the speakers exhibited deviant vocal quality. D'Antonio et al. (1988) determined the occurrence of either vocal dysphonia or laryngeal abnormalities in a sample of 85 patients, also including children, diagnosed with VPI. They reported that 41% of the speakers exhibited "laryngeal abnormalities, abnormal vocal quality, or both."

The reason for voice disorders in speakers with cleft palate and VPI is unclear. It may occur due to increased respiratory effort or hyperfunctional use of the voice. Curtis (1968) suggested that speakers with cleft palate and VPI may need to exert greater respiratory effort to achieve a given intensity level because of acoustic damping by the nasal cavity. Indeed, Bernthal and Beukelman (1977) reported a reduction in the overall intensity of vowels when oronasal coupling occurs. Hamlet (1973) reported that the glottal open quotient was reduced for nasalized vowels indicating "strong muscular adductory forces" and "glottal tightness." Hamlet suggested that these particular features of vocal-fold vibration might contribute to vocal abuse in speakers with VPI. Warren (1986) speculated that speakers with VPI might employ glottal compensations to regulate the aerodynamic requirements for speech. He suggested

that glottal resistance might be increased to maintain subglottal air pressure in the face of a defective velopharyngeal valve. Warren cited the use of glottal stops as an example of a compensatory response that allows a speaker with VPI to control vocal tract air pressure.

Zajac and Milholland (2014) investigated laryngeal engagement in children with repaired cleft palate who had adequate velopharyngeal function. Laryngeal engagement is the time required to adduct the vocal folds and begin voicing in a voiceless consonant-vowel sequence. Zajac and Milholland obtained oral airflow and sound pressure level (SPL) measures of children with and without cleft palate during counting. An index of laryngeal engagement was determined as the maximum declination in oral airflow following release of a voiceless plosive in a consonant-vowel syllable. Zajac and Milholland reported that children with cleft palate exhibited abrupt laryngeal engagement compared to children without cleft palate. This means that they adducted the vocal folds faster than children without cleft palate. In addition, there was a negative correlation between laryngeal engagement and SPL among all children. Zajac and Milholland suggested that children with cleft palate might use abrupt laryngeal engagement to increase SPL, facilitate velopharyngeal closure, or both. Abrupt laryngeal engagement, however, might also lead to vocal dysfunction and perceptual symptoms such as hoarseness and harshness.

Fluency

It was stated in the introduction to the chapter that children born with cleft palate are not immune to other developmental or organic communication disorders. Clinical observations, however, have long noted a relatively low incidence of stuttering. Dalston, Martinkosky, and Hinton (1987) reviewed the clinic records of 534 patients either having or suspected to have palatal anomalies. The patients ranged in age from 3 to 66 years. They reported that only a single patient was identified whose speech was characterized by stuttering. Dalston et al. noted that the prevalence rate of 1.87 per 1,000 was less than the typically reported prevalence rate of 7 per 1,000 for the general population (Andrews, Craig, Feyer, Hoddinott, Howie, & Neilson, 1983; Young, 1975). Although additional information on the prevalence of stuttering in speakers with cleft palate has not been reported, it has been our clinical observation that stuttering is rare.

Dalston et al. (1987) speculated that stuttering might be expected to occur more frequently in individuals with cleft palate. This is because stuttering has been reported to occur more often in individuals with central nervous system disorders (Andrews et al., 1983), and children with facial clefts might be more susceptible to subtle brain anomalies (Nopoulos, Berg, Canady, et al., 2000). Because embryologic development of the face and brain are closely related both temporally and spatially, structural anomalies associated with the face might also be more likely to occur in the brain. Dalston et al. pointed out that generally high rates of learning disabilities and other cognitive deficits have been reported among children with cleft lip and palate (e.g., Richman, 1980; Richman & Eliason, 1984; see Chapter 10 also).

Dalston et al. (1987) offered two plausible explanations for the finding of low stuttering in children with cleft palate. First, parents of children born with cleft lip and palate are acutely aware that their child may have speech and language delays. To be sure, as reviewed in Chapter 7, one of the early primary functions of the SLP is to counsel parents regarding speech and language development and model parent-child interactions that facilitate development of speech and language. Dalston et al. suggested, therefore, that parents might be more accepting and tolerant of early speech attempts by their children, thus reducing communicative pressure as a potential environmental trigger to stuttering. This view is consistent with a conceptual model of stuttering described by Starkweather (1997), called the demands and capacities model. In this model, stuttering develops when environmental pressures on a child for fluent speech exceed the child's linguistic, motor, emotional, and cognitive capacities. Second, Dalston et al. speculated that inadequate velopharyngeal closure might cause respiratory, aerodynamic, or temporal changes in speech that might reduce the likelihood of stuttering. They noted, for example, that slowing the rate of speech is a therapeutic strategy for reducing stuttering and that some research has suggested that children with cleft palate tend to prolong speech segments (e.g., Forner, 1980).

It is also possible that normal developmental dysfluency might be reduced in children with cleft palate for the same reasons discussed above. Children typically experience a period of dysfluency roughly between 2½ and 3½ years of age when rapidly expanding linguistic ability may outpace more slowly developing speech motor-control skills. At this time, children usually exhibit easy repetition of words, usually at the beginning of sentences. The period of developmental dysfluency varies from child to child and usually lasts a relatively short time, presumably until motor skills catch up to language skills.

Intelligibility

Kent, Weismer, Kent, and Rosenbek (1989) defined intelligibility as "the degree to which the speaker's intended message is recovered by the listener" (p. 483). As such, intelligibility is dependent on the speaker, the situation, and the listener. As reviewed by McWilliams et al. (1990), early studies that investigated intelligibility in children with repaired cleft palate employed transcription or write-down techniques (Fletcher, 1978; Prins & Bloomer, 1965, 1968). In general, these studies indicated (a) clear differences in intelligibility between speakers with and without cleft palate; (b) a tendency for articulation and intelligibility scores to be correlated, especially errors involving stop consonants; and (c) a tendency for intelligibility and velopharyngeal function to be correlated.

Intelligibility in children with repaired cleft palate may be affected by many speech production factors including articulation, resonance, nasal air emission, speaking rate, and prosody. Children who exhibit maladaptive articulations, moderate to severe hypernasality, frequent audible nasal air emission, reduced oral air pressure, and reduced loudness may be especially difficult to understand, even at the single word level. In connected speech, intelligibility may be further reduced due to a fast speaking rate and obligatory dental-occlusal distortions.

As indicated in the next chapter, assessment of speech intelligibility in children with cleft palate typically is done via perceptual rating scales during connected speech. A few studies, however, have used a single-word approach. Whitehill and Chau (2004) investigated Cantonese speakers with repaired cleft palate using a multiple-choice word test based on 13 phonetic contrasts that were identified as being problematic for speakers with cleft palate. The contrasts that most contributed to reduced intelligibility were place of articulation for stops and nasals, stop versus fricative, and stop versus affricate. Whitehill and Chau reported that single-word intelligibility could be predicted with 87% accuracy using two contrasts, stop versus fricative and initial consonant versus null. The investigators also noted that some speakers had similar intelligibility scores but very different phonetic contrast error profiles. They suggested that this occurred due to different underlying causes of unintelligibility.

Hodge and Gotzke (2007) used an open-set, single-word transcription task to determine intelligibility of five children with cleft palate and 10 children without cleft palate. An open-set task means that listeners simply wrote down the word they heard from audio recordings; the intelligibility score was the percentage of correctly transcribed words. Hodge and Gotzke reported a mean single-word intelligibility score of 54.6% for the children with cleft palate and a mean of 79.1% for the children without cleft palate.

Similarly, Zajac, Plante, Lloyd, and Haley (2011) used a computer-mediated, single-word intelligibility test to assess 22 children with repaired cleft palate and 16 controls. All children were 4 to 9 years of age. Zajac et al. constructed 50 sets of phonetically similar words from a larger corpus of 510 words determined to be familiar to young children. A computer program randomly selected a word from each of the 50 sets, and the children simply repeated the word while being audio recorded. Each child was assessed using two different 50-word tests. Twenty adult listeners used orthographic transcription to identify the recorded words. Zajac et al. reported high intra- and interlistener reliability of the test, and no significant difference between intelligibility scores of the two consecutively administered tests. Overall, the mean single-word intelligibility scores, adjusted for age of the children, were 85% for controls and 67% for children with repaired cleft palate. The relatively low intelligibility for controls (i.e., under 90%) was due to developmental articulation errors exhibited by some of the children.

Zajac et al. (2011) also compared children with cleft palate who had adequate velopharyngeal closure ($n = 15$) to those who exhibited some degree of VPI ($n = 7$). Velopharyngeal status was determined by pressure-flow assessment during production of "hamper." Mean intelligibility of the children with adequate closure was 71% compared to 66% for those with some degree of VPI. The difference, however, was not statistically significant.

As part of unpublished research, we have also determined single-word intelligibility of 20 children with repaired cleft lip and palate (CLP) and 10 controls using a 154-word test. Mean age of all children was 8 years. Most of the children had not undergone alveolar bone grafting or orthodontic treatment such as maxillary expansion. The test consisted of seven minimum word pairs that targeted 11 phonetic contrasts (154 total words) considered problematic for children with cleft palate. Table 8–3 lists the 11 phonetic contrasts and examples of minimum word pairs. The children were recorded using

Table 8–3. Eleven Phonetic Contrasts Targeted in a 154 Single-Word Intelligibility Test Developed for Children With Repaired Cleft Lip and Palate

Contrast	Minimal Pair Example
Alveolar–velar stop	tap–cap
Initial consonant–null	pat–at
Alveolar–palatal fricative	see–she
Cluster–singleton	stop–top
Fricative–affricate	ship–chip
Stop–nasal	bop–mop
High–low vowel	beat–bit
Liquid–glide	ray–way
Stop–fricative/affricate	base–vase
Front–back vowel	fill–full
Voiced–voiceless stop	big–pig

the computer program and procedures described by Zajac et al. (2011). Fifty additional, common words were randomly selected and recorded for each child as distractors to reduce the possibility of listeners remembering the target words. Mean single-word intelligibility for the control children was 93% (SD = 3) compared to 78% (SD = 12) for the children with CLP (*p* < .001). The phonetic contrasts most in error for the children with CLP were alveolar-velar stop, alveolar-palatal fricative, fricative-affricate, and liquid-glide.

The above single-word intelligibility results are noteworthy for two reasons. First, the majority of the children with CLP had adequate velopharyngeal function. Thus, few errors occurred due to phonetic contrasts that might be susceptible to VPI such as nasal-stop. Second, three of the four contrasts most in error for children with CLP involved articulation placements at the alveolar ridge or palate, with the alveolar-velar contrast being the most frequent in error. This finding suggests that anterior structural anomalies such as maxillary collapse may affect single-word intelligibility. The findings also reinforce the point made by Whitehill and Chau (2004) in that there may be different underlying anatomical reasons for reduced intelligibility in children with repaired cleft palate.

CHAPTER SUMMARY

School-aged children with repaired cleft lip and palate can present with resonance, nasal emission, articulation, and voice problems. Some of these problems are directly related to the cleft condition, and others are actively learned as compensations. Resonance can be hypernasal due to inadequate velopharyngeal function, or, in some cases, to large oronasal fistulae. Resonance can also be hyponasal due to posterior or anterior nasal airway obstruction. Passive audible nasal air emission and nasal turbulence with or without velopharyngeal tissue flutter can occur due to incomplete velopharyngeal closure. Active (learned) nasal fricatives can occur that may sound similar to passive symptoms. Although most clinicians have traditionally assumed that active articulations such as posterior nasal fricatives are compensatory to velopharyngeal inadequacy, there are reasons to question this assumption. Some children with repaired cleft lip and palate may also exhibit obligatory articulation distortions due to dentition or occlusal status. Both obligatory and learned speech symptoms can reduce overall intelligibility or create social stigmata.

REFERENCES

Abdel-Aziz, M. (2012). Hypertrophied tonsils impair velopharyngeal function after palatoplasty. *Laryngoscope, 122*(3), 528–532.

Andrews, G., Craig, A., Feyer, A. M., Hoddinott, S., Howie P., & Neilson, M. (1983) Stuttering: A review of research findings and theories circa 1982. *Journal of Speech and Hearing Disorders, 48,* 226–246.

Angle, E. H. (1899). Classification of maloccasion. *Dental Cosmos, 41,* 248–264, 350–357.

Baken, R. J., & Orlikoff, R. F. (2000). *Clinical measurement of speech and voice* (2nd ed.). San Diego, CA: Singular.

Bernthal, J., & Beukelman, D. (1977). The effect of changes in velopharyngeal orifice area on vowel intensity. *Cleft Palate Journal, 14,* 63–77.

Bloomer, H., & Peterson, G. (1955). A spectrographic study of hypernasality. *Cleft Palate Bulletin, 5,* 5–6.

Bundy, E., & Zajac, D. J. (2006). Estimation of transpalatal Nasalance during production of voiced stop consonants by non-cleft speakers using an oral-nasal mask. *Cleft Palate-Craniofacial Journal, 43*(6), 691–701.

Carney, P. J., & Sherman, D. (1971). Severity of nasality in three selected speech tasks. *Journal of Speech and Hearing Research, 14*(2), 396–407.

Chapman, K. L., & Hardin, M. A. (1992). Phonetic and phonologic skills of two-year-olds with cleft palate. *Cleft Palate-Craniofacial Journal, 29* 435–443.

Curtis J. (1968). Acoustics of speech production and nasalization. In C. Spriesterback & D. Sheman (Eds)., *Cleft palate and communication* (pp. 27–60). New York, NY: Academic Press.

Dalston, R. M., Martinkosky, S. J., & Hinton, V. A. (1987). Stuttering prevalence among patients at risk for velopharyngeal inadequacy: A preliminary investigation. *Cleft Palate Journal, 24*(3), 233–239.

D'Antonio, L., Muntz, H., Providence, M., & Marsh, J. (1988). Laryngeal/voice findings in patients with velopharyngeal dysfunction. *Laryngoscope, 98*, 432–438.

Dickson, D. R. (1962). An acoustic study of nasality. *Journal of Speech and Hearing Research, 5*, 103–111.

Dickson, D. R., & Maue-Dickson, W. (1982). *Anatomical and physiological bases of speech.* Boston, MA: Little, Brown and Company.

Dotevall, H., Ejnell, H., & Bake, B. (2001). Nasal airflow patterns during the velopharyngeal closing phase in speech in children with and without cleft palate. *Cleft Palate-Craniofacial Journal, 38*(4), 358–373.

Dwyer, C. H., Robb, M. P., O'Beirne, G. A., & Gilbert, H. R. (2009). The influence of speaking rate on nasality in the speech of hearing-impaired individuals. *Journal of Speech Language and Hearing Research, 52*(5), 1321–1333.

Eshghi, M., Zajac, D. J., Bijankhan, M., & Shirazi, M. (2013). Spectral analysis of word-initial alveolar and velar plosives produced by Iranian children with cleft lip and palate. *Clinical Linguistics and Phonetics, 27*(3), 213–219.

Fletcher, S. G. (1978). *Diagnosing speech disorders from cleft palate.* New York, NY: Grune & Stratton.

Fletcher, S. G. (1992). *Articulation: A physiological approach.* San Diego, CA: Singular.

Forner, L. (1980). Speech segment durations produced by five and six year old speakers with and without cleft palates. *Cleft Palate Journal, 20*, 185–198.

Gibbon, F. E., Ellis, L., & Crampin, L. (2004). Articulatory placement for /t/, /d/, /k/ and /g/ targets in school age children with speech disorders associated with cleft palate. *Clinical Linguistics and Phonetics, 186*(8), 391–404.

Gildersleeve-Neumann, C. E., & Dalston, R. M. (2001). Nasalance scores in noncleft individuals: Why not zero? *Cleft Palate-Craniofacial Journal, 38*(2), 106–111.

Golding-Kushner, K. J. (1995). Treatment of articulation and resonance disorders associated with cleft palate and VPI. In R. J. Shprintzen, & J. Bardach (Eds.), *Cleft palate speech management: A multidisciplinary approach.* St. Louis, MO: Mosby.

Hamlet, S. (1973). Vocal compensation: An ultrasonic study of vocal vibration in normal and nasal vowels. *Cleft Palate Journal, 10*, 267–285.

Hardin-Jones, M. A., & Chapman, K. L. (2015). *The significance of nasal substitutions in the early phonology of toddlers with repaired cleft palate.* Poster presented at the Annual Meeting of the American Cleft Palate-Craniofacial Association, Palm Springs, CA.

Harding, A., & Grunwell, P. (1998). Active versus passive cleft-type speech characteristics. *International Journal of Language and Communication Disorders, 33*(3), 329–352.

Henningsson, G. E., & Isberg, A. M. (1986). Velopharyngeal movement patterns in patients alternating between oral and glottal articulation: A clinical and cineradiographical study. *Cleft Palate Journal, 23*(1), 1–9.

Hess, D. A. (1959). Pitch, intensity and cleft palate voice quality. *Journal of Speech and Hearing Research, 2*, 113–125.

Hixon, T. J., Weismer, G., & Hoit, J, D. (2008). *Preclinical speech science: Anatomy physiology acoustics perception.* San Diego, CA: Plural.

Hodge, M., & Gotzke, C. L. (2007). Preliminary results of an intelligibility measure for English-speaking children with cleft palate. *Cleft Palate-Craniofacial Journal, 44,* 163–174.

House, A. S., & Stevens, K. N. (1956). Analog studies of the nasalization of vowels. *Journal of Speech and Hearing Disorders, 21,* 218–232.

Jones, D. L., Folkins, J. W., & Morris, H. L. (1990). Speech production time and judgments of disordered nasalization in speakers with cleft palate. *Journal of Speech and Hearing Research, 33*(3), 458–466.

Kent, R. D., Weismer, G., Kent, J. F., & Rosenbek, J. C. (1989). Toward phonetic intelligibility testing in dysarthria. *Journal of Speech and Hearing Disorders, 54,* 482–499.

Kummer, A. W. (2014). *Cleft palate and craniofacial anomalies: Effects on speech and resonance* (3rd ed.). Clifton Park, NY: Cengage Learning.

Kummer, A. W., Briggs, M., & Lee, L. (2003). The relationship between the characteristics of speech and velopharyngeal gap size. *Cleft Palate-Craniofacial Journal, 40,* 590–596.

Kummer, A. W., Curtis, C., Wiggs, M., Lee, L., & Strife, J. L. L. (1992). Comparison of velopharyngeal gap size in patients with hypernasality, hypernasality and audible nasal emission, or nasal turbulence (rustle) as the primary speech characteristic. *Cleft Palate Journal, 29,* 152–156.

Lach, R., Ling, D., Ling, A. H., & Ship, N. (1970). Early speech development in deaf infants. *American Annals of the Deaf, 115*(5), 522–526.

Lee, A., Gibbon, F. E., & Oebels, J. (2015). Lateral bracing of the tongue during the onset phase of alveolar stops: An EPG study. *Clinical Linguistics and Phonetics, 29*(3), 236–245.

Lintz, L. B., & Sherman, D. (1961). Phonetic elements and perception of nasality. *Journal of Speech and Hearing Research, 4,* 381–396.

Mandulak, K. C., & Zajac, D. J. (2009). Effects of altered fundamental frequency on nasalance during vowel production by adult speakers at targeted sound pressure levels. *Cleft Palate-Craniofacial Journal, 46,* 39–46.

Marks, C., Barker, K., & Tardy, M. (1971). Prevalence of perceived acoustic deviations related to laryngeal function among subjects with palatal anomalies. *Cleft Palate Journal, 8,* 201–210.

McWilliams, B. J., Bluestone, C., & Musgrave, R. (1969). Diagnostic implications of vocal cord nodules in children with cleft palate. *Laryngoscope, 79,* 2072–2080.

McWilliams, B. J., Morris, H. L., & Shelton, R. (1990). *Cleft palate speech* (2nd ed.). St. Louis, MO: Mosby.

Moll, K. L. (1960). Cinefluorographic techniques in speech research. *Journal of Speech and Hearing Research, 3,* 227–241.

Moll, K. L., & Shriner, T. (1967). Preliminary investigation of a new concept of velar activity during speech. *Cleft Palate Journal, 4,* 58–69.

Nopoulos, P., Berg, S., Canady, J., Richman, L., Van Demark, D., & Andreasen, N. C. (2000). Abnormal brain morphology in patients with isolated cleft lip, cleft palate, or both: A preliminary analysis. *Cleft Palate-Craniofacial Journal, 37,* 441–446.

Okazaki, K., Kato, M., & Onizuka, T. (1991). Palate morphology in children with cleft palate with palatalized articulation. *Annals of Plastic Surgery, 26,* 156–163.

Peterson, S. J. (1975). Nasal emission as a component of the misarticulation of sibilants and affricates. *Journal of Speech and Hearing Disorders, 40*(1), 106–114.

Peterson-Falzone, S. J. (1990). A cross-sectional analysis of speech results following palatal closure. In J. Bardach & H. L. Morris (Eds.), *Multidisciplinary management of cleft lip and palate.* Philadelphia, PA: W.B. Saunders.

Peterson-Falzone, S. J., & Graham, M. S. (1990). Phoneme-specific nasal emission in children with and without physical anomalies of the velopharyngeal mechanism. *Journal of Speech and Hearing Disorders, 55*(1), 132–139.

Peterson-Falzone, S. J., Hardin-Jones, M. A., & Karnell, M. P. (2001). *Cleft palate speech* (3rd ed.). St. Louis, MO: Mosby.

Peterson-Falzone, S. J., Hardin-Jones, M. A., & Karnell, M. P. (2010). *Cleft palate speech* (4th ed.). St. Louis, MO: Mosby.

Peterson-Falzone, S. J., Trost-Cardamone, J. E., Karnell, M. P., & Hardin-Jones, M. A. (2006). *The clinician's guide to treating cleft palate speech.* St Louis, MO: Mosby Elsevier.

Prins, D., & Bloomer, H. (1965). A word intelligibility approach to the study of speech change in oral cleft patients. *Cleft Palate Journal, 2,* 357–368.

Prins, D., & Bloomer, H. (1968). Consonant intelligibility: A procedure for evaluating speech in oral cleft subjects. *Journal of Speech and Hearing Research, 11,* 128–137.

Proctor, D. F. (1982). The upper airway. In D. F. Proctor & I. B. Anderson (Eds.), *The nose: Upper airway physiology and the atmospheric environment.* New York, NY: Elsevier Biomedical Press.

Richman, L. C. (1980). Cognitive patterns and learning disabilities in cleft palate children with verbal deficits. *Journal of Speech and Hearing Research, 23,* 447–456.

Richman, L. C., & Eliason, M. (1984). Type of reading disability related to cleft type and neuropsychological patterns. *Cleft Palate Journal, 21,* 1–6.

Santelmann, L., Sussman, J., & Chapman, K. (1999). Perception of middorsum palatal stops from the speech of three children with repaired cleft palate. *Cleft Palate-Craniofacial Journal, 36,* 233–241.

Schwartz, M. F. (1968). Acoustics of normal and nasal vowel production. *Cleft Palate Journal, 5,* 125–138.

Searl, J., & Knollhoff, S. (2013). Oral pressure and nasal flow on /m/ and /p/ in 3- to 5-year-old children without cleft palate. *Cleft Palate Craniofacial Journal, 50,* 40–50.

Sell, D., Harding, A., & Grunwell, P. (1999). GOS.SP.ASS.'98: An assessment for speech disorders associated with cleft palate and/or velopharyngeal dysfunction (Revised). *International Journal of Language and Communication Disorders, 34*(1), 17–33.

Smith, C. R. (1975). Interjected sounds in deaf children's speech. *Journal of Communication Disorders, 8*(2), 123–128.

Spriestersbach, D. C., & Powers, G. R. (1959). Nasality in isolated vowels and connected speech of cleft palate speakers. *Journal of Speech and Hearing Research, 2*(1), 40–45.

Starkweather, C. W. (1997). Therapy for younger children. In R. F. Curlee & G. M. Siegel (Eds.), *Nature and treatment of stuttering: New directions* (2nd ed.). Boston, MA: Allyn & Bacon.

Stoel-Gammon, C. (1982). The acquisition of segmental phonology by normal and hearing-impaired children. In I. Hochberg, H. Levitt, & M. Osberger (Eds.), *Speech and the hearing impaired: Research, training, and personnel preparation.* Baltimore, MD: University Park Press.

Trost, J. E. (1981). Articulatory additions to the classical description of the speech of persons with cleft palate. *Cleft Palate Journal, 18,* 193–203.

Vallino, L. D., Peterson-Falzone, S. J., & Napoli, J. A. (2006). The syndromes of Treacher Collins and Nager. *Advances in Speech-Language Pathology, 8,* 34–44.

Vallino, L. D., & Thompson, B. (1993). Perceptual characteristics of consonant errors associated with malocclusion. *Journal of Oral and Maxillofacial Surgery, 51*(8), 850–856.

Vorperian, H.K., Wang, S., Chung, M.K., Schimek, E.M., Durtschi, R.B., Kent, R.D., . . . Gentry, L. R. (2009). Anatomic development of the oral and pharyngeal portions of the vocal tract: An imaging study. *Journal of the Acoustical Society of America, 125*(3), 1666–1678.

Warren, D. W. (1986). Compensatory speech behaviors in individuals with cleft palate: A regulation/control phenomenon? *Cleft Palate Journal, 23,* 251–260.

Whitehill, T. L., & Chau, C. H. (2004). Single-word intelligibility in speakers with repaired cleft palate. *Clinical Linguistics & Phonetics, 18*(4–5), 341–355.

Young, M. A. (1975). Onset, prevalence, and recovery from stuttering. *Journal of Speech and Hearing Disorders, 40,* 49–58.

Zajac, D. J. (2000). Pressure-flow characteristics of /m/ and /p/ production in speakers without cleft palate: Developmental findings. *Cleft Palate-Craniofacial Journal, 37,* 468–477.

Zajac, D. J. (2003). *Pressure-flow characteristics of speakers with repaired cleft palate.* Paper presented at the Annual Meeting of the American Cleft Palate-Craniofacial Association, Asheville, NC.

Zajac, D. J. (2015a). The nature of nasal fricatives: Articulatory-perceptual characteristics and etiologic considerations. *SIG 5 Perspectives on Speech Science and Orofacial Disorders, 25,* 17–28.

Zajac, D. J. (2015b). Velopharyngeal function in speech production: Some developmental and structural considerations. In M. A. Redford (Ed.), *Handbook of speech production* (pp. 109–130). Malden, MA: Blackwell.

Zajac, D. J., Cevidanes, L., Shah, S., & Haley, K. (2012). Maxillary arch dimensions and spectral characteristics of children with cleft lip and palate who produce middorsum palatal stops. *Journal of Speech, Language, and Hearing Research, 55,* 1876–1886.

Zajac, D. J., Mayo, R., Kataoka, R., & Kuo, J. (1996). Aerodynamic and acoustic characteristics of a speaker with turbulent nasal emission: A case report. *Cleft Palate-Craniofacial Journal, 33,* 440–444.

Zajac, D. J., & Milholland, S. (2014). Abrupt laryngeal engagement during stop plosive-vowel transitions in children with repaired cleft palate and adequate velopharyngeal closure: Aerodynamic and sound pressure level evidence. *Cleft Palate-Craniofacial Journal, 51,* 98–104.

Zajac, D. J., Plante, C., Lloyd, A., & Haley, K. (2011). Reliability and validity of a computer mediated single-word intelligibility test: Preliminary findings for children with repaired cleft lip and palate. *Cleft Palate-Craniofacial Journal, 48,* 538–549.

Zajac, D. J., & Preisser, J. (2015). Influence of age and phonetic context on velar flutter as a component of nasal turbulence in children with repaired cleft palate. *Cleft Palate-Craniofacial Journal.* Advance onine publication.

Zajac, D. J., Preisser, J., Drake, A., Eshghi, M., McGee, J., Vivaldi, D., & Feldbaum, M. (2015, April). *Longitudinal analysis of hypernasality in school-aged children with repaired cleft palate.* Paper presented at the Annual Meeting of the American Cleft Palate-Craniofacial Association, Palm Springs, CA.

9

Assessment of Speech and Velopharyngeal Function

INTRODUCTION

The primary goal of the speech-language pathologist (SLP) in assessing the school-aged child with repaired cleft palate is to determine the adequacy of velopharyngeal function for speech production. Perceptual assessment is the gold standard to achieve this goal. Perceptual findings determine the need for and type of subsequent instrumental assessment. Instrumental assessments are vital not only to confirm a diagnosis but also to monitor velopharyngeal function over time, especially during the rapid growth period of puberty, and provide postmanagement data to objectively evaluate outcomes. In the case of imaging studies, information is also provided to help guide the type of surgical or prosthetic intervention (see Chapter 11). The purpose of this chapter is to describe some common perceptual and instrumental procedures to assess speech characteristics and velopharyngeal function of the school-aged child with or without repaired cleft palate.

A PROTOCOL TO GUIDE CLINICAL ASSESSMENT

Figure 9–1 presents a protocol to guide perceptual and instrumental evaluation of the school-aged child (also applicable to older patients). The case history is often a neglected but essential component of the diagnostic process. The SLP must know the history of the child, especially past and current surgical and behavioral interventions, to effectively plan the evaluation. An oral examination is also essential to confirm previous surgeries and determine current structural function. The heart of the diagnostic process is perceptual assessment of speech characteristics. Based on perceptual findings, the SLP makes a preliminary diagnosis of velopharyngeal status. If velopharyngeal function is adequate, recommendations are made regarding any atypical findings that are not related to palatal function (e.g., phonological disorders, language delay). If velopharyngeal function is questionable or inadequate, then referral

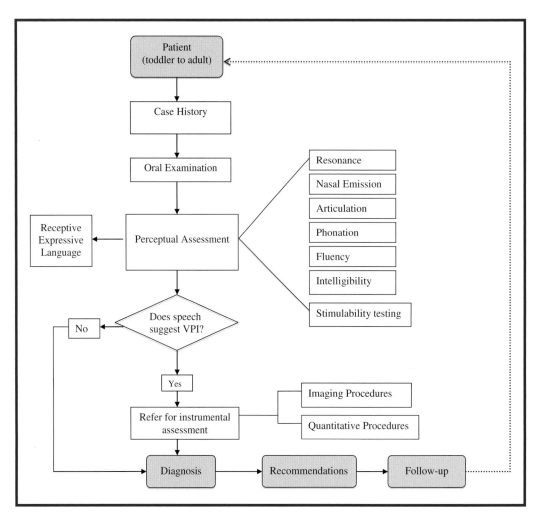

Figure 9–1. Protocol for clinical assessment of patients. Republished with permission of American Speech-Language-Hearing Association, from Assessing Communication in Cleft and Craniofacial Disorders: A Process Model for the Practitioner, Linda Vallino-Napoli, Vol. 11, December 2004; permission conveyed through Copyright Clearance Center, Inc.

for appropriate instrumental assessment occurs. A child should be referred for some types of instrumental assessments even if velopharyngeal function is judged adequate by perceptual means. It is our philosophy that noninvasive procedures such as pressure flow should be done routinely beginning at 5 or 6 years of age when most children become cooperative. It is important to obtain baseline information on physiologic parameters that change with age, such as oral air pressure during consonant production and resistance of the nasal airway during quiet breathing. In addition, Mason and Warren (1980) have shown that aerodynamic estimates of velopharyngeal gap size during speech—along with lateral radiographic information on adenoid size—can identify children who are at risk for the development of hypernasality well before they exhibit perceptual symptoms.

A form to document outcomes of the clinical evaluation appears in Appendix 9–A. This form, developed at the Craniofacial Center of the University of North Carolina at Chapel Hill, covers all components of the assessment protocol shown in Figure 9–1 except for instrumental imaging studies, which may be done at times other than the perceptual evaluation. The form can be modified, however, to better fit the needs of particular clinicians and clinics.

Case History

Obtaining a case history is essential to understanding past treatments, current conditions, and to guide the evaluation. Case history information should include (a) ages that lip and palate surgeries were done and type of surgery (e.g., two-flap palatoplasty or double-opposing Z-plasty), (b) ages and number of myringotomies and ventilation tubes, (c) number and type of secondary palatal procedures (e.g., pharyngeal flap, sphincter pharyngoplasty, posterior pharyngeal wall augmentation—see Chapter 11), and (d) the type and duration of previous and current intervention services. If a child is new to the SLP or team, such information should be obtained prior to the evaluation.

The importance of obtaining complete case history information cannot be overemphasized. Because of the multiple dental-surgical procedures that a child may undergo at varying chronological ages, the SLP must be aware of all procedures that could potentially impact the evaluation. An example is a school-age child who previously had a pharyngeal flap procedure. A pharyngeal flap may not be visible on oral examination. If the SLP or team is not aware of this history, then they may be puzzled by speech symptoms such as hyponasality and may even refer the child for unneeded diagnostic procedures.

Oral Examination

The oral examination is an essential element of the total speech assessment. Specific to the child with a cleft lip/palate and craniofacial condition, the goal is to examine for structural abnormalities that may have an adverse affect on speech function. The examination has three components: (a) preparing the child for the examination, (b) assessing oral structures, and (c) assessing function as it relates to structure. The components are summarized here and shown in Appendix 9–B.

Preparing the Child

A careful examination of the oral cavity should be done using a tongue depressor, flashlight, procedure mask, and nonlatex gloves. Because the sight of a mask, gloves, or tongue depressor might alarm a young child, it is helpful if the SLP asks the caregiver about the child's past reactions to such examinations and offers a simple reassurance to the child that the SLP is only looking into the mouth. Allowing the child to first watch the SLP examine a parent's mouth or the mouth of a puppet or stuffed animal can sometimes reassure a hesitant child.

Examining Structure

The structures to be examined include the nose, lips, teeth, occlusion, and palate. The size of the tonsils should be noted. Missing or extra teeth, dental occlusal defects (i.e., crossbite), and type of malocclusion should be documented. Examination of the palate should note the presence and approximate size of any oronasal fistula (ONF). The upper lip should be lifted with the tongue depressor to check for ONFs that extend into the nasal cavity. Although labial (or buccal) ONFs may be symptomatic for nasal reflux of liquids and soft foods, they typically are not symptomatic for nasal air emission during speech.

Examining Function

Functional adequacy of the lips, tongue, jaw, and soft palate should be assessed in both speech and nonspeech tasks. Extent and symmetry of velar movement during phonation and formation of a Passavant's pad, if visible, should be noted (see Figure 9–25 later in the chapter). Although no one likes to be gagged, the SLP should attempt to elicit a gag reflex, especially in cases of known or suspected motor dysfunction.

Clinicians who work on a craniofacial team may benefit from the expertise of other team members regarding confirmation of oral findings. Clinicians should be aware, however, that these are subjective judgments that typically vary among specialists. It is not uncommon, for example, to hear widely varying descriptions of the length and mobility of a child's soft palate at craniofacial team meetings.

Perceptual Assessments

Resonance

Because resonance is an acoustic-perceptual phenomenon, clinical assessment primarily involves perceptual judgments. Graduate students in speech-language pathology often express concern relative to identifying the type of resonance that they hear—normal, hypernasal, hyponasal, mixed hyper-/hyponasal, or cul-de-sac—let alone assigning a level of severity to a specific type. To be sure, this can be a formidable task. As indicated in the previous chapter, numerous factors can affect per-

ceived nasality. Because of this, perceptual assessment should begin by engaging the child in conversational speech. By eliciting conversational speech, phonetic variability relative to vowel type and nasal consonants will be mostly controlled, and the SLP can make a global judgment of the predominate type and severity of resonance. Although factors such as loudness, pitch, and speaking rate may vary during conversation, the effects of these parameters can be noted and further evaluated in additional speaking tasks such as counting, repeating sentences, and prolonging vowels (Table 9–1). Obviously, eliciting conversational speech may be difficult with some young school-aged children. We have found that tasks such as counting from "one" to "ten" are often successful with children as young as 3 years of age. Imitation of short phrases such as "puppy dog," "teddy bear," and "kitty cat" is also successful with young children relative to eliciting connected, conversational-like speech. For older children, counting from 80 to 90 and from 90 to 100 may facilitate evaluation of hypernasality and hyponasality, respectively. Older children are also more likely to repeat sentences and prolong vowels that can help evaluate resonance. Vowels should target high and low tongue placement to evaluate consistency and severity of hypernasality. If a child is excessively loud or soft or excessively fast or slow during conversational or elicited speech samples, then the SLP can attempt to modify these parameters as part of stimulability testing to assess any change in resonance. Table 9–1 summarizes the rationale and protocol for perceptual evaluation of resonance with school-aged children.

The "cul-de-sac" test may be helpful to evaluate hypernasality (Bzoch, 1979). The test consists of 10 simple words begin-

Table 9–1. Evaluation Rationale and Protocol for Resonance

Parameter of Speech	Rationale for Evaluation	Protocol
Resonance	To determine presence of a resonance disorder	Listen for hypernasality, hyponasality, or mixed resonance using:
	To identify type of resonance disorder—hypernasal, hyponasal, mixed	Conversational speech Counting from 1 to 10, 60 to 70, 80 to 90 Counting from 90 to 100 (listen for hyponasality)

	To determine the degree of severity of the resonance disorder	Sentence elicitation:
		  Put the baby in the buggy.
		  Kindly give Kate the cake.

	To determine consistency of resonance disorder and the phonetic contexts within which the resonance disorder is perceived	Sissy sees the sun in the sky. Joe and Charlie chew food. The ship goes in shallow water. Mama made lemon jam. (listen for hyponasality)
		Prolonged vowels: /i/ /u/ /a/
		Rate resonance using rating scales
		Use cul-de-sac test to alternately open and close the nostrils to determine if there is a difference in resonance

ning with /b/ that do not contain nasal consonants. The child is asked to repeat a word normally followed by repeating the word with the nostrils occluded. The clinician listens for a change in resonance when the nostrils are occluded. If a perceptible change occurs (i.e., less nasality with nostrils occluded), then it is assumed that velopharyngeal inadequacy (VPI) is present to some extent. Bzoch recommended that the percentage of words scored as hypernasal be used as a severity index and to document change with treatment. The cul-de-sac procedure can also be done by having the child prolong vowels, especially high vowels, and not-

ing if a change in resonance occurs when the nostrils are occluded.

Perceptual Rating Scales

Commonly, clinicians use either relatively simple descriptive terms (e.g., normal, mild, moderate, severe) or ordinal or interval scales to rate and document resonance in children (Kuehn & Moller, 2000). Equal-appearing interval (EAI) scales may consist of as few as three to four intervals to as many as seven to nine intervals. A critical assumption of all EAI scales is that the perceptual distance between scale points is the same across the scale.

This means that an increase from scale point 1 to 2 represents the same increase as from scale point 6 to 7 on a 7-point scale. As discussed later, however, this assumption may not be valid when rating hypernasality.

Several perceptual rating scales have been described to assess hypernasality. Lohmander, Willadsen, Persson, Henningsson, Bowden, and Hutters (2009) used a 5-point ordinal scale in a pilot study assessing surgical outcomes of 50 children with repaired cleft palate across five languages—Danish, English, Finnish, Norwegian, and Swedish. A clinician of each language rated hypernasality in connected speech using the following ordinal scores and descriptors: 0 = absent, 1 = slight/minimal, 2 = mild (evident on high vowels), 3 = moderate (evident on high and low vowels), 4 = severe (evident on vowels and voiced consonants). Lohmander et al. reported high intraobserver agreement among the five speech clinicians with four having exact repeat ratings and one falling within one scale point. No interobserver reliability was reported in this pilot study.

Henningsson and colleagues (2008) described a 4-point EAI scale to rate hypernasality as part of a universal reporting protocol to document speech outcomes across centers. The scale, similar to the one used by Lohmander et al. (2009), consisted of four scores and descriptors: 0 = within normal limits, 1 = mild, 2 = moderate, and 3 = severe. Hypernasality was assessed separately for single words and sentences, selected to contain high and low vowels. These stimuli, rather than conversation, were used to control phonetic variability across different languages.

Kuehn et al. (2002) developed an 8-point EAI scale to rate hypernasality as part of a study investigating the effects of continuous positive airway pres-

sure (CPAP) therapy (see Chapter 11). Scale point 1 represented resonance that was "normal"; scale point 8 represented "extremely severe" hypernasality. The investigators developed three sets of reference samples for this scale using recordings obtained from children, men, and women. The reference samples were selected "so that the differences in perceived nasality between adjacent sample pairs within the set were similar, thus producing an equal-appearing interval scale" (p. 270). As part of the study's procedures, experienced SLPs were trained to rate hypernasality using the three sets of reference samples. Following training, they blindly rated audio samples obtained from the participants before and after CPAP therapy. For each participant, the SLPs made successive pair-wise comparisons to an appropriate reference sample (children, men, or women) beginning with the normal sample until a final scale rating was achieved. That is, ratings were continued until the participant was perceived to be greater in nasality than a given reference sample but less than the next reference sample. The final rating was assigned as the lesser of the two consecutive reference scale points.

The three sets of reference samples developed by Kuehn et al. (2002) are available on the American Cleft Palate-Craniofacial Association website. In clinical practice, an SLP could use the reference samples in the same fashion as Kuehn et al. by making pair-wise comparisons of a recorded patient and the reference samples. Or, an SLP could simply use the reference samples for training and calibration. As discussed next, however, hypernasality is a perceptual dimension that may not be amendable to EAI scaling procedures.

Validity of Perceptual Rating Scales. Although Kuehn et al. (2002) attempted to select reference samples that conformed to a true EAI scale, this may be difficult, if not impossible, due to the nature of hypernasality as a psychophysical construct. Investigations have shown that hypernasality is a *prothetic* dimension (Whitehill, Lee, & Chun, 2002; Zraick & Liss, 2000). A prothetic dimension varies according to quantity or magnitude and is considered additive (Stevens, 1975). *Metathetic* dimensions, on the other hand, vary according to quality and are considered substitutive. Stevens (1975) cites pitch as an example of a metathetic dimension in that as pitch changes, listeners perceive a change in quality rather than magnitude. Stevens (1974) has shown that metathetic dimensions can be judged using EAI scales because listeners can perceptually divide the continuum into equal intervals. Such is not the case for prothetic dimensions. That is, listeners tend to subdivide the lower end of a prothetic dimension into smaller subunits relative to the upper end (Stevens, 1974). This results in a continuum that is not equal and violates the assumption of an EAI scale.

Zraick and Liss (2000) and Whitehill et al. (2002) demonstrated that hypernasality is a prothetic dimension, not amendable to scaling by EAI methods. They had listeners make judgments of hypernasality using both EAI and direct magnitude estimation (DME) methods. In DME procedures, listeners judge hypernasality of a sample by either comparing it to a reference sample assigned some arbitrary value (called a modulus) or to each subsequent sample (a modulus-free condition). In a modulus condition, listeners are instructed to judge the sample relative to the modulus on a ratio scale. That is, if the modulus is assigned an arbitrary value of 100, then the listener would assign a value of 200 to the sample if he or she judged it to be twice as nasal as the

modulus. Conversely, the listener would assign a value of 50 if he or she judged it to be half as nasal as the modulus. Because DME ratings are typically expressed using geometric rather than arithmetic means, listeners are instructed not to assign either a zero or negative value to a sample. Both Zraick and Liss (2000) and Whitehill et al. (2002) reported a curvilinear relationship when EAI and DME ratings were plotted against each other (Figure 9–2). This means that listeners could not assign hypernasality to equal-appearing intervals and that hypernasality was a prothetic dimension.

Figure 9–2 shows a curvilinear relationship between EAI and DME scales for hypernasality. The listeners were graduate students in a craniofacial course at the University of North Carolina at Chapel Hill. They were instructed on DME procedures, and the fourth reference sample of children from Kuehn et al. (2002) was used as a modulus and assigned a value of 100. The students then judged the nasality of reference samples 1, 2, 3, 5, 6, and 7 from Kuehn et al. in a quasi-random order. The students were not told that the modulus or the six speech samples were taken from Kuehn et al. and represented an EAI scale. The DME values plotted in Figure 9–2 are geometric means of the class. As shown in the figure, there is a curvilinear relationship between DME and EAI values. Although there is fair correspondence between the two scaling methods at the lower end of the EAI scale (intervals 1–3), the relationship becomes nonlinear at the higher end of the scale (intervals 5–7). This classroom exercise has been conducted for over 8 years by one of the authors (DJZ). Every class has demonstrated similar results as shown in Figure 9–2, consistent with the psychophysical principle that a prothetic dimension such as hypernasality cannot be evenly divided along a continuum.

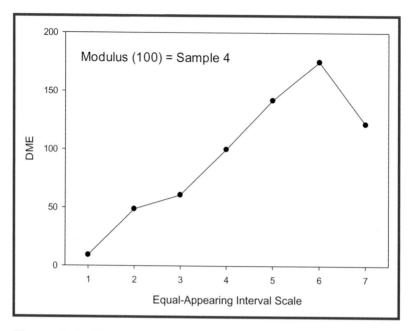

Figure 9–2. Plot showing nonlinear relationship between direct magnitude estimation (DME) and equal-appearing interval ratings of hypernasality for reference samples provided by Kuehn et al. (2002).

Zraick and Liss (2000) recommended that researchers use DME procedures to overcome the psychophysical scaling problems for hypernasality. They noted that DME does not assume a linear continuum, and listeners are not constrained to using fixed minimum and maximum end points. DME procedures, however, are typically not used clinically due to complexity and time constraints. A similar scaling method, called visual analog scaling (VAS), was recently recommended by Baylis, Chapman, Whitehill, et al. (2014). In VAS, a listener simply marks a point along a line, usually 100 mm in length, to reflect his or her judgment of perceived nasality. The hypernasality score is the measured distance from the beginning of the line to the marked point. VAS is similar to DME in that discrete equal-appearing intervals are not used. Baylis et al. reported that VAS of hypernasality was a

reliable procedure and relatively easy to use in the clinical setting.

Nasal Air Emission

Perceptual assessment of nasal air emission should also begin by eliciting conversational speech. The SLP should make a global assessment of the type—audible, turbulent, or both—and frequency of nasal air emission. As noted in Chapter 8, some children may grimace the nose if nasal air emission is present. The SLP should not only note the occurrence of nasal grimacing but also attempt to determine if it occurs across all obstruent consonants or is limited to fricatives, as grimacing is sometimes associated with production of active nasal fricatives.

Following conversational assessment, the SLP should elicit consonant-vowel

(CV) syllables and sentences loaded with obstruent consonants to further probe for nasal air emission. Syllables incorporating voiceless stops and fricatives should be elicited using both high and low vowels (e.g., /pi/, /pa/, /si/, /sa/). Sentences that contain stops, fricatives, and affricates should also be elicited. Table 9–2 lists some useful syllables and sentences. As in conversation, the clinician should note the occurrence of nasal air emission and grimacing.

Table 9–2. Evaluation Rationale and Protocol for Nasal Air Emission

Parameter of Speech	Rationale for Assessment	Protocol
Nasal air emission	To identify the appropriate presence or absence of nasal air emission occurring on nasal and non-nasal consonants To determine if nasal emission is visible or audible To determine appropriateness and sources of nasal emission on non-nasal consonants and nasal consonants	Listen for audible or turbulent nasal air emission and look for nasal grimacing: Conversational speech Repetition of CV syllables: /pi/, /pa/ /si/, /sa/ /ki/, /ka/* Sentence elicitation: Put the baby in the buggy. Kindly give Kate the cake. Sissy sees the sun in the sky. Joe and Charlie chew food. The ship goes in shallow water. Hold mirror under client's nose while he or she repeats CV syllables and sentences. Look for inappropriate mirror fogging. *Include /ki/ and /ka/ if anterior oronasal fistula is present. Include /mi/, /ma/, and "Momma made lemon jam" to assess appropriate nasal air emission. Document if nasal emission is present or absent. In most individuals without VPI, nasal emission should be absent on CV syllables and sentences loaded with non-nasal consonants and present on those with nasal consonants. If absent on nasal consonants, consider nasal blockage. If an oral nasal fistula is present and suspected as causative factor, obturate fistula and note any change in nasal emission.

After listening for nasal air emission, the SLP should have the child repeat syllables and sentences while looking for visible nasal air escape. We recommend that the SLP do this after listening, as we believe that a clinician may be more primed to hear very mild nasal air emission after seeing it. Evaluation of visible nasal air escape is easily done using a small dental mirror or detail reflector. We prefer a detail reflector as these are usually larger than a dental mirror and can detect nasal air emission from both nostrils simultaneously. The detail reflector is simply held beneath the nostrils of the child while he or she first exhales through the nose and then repeats syllables and sentences (Figure 9–3). Fogging on the detail reflector during exhalation indicates patency of the nostrils. Fogging during production of oral pressure consonants indicates visible nasal air escape as a result of incomplete velopharyngeal closure. The hard surface of the detail reflector may also amplify very mild audible nasal air escape that was not detected previously. If this occurs, the clinician should determine if audible nasal air emission is still perceptible when the reflector is removed. Either

a dental mirror or detail reflector is easily cleaned with alcohol or disinfectant wipes.

An oronasal fistula in the anterior hard palate may also cause fogging on a detail reflector (Figure 9–4). In some cases, the clinician may be able to confirm that an anterior oronasal fistula is the source of visible nasal air emission by eliciting the velar stop /k/. Because oral stopping of airflow during production of /k/ occurs posterior to the oronasal fistula, visible nasal air escape will be eliminated if velopharyngeal closure is complete. A clinician may also have the child attempt to occlude the fistula with chewing gum and repeat nasal emission testing. Table 9–2 summarizes the diagnostic protocol for the evaluation of nasal air emission.

Although use of a detail reflector (or mirror) is straightforward, the clinician must be alerted that nasal air emission may occur at the onset and offset of an utterance due to normal movement of the velum for respiration. To avoid misinterpreting these normal respiratory events, the clinician should bring the detail reflector to the nose after the child has started the speech sample and disregard the significance of any nasal air escape at the end

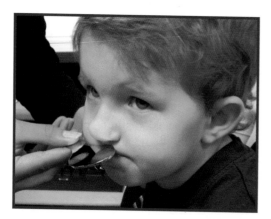

Figure 9–3. Detail reflector used to detect visible nasal air escape during speech and breathing.

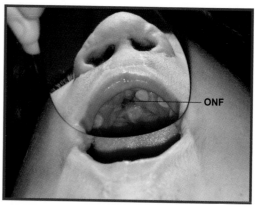

Figure 9–4. Teenager with repaired cleft lip and palate and anterior oronasal fistula (ONF).

of the utterance. The clinician should also ensure that the child uses a single breath to produce the speech sample. If the child speaks slowly and takes a new breath for each syllable or word, then multiple respiratory onsets and offsets may occur that are difficult to interpret.

Clinical Documentation. The occurrence of nasal air emission can be documented using simple checklists and obtaining frequency counts during elicitation of syllables, words, sentences, or conversation.

The presence or absence of nasal air emission via mirror testing can be recorded for each nostril using the clinical assessment form presented in Appendix 9–A. The occurrence of nasal grimacing or active nasal air emission associated with production of nasal fricatives can also be indicated on the form. McWilliams and Philips (1979) described a similar nasal emission checklist. That checklist, part of a larger evaluation protocol called The University of Pittsburgh Weighted Values for Speech Symptoms Associated with VPI, is used by some centers.

Nasal air emission can also be counted from either live assessment or audio recordings of a child. Diacritic symbols can be used to mark the occurrence of nasal air emission during standardized articulation testing. The nasometer can be used to record children during articulation testing and production of a speech sample consisting of CV syllables. The nasal audio signal can be examined to determine percentage of consonants produced with audible and turbulent nasal air emission. A protocol for this type of assessment is described later in the chapter.

Caveats Regarding Low-Tech Assessment of Nasal Air Emission. There are a number of devices that can be used to detect visible and audible nasal air emission. These include common objects such as mirrors, feathers, and strips of paper or tissue (sometimes called air paddles) held beneath the nose. There are also commercial devices such as the See-Scape (Figure 9–5) and various listening tubes to hear nasal air emission. Even though these low-tech devices are certainly useful to detect nasal air emission and screen velopharyngeal function, all have major limitations that prevent use as definitive diagnostic tools (Lass & Pannbacker, 2015).

First, these devices provide no information regarding size of the velopharyngeal port. Clinicians cannot assume that there is a direct correspondence between height of the See-Scape float or amount of fogging on a mirror and size of the velopharyngeal opening. Second, as indicated above, clinicians may misinterpret normal respiratory events as velopharyngeal dysfunction. Initiation of an utterance involves movement of the velum from rest to an elevated position. This period of movement can be associated with a burst of nasal airflow prior to the actual production of the utterance. Likewise, the offset of an utterance involves lowering of the velum in anticipation of nasal breathing and is also associated with expiratory nasal airflow. Moll (1960) reported that end-of-utterance velar lowering actually begins slightly before termination of voicing for some utterances. Thus, either onset or offset nasal airflow due to normal respiratory phenomena may be easily misidentified as inappropriate oral-nasal coupling when using low-tech devices.

Third, some speakers may exhibit nasal airflow during an utterance in the presence of airtight velopharyngeal closure due to *velar bounce* (see Figure 9–15 below). This is a slight up and down movement of the elevated soft palate against the posterior pharyngeal wall due

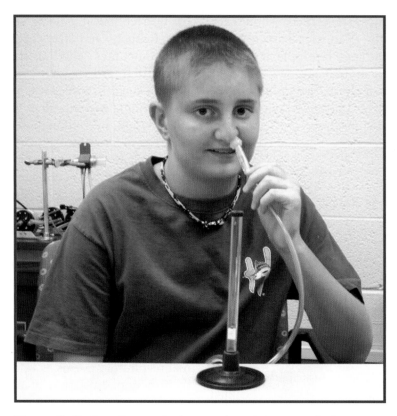

Figure 9–5. See-Scape device used to detect nasal air escape during speech and breathing.

to contractions of the levator muscle. The upward movement of the velum will displace the volume of air in the nasal cavity and cause slight fogging on a mirror or detail reflector. The downward movement of the velum will draw air into the nasal cavity. Because a mirror or detail reflector will detect only the outward nasal airflow, it may be misinterpreted as a velopharyngeal opening.

Finally, even when there is true oral-nasal coupling, all low-tech devices suffer from poor temporal resolution that makes identification of specific speech segments affected by nasal air emission difficult. As discussed later, pressure-flow instrumentation circumvents all of the above problems.

Articulation

Informal assessment of articulation should start as part of listening for hypernasality and nasal air emission. As reviewed in Chapter 10, a formal assessment of articulation should be done using any standardized articulation test. Most articulation tests require only two-way (correct, incorrect) or five-way (correct, omissions, additions, substitutions, distortions) scoring (see Shriberg and Kent, 2003), but the SLP may wish to use phonetic transcription and the International Phonetic Alphabet (IPA). Phonetic transcription promotes concise and accurate documentation of errors and may reveal patterns of unusual articulation, especially if diacritic symbols are used. Disadvantages of phonetic transcription, however, are that many SLPs are not well trained in transcription practices, and some articulations used by children with cleft palate are not easily transcribed using standard symbols and diacritics (e.g., active nasal fricatives).

Formal articulation assessment of the child should always be audio (if not video) recorded. With the low-cost and widespread availability of digital audio and video recording devices—even on smartphones—speech recordings should be standard practice (Figure 9–6). Audio recordings can be used to confirm live assessment decisions, facilitate training of graduate students, and, if archived, monitor changes in speech and articulation of the child over time and evaluate intervention outcomes.

As indicated in Chapter 8, perceptual identification of some maladaptive articulations can be difficult, even for experienced clinicians. Posterior and anterior nasal fricatives can sound identical to passive nasal air escape during production of oral fricatives. The relatively loud nasal turbulence of posterior nasal fricatives is likely to mask the low-intensity oral stop component and make perceptual identification difficult. If a child cannot produce /s/ when the nose is occluded, this may signal the presence of a nasal fricative as all airflow will be stopped due to the oral component. A more reliable technique, however, to differentiate active nasal fricatives from passive nasal air emission is the use of nasometric recordings. As described later in the chapter, this technique allows the SLP to acoustically identify the oral stopping component of an active nasal fricative. Finally, because mid-dorsum palatal stops are nonphonemic in English, auditory-perceptual identification is difficult. To facilitate identification, SLPs should carefully watch for a pattern of tongue-tip down and middle-of-the-tongue up during articulation of words targeting /t/ and /d/ in addition to listening.

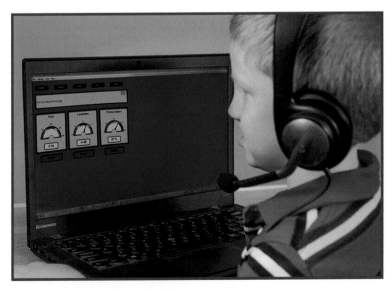

Figure 9–6. School-age child being audio recorded during perceptual speech evaluation.

Phonation

Vocal quality should be assessed during conversation, elicited sentences, counting from 80 to 85, and prolonged vowels. The SLP needs to make a global judgment of voice as normal, hyperfunctional, or hypofunctional (see Appendix 9–A). It should be noted if the child is habitually too soft or too loud. If the child is excessively soft spoken during the evaluation, the SLP should ask parents if this is typical of other situations. If excessively loud, the SLP should query parents regarding current status of middle ear function and ventilation tubes. The child's vocal quality should be recorded as breathy, harsh (or strained), hoarse, or aphonic. Hard glottal attacks should be noted. A child with moderate to severe vocal symptoms, especially in the absence of VPI, should be referred for an ear, nose, and throat (ENT) evaluation.

As indicated in Chapter 8, hoarseness and breathiness might make perceptual assessment of resonance difficult and may actually be a symptom of VPI. A child might use excessive loudness or abrupt laryngeal engagement (i.e., hard glottal attack) to compensate for marginal VPI. That is, to overcome reduced vocal intensity due to hypernasality, the child may speak more loudly, resulting in hoarseness. Conversely, a child might use hypofunctional behaviors such as reduced loudness or excessive breathiness to camouflage or mask symptoms of VPI. Asking the child to speak louder may uncover symptoms. The SLP, therefore, must be cognizant of different vocal strategies to compensate for and camouflage VPI.

Fluency

Stuttering does not occur often in children with repaired cleft palate (Dalston, Martinkosky, & Hinton, 1987). Nevertheless, the SLP should screen for stuttering. A potential problem is that onset of stuttering in young children tends to be episodic in nature. Therefore, even though a child may be an incipient stutterer, the SLP might not encounter evidence of it. If parents report stuttering but the child does not exhibit disfluencies during the evaluation, then the SLP should either schedule the child for a follow-up evaluation or refer to another SLP with expertise in fluency.

Conture (1997) states that the objectives of evaluation with the young child are to determine if the child is a stutterer, the severity of stuttering, and the risk for continued stuttering. Although most SLPs —indeed, even laypeople—can accomplish the first and second objectives, accomplishing the third may be beyond the expertise of most SLPs unless they have experience with stuttering. Conture cites the following indicators of childhood stuttering: (a) three or more within word disfluencies per 100 words of conversational speech, (b) 25% or more of total disfluencies that are sound prolongations, (c) speaking rate of the mother that averages two or more syllables per second faster than the child, (d) presence of any two-element disfluency clusters within a word, and (e) eyeball movements to the side or eyelid blinking during stuttering. According to Conture, these indicators are additive in that the greater number a child displays, the higher the risk for stuttering to continue.

Intelligibility

Yorkston and Beukelman (1978) state that intelligibility is the most important measure of a speech disorder. Undeniably, improved intelligibility is the implicit goal of all therapy interventions. Even so,

Kent, Weismer, Kent, and Rosenbek (1989) noted, "intelligibility assessment tends to be one of the most variable components in assessment protocols" (p. 483). Whitehill (2002) confirmed this observation regarding individuals with cleft palate. Whitehill reviewed 57 published articles between 1960 and 1998 and reported that intelligibility was assessed by various methods, including global judgments (15.8%), rating scales (47.4%), articulation test scores (8.8%), transcription tasks (14.0%), other means (5.3%), and unspecified (8.8%). In addition, Whitehill expressed concern that the majority of studies employed EAI scales that research has shown to be less valid measures of speech intelligibility. Schiavetti (1992), for example, demonstrated that intelligibility, like hypernasality, is a prothetic dimension.

SLPs will undoubtedly continue to use global judgements and rating scales to assess intelligibility, as these are relatively easy methods. The use of single-word intelligibility tests as described in Chapter 8, however, should be encouraged for several reasons. First, these tests use a common corpus of words and can be standardized regarding elicitation and recording procedures. Second, administration time is minimal. A single child, for example, can be recorded saying 50 words in less than 10 minutes. Likewise, a single listener can orthographically transcribe 50 words in a similar amount of time. Last, and most important, single-word tests are more valid measures of speech intelligibility than EAI scales. Some disadvantages of single-word tests are that initial test construction may be time-consuming, and listeners may become familiar with test words over time. Morris, Wilcox, and Schooling (1995), however, suggested that a single clinician could make reliable estimates of intelligibility, even of the same speaker over time, using randomly generated tests of 50 words. Ultimately, the use of automatic speech recognition systems may eliminate the need for human listeners entirely (e.g., Schuster et al., 2006).

Instrumental Assessment of Velopharyngeal Function

Velopharyngeal function can be assessed by direct and indirect instrumental procedures. Lubker and Moll (1965) state that direct methods provide actual observations of the articulatory structure. Common direct methods to assess velopharyngeal structure and function include radiographic imaging and fiberoptic nasoendoscopy. Indirect methods provide information on some effect or consequence of the articulatory structure, with function being inferred. Common indirect procedures involve acoustics and aerodynamics. There are many instrumental procedures to assess velopharyngeal function. The following discussion, therefore, is limited to those commonly used in a clinical setting.

Indirect Methods

Acoustics: Nasometry. The nasometer is an acoustic device that uses two microphones to detect nasal sound energy in relation to oral sound energy produced during speech. Fletcher (1970, 1976) originally developed the concept for the nasometer and called early models Tonar (The Oral-Nasal Acoustic Ratio). Currently, the nasometer is commercially available from Kay Pentax Corporation (Lincoln Park, New Jersey). It consists of two microphones separated by a metal plate that provides 25 dB sound separation. A head harness positions the sound barrier to rest on the upper lip beneath the nose (Figure 9–7). Newer versions of the nasometer provide a handheld option that eliminates

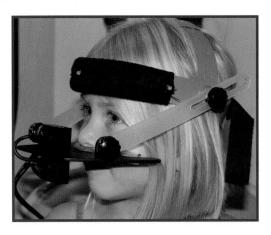

Figure 9–7. Head-mounted nasometer. Two microphones are used to detect oral and nasal sound energies during speech. Output of the nasometer is a measure called nasalance.

the need for a head harness. The outputs of each microphone are band-pass filtered at 350 to 650 Hz, are digitized to a computer, and percent nasalance is displayed during running speech and prolongation of vowels. Percent nasalance is calculated as nasal intensity divided by oral plus nasal intensity multiplied by 100.

For older children and adults, nasalance is determined during reading of passages devoid of nasal consonants (e.g., the "Zoo" passage) and sentences loaded with nasal consonants. Fletcher, Adams, and McCutcheon (1989) provided norms for several passages. They studied 117 children without cleft palate between 5 and 12 years of age. The children read the Zoo passage, the Rainbow passage (11% nasal consonants), and sentences containing 35% nasal consonants. Fletcher et al. reported that nasalance was 15.5% (±4.9) for the Zoo passage, 35.5% (±5.2) for the Rainbow passage, and 61.0% (±6.9) for nasal sentences.

Younger children can either repeat the above passages or repeat simple CV

syllables. MacKay and Kummer (1994) developed the Simplified Nasometric Assessment Procedures (SNAP) test for young children. The test consists of CV syllables that include voiceless stops and fricatives combined with high and low vowels. MacKay and Kummer provided nasalance norms for the SNAP test obtained from a group of children 3 to 9 years of age. Of interest, the SNAP test uses only voiceless consonants. This could be problematic if a child exhibits nasal turbulence with velar flutter. As illustrated in Figure 9–10 later in this chapter, velar flutter produces low-frequency, quasi-periodic noise that is readily detected by the nasometer. Because nasal turbulence and flutter are likely to occur during voiceless oral pressure consonants, the SNAP test may inflate nasalance scores for some children.

Numerous studies have reported nasalance data for speakers with cleft palate of various languages (see Baken & Orlikoff, 2000, for a review). These studies have shown that nasalance appears to be a fairly sensitive indicator of perceived hypernasality and hyponasality. Dalston, Warren, and Dalston (1991a), for example, reported that nasalance scores of 32% or greater during reading of the Zoo passage had a sensitivity of 0.89 and a specificity of 0.95 in identifying speakers with at least mild hypernasality. Vallino-Napoli and Montgomery (1997) reported similar findings for the Zoo passage. Sensitivity is the proportion of individuals who test positive for a condition, who actually have the condition; specificity is the proportion of individuals who test negative for a condition, who actually do not have the condition. In another study, Dalston, Warren, and Dalston (1991b) reported that nasalance scores of 50% or less during reading of sentences loaded with nasal consonants had a sensitivity of 0.48 and a specificity of 0.79 in identifying speakers with perceived hyponasality. The researchers noted that the relatively low sensitivity increased to 1 (perfect agreement) when speakers who exhibited audible nasal emission during voiceless consonants were omitted from analysis.

In addition to the nasometer, several similar devices are commercially available. One is the Nasalance Visualization System (NAS), available from Glottal Enterprises (Syracuse, New York). The NAS uses either a dual-chambered, circumferentially vented mask with microphones built into the handle (Figure 9–8) or a handheld separator plate with microphones to obtain nasalance. The NAS uses preset filters that calculate nasalance based on the fundamental frequency of the speaker—children, women, or men. Glottal Enterprises claim that this filtering method provides nasalance scores that are less influenced by vowel type than band-pass filtering at a frequency near the first formant, as done by the nasometer.

Plante, Zajac, Queiros, and Vallino (2011) provided support for the above claim. They obtained nasalance scores from 15 children with repaired cleft palate and varying degrees of hypernasality using both the nasometer and the mask model of the NAS during the same session. Plante et al. reported that mean nasalance obtained for /i/ by both devices was 35%. Mean nasalance for /a/ was 24% from the NAS and 13% from the nasometer. Plante et al. suggested that the reduced nasalance for /a/ from the nasometer was due to relatively low band-pass filtering that missed the higher first formant of the vowel. It must be noted that Plante et al. did not conduct perceptual evaluations of the children. It is not known, therefore, if differences between the two systems relative to /a/ are meaningful.

Advantages and Limitations. Acoustic nasometry is a relatively low-cost instrument that is easily tolerated by even young children. Normative data have been reported for several languages.

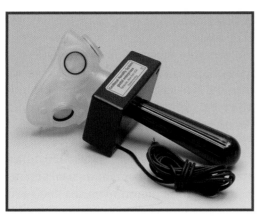 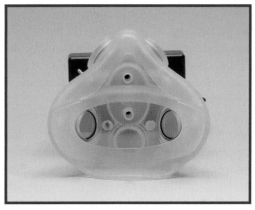

A   B

Figure 9–8. Nasalance Visualization System (NAS). NAS consists of a dual-chambered, circumferentially vented mask with microphones built into the handle. **A.** Side view showing mask, handle, and wiring. **B.** Front view showing dual-chambered mask and ports for microphones.

There are several limitations, however, that clinicians must be aware of when interpreting nasalance scores.

First, nasalance scores are not necessarily an index of actual oral-nasal coupling. Because the sound separation between the oral and nasal microphones is limited, a nasalance score of 0% will never occur during non-nasal sounds even though a speaker may achieve complete velopharyngeal closure (Gildersleeve-Neumann & Dalston, 2001). Sympathetic excitation of the nasal air mass also may occur as described in Chapter 8. This will further contribute to nonzero nasalance scores (Bundy & Zajac, 2006). There are also substantial vowel effects associated with nasalance scores—at least for the nasometer—that are not due to direct oral-nasal coupling. Gildersleeve-Neumann and Dalston (2001), for example, reported almost doubling of nasalance scores for /i/ versus /a/ in normal speakers. This occurs due to greater impedance of oral sound transmission for high versus low vowels (in addition to band-pass filtering as noted above). Clearly, because of limitations with the device and natural oral impedance differences of vowels, nasalance scores should be considered as correlates of perceived nasality, *not* direct oral-nasal coupling. In other words, it may be tenuous to accept nasalance scores as acoustic indicators of velopharyngeal dysfunction.

A second limitation of nasalance scores relates to possible differences across devices. Because the nasometer uses two microphones, there may be subtle mismatches in the sensitivities as a function of frequency response. Users of both the original Tonar and the current nasometer have been cautioned relative to this possibility (Weinberg, Noll, & Donohue, 1979; Zajac, Lutz, & Mayo, 1996, respectively). If mismatches in microphone sensitivity exist, then discrepancies in nasalance scores may occur as a function of different nasometers, and comparisons across centers may be problematic. Zajac et al. (1996) suggested that clinicians tolerate at least a range of plus or minus 7% when comparing a given nasalance score to published norms as differences may exist across different nasometers.

Nasometric Identification of Nasal Air Emission. Although the nasometer is intended to assess hypernasality, it can also be used to identify audible nasal air emission. As discussed in Chapter 8, nasal air emission occurs across a continuum from visible only to audible to turbulent. In addition, turbulent nasal air emission can be accompanied by tissue flutter occurring at the velopharyngeal port. Acoustic and spectral analyses are well suited to help the clinician distinguish different types of nasal air emission, especially flutter given the nature of its quasi-periodic vibration.

Zajac and Preisser (2015) described a nasometric recording protocol that can be used for clinical assessment of nasal air emission. The protocol involves using the headset and microphones of the nasometer, either models 6200 or 6450, to record the separate oral and nasal acoustic signals of a speaker. If model 6200 is used, then the oral and nasal outputs of the unit must be input into another multichannel recording device (e.g., Computerized Speech Lab, model 4500, Kay Pentax). The newer nasometer, model 6450, automatically saves the oral and nasal signals to an audio file, circumventing the need for an additional device. Clinicians who use model 6450, however, may want to change the default sampling rate from 11 kHz to either 22.05 or 44.1 kHz to capture higher frequencies associated with turbulent nasal air emission.

As part of the protocol, speakers produce eight CV syllables while recorded with the nasometer. The syllables are /pi/, /pʌ/, /fi/, /fʌ/, /ti/, /tʌ/, /si/, and /sʌ/ and are produced three times in the carrier phrase, "Say ___ ___ ___ again." Thus, each speaker produces 24 syllables that contrast bilabial plosives with labial fricatives in high-front and mid-low vowel contexts and alveolar plosives with alveolar fricatives in high-front and mid-low vowel contexts. Only voiceless consonants are used, as these are produced with greater oral air pressure than voiced consonants (Arkebauer, Hixon, & Hardy, 1967; Subtelny, Worth, & Sakuda, 1966). The order of the syllables is randomized, and speakers produce the eight syllables in the same randomized order.

TF32 software (Milenkovic, 2000) is used to perceptually and spectrally examine the recorded syllables for evidence of audible and turbulent nasal air emission. The software is configured to display both the oral and nasal acoustic waveforms and the spectrogram of the nasal waveform. Audible or turbulent nasal air emission is identified by using the cursors of TF32 to isolate each consonant segment in the oral waveform and listening to the audio from the nasal waveform. The spectrogram of the nasal signal is examined for evidence of either aperiodic noise (i.e., turbulence) or quasi-periodic flutter.

Figure 9–9 illustrates an example of obligatory audible nasal air emission identified by the above method. The speaker was a child with repaired cleft palate who said, "Say pea pea pea again." The three /pi/ syllables are labeled in the figure with vertical cursors indicating the stop gap and release burst of the second /p/ segment. As seen in the figure, the oral waveform shows a silent stop-gap, and the nasal waveform shows evidence of low-amplitude noise. Playback of the stop-gap segment from the nasal waveform reveals a frication-like noise. Inspection of the nasal spectrogram reveals diffuse aperiodic energy from approximately 5 to 12 kHz consistent with a frication or turbulent-like noise.

Conversely, Figure 9–10 illustrates an example of obligatory nasal turbulence with flutter. The speaker was also a child with repaired cleft palate who said, "Say pea pea pea again." As seen in the figure, there is evidence of noise on the nasal waveform during the stop gap of the first /p/ segment. Compared to Figure 9–9, however, there are two differences. First, although the input gain was the same for both recordings, the amplitude of the noise on the nasal waveform is greater in Figure 9–10. Second, there is a quasi-periodic, low-frequency component present in the nasal spectrogram as indicated by regularly spaced vertical striations. Playback of this segment of the nasal waveform indicates a distinctive, raspberry-like sound, consistent with tissue flutter.

As mentioned previously, nasometric recordings can also facilitate identification of active nasal fricatives. Figure 9–11 illustrates the oral and nasal recordings of a 7-year-old boy without cleft palate who substituted posterior nasal fricatives for /s/ as part of phoneme-specific nasal air emission. The boy repeated the syllable /sa/ four times. As seen in the oral waveform, there are stop gaps—and release bursts—instead of frication noise for each /s/ segment, consistent with oral occlusion. Conversely, acoustic energy is present in each /s/ segment of the nasal waveform, the second /s/ is indicated by vertical cursors. The nasal spectrogram reveals evidence of both aperiodic noise associated with turbulence and quasi-periodic vibrations associated with tissue flutter.

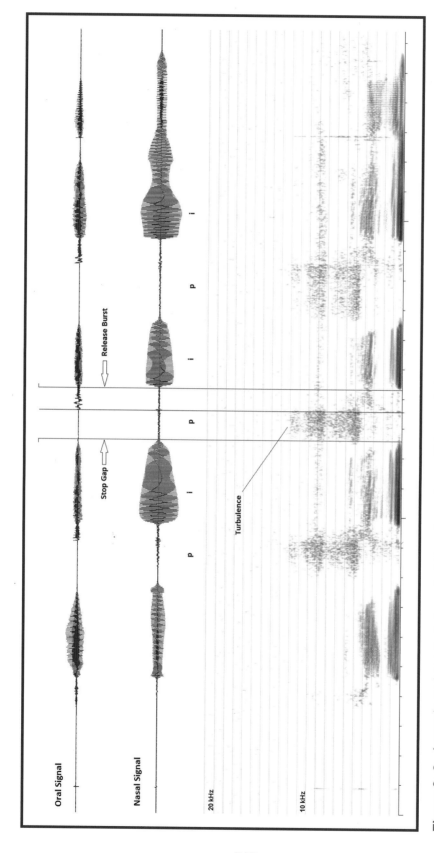

Figure 9–9. Acoustic and spectral characteristics of passive audible nasal air emission. Shown are oral and nasal microphone signals from nasometer (*top*) and spectrogram of nasal microphone signal (*bottom*). Speech sample was "Say pea pea pea again." Stop-gap and release burst of second /p/ segment are illustrated. Aperiodic noise (turbulence) is present during the stop-gap.

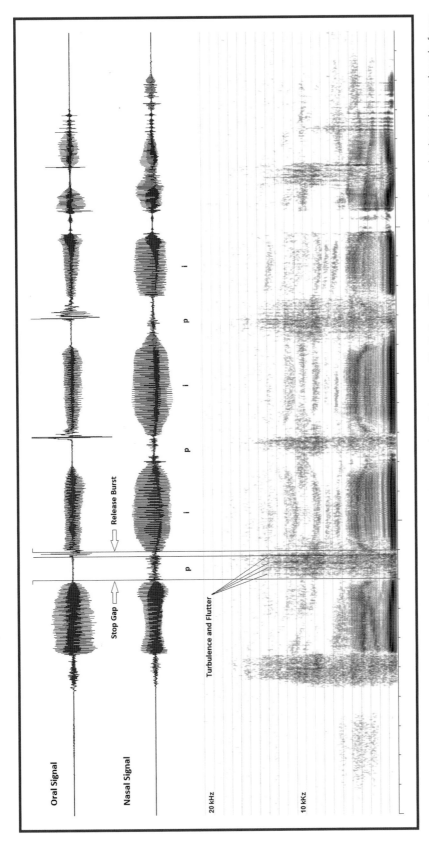

Figure 9–10. Acoustic and spectral characteristics of passive nasal turbulence with flutter. Shown are oral and nasal microphone signals from nasometer (*top*) and spectrogram of nasal microphone signal (*bottom*). Speech sample was "Say pea pea pea again." Stop-gap and release burst of first /p/ segment are illustrated. Aperiodic noise (turbulence) and flutter are present during the stop-gap. Flutter is characterized by periodic vertical striations that modulate the aperiodic noise.

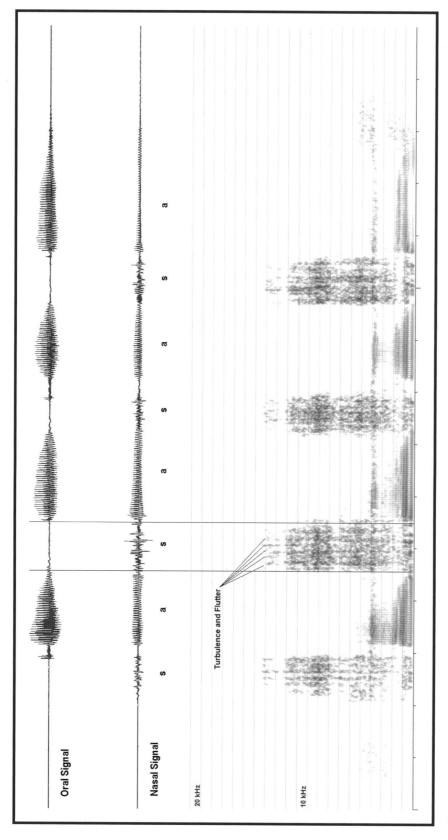

Figure 9–11. Acoustic and spectral characteristics of active posterior nasal fricative. Shown are oral and nasal microphone signals from nasometer (*top*) and spectrogram of nasal microphone signal (*bottom*). Speech sample was "sah sah sah sah." The second /s/ segment shows a stop-gap on the oral waveform and frication noise on the nasal waveform. Aperiodic noise (turbulence) and flutter are present during the /s/ segment.

Of interest, the spectral pattern for the posterior nasal fricative shown in Figure 9–11 is quite similar to the spectral pattern for obligatory nasal turbulence with flutter shown in Figure 9–10. Because of the perceptual similarities, some clinicians will refer to obligatory nasal turbulence with flutter as a "passive posterior nasal fricative" (e.g., Peterson-Falzone, Trost-Cardamone, Karnell, and Hardin-Jones, 2006).

Clinical use of the nasometer as a recording tool can provide an index of the type and consistency of nasal air emission that may guide diagnostic and management decisions. A child, for example, who exhibits obligatory audible nasal air emission is likely to have relatively large velopharyngeal gaps. If the audible nasal air emission is consistent (i.e., occurring on a high percentage of syllables), then the child should be referred for imaging procedures to determine the need for secondary surgical management. Conversely, a child who exhibits obligatory nasal turbulence with flutter is likely to have small velopharyngeal gaps. If the nasal turbulence or flutter is inconsistent (i.e., occurring on relatively few syllables), then the child may be a candidate for trial behavioral therapy that attempts to change articulatory parameters such as contact pressure and segment duration.

Advantages and Limitations. Nasometric recording of a child to identify the type and frequency of audible nasal emission is a promising clinical tool. It is especially well suited to help clinicians identify the stop component of active nasal fricatives. Because the nasal microphone of the nasometer is positioned close to the nose, however, it is likely to detect even very mild audible nasal air emission. Clinicians, therefore, also need to determine the perceptual significance of a child's nasal air emission.

Aerodynamics: Pressure-Flow Method. Warren and colleagues were the first researchers to apply aeromechanical principles to estimate velopharyngeal orifice area during speech (Warren, 1964a, 1964b; Warren & DuBois, 1964). Warren and DuBois (1964) used a plastic model of the upper vocal tract to show that the minimal cross-sectional area of the velopharyngeal port could be estimated by simultaneously measuring the pressure drop across the port along with the volume rate of airflow through the port. They calculated area using a modification of Bernoulli's equation that included a correction factor (k) for unsteady or turbulent airflow:

$$\text{orifice area (cm}^2) = V/k[2(p_1 - p_2)/D)]^{\frac{1}{2}}$$

where V is rate of airflow in milliliters per second (mL/s); $k = 0.65$; p_1 is the upstream stagnation pressure in dynes per square centimeters (dynes/cm^2); p_2 is the downstream stagnation pressure in dynes per square centimeters (dynes/cm^2); and D is the density of air (0.001 g/cm^3).

Yates, McWilliams, and Vallino (1990) noted that accuracy of the pressure-flow method is dependent on the value of the flow coefficient k, used to correct for turbulent airflow. Warren and Dubois selected a value of 0.65 based upon model tests that used short tubes ranging in area from 2.4 to 120.4 mm^2. The k value was an average value derived from all tubes. The value of k, however, also varies as a function of inlet geometry of the orifice. Sharp-edge orifices such as thin plates and short tubes create greater turbulence than rounded orifices. Yates et al. pointed out that a k value approaching 0.99 may be more representative of rounded inlets that are likely to be present in the velo-pharyngeal anatomy. If so, then estimates of orifice size may be overestimated when using 0.65 as the value of *k*. Yates et al. did not suggest a change in the value of *k* because the exact shape of the velopharyngeal port is unlikely to be determined for a given speaker. If the exact shape was known, there would be no need to estimate orifice size.

Clinical application of the pressure-flow method is straightforward (Figure 9–12). Three measures are needed to estimate velopharyngeal orifice area: oral air pressure (upstream pressure), nasal air pressure (downstream pressure), and nasal airflow. Oral air pressure is detected by placing the open end of a small catheter behind the lips. The catheter is connected to a calibrated differential air-pressure transducer. Nasal air pressure is detected by passing another small catheter through a foam plug that is secured in one nostril of the speaker. The nasal catheter is attached to a second calibrated differential air-pressure transducer. By occluding the nostril, a stagnation pressure is created in the nasal cavity that is continuous with pressure directly downstream of the velopharyngeal port. Differential pressure across the velopharyngeal port is simply determined as the difference between oral and nasal air pressure. The volume rate of airflow through the port is obtained by inserting a snug-fitting tube into the other nostril of the speaker. The nasal flow tube is coupled to a heated and calibrated pneumotachometer.

The pressure-flow method is ideally suited to studying the voiceless bilabial stop /p/ in CV syllables and words. No special orientation of the pressure-detecting

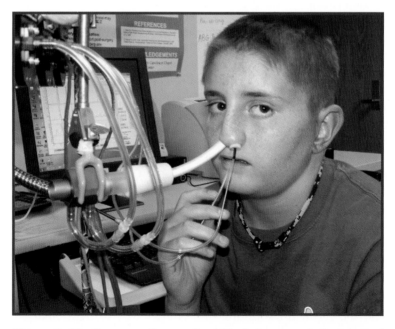

Figure 9–12. Pressure-flow method. Oral air pressure is detected by a catheter placed in the mouth, nasal air pressure is detected by a foam catheter inserted into one nostril, and nasal airflow is detected by a flow tube that is inserted into the other nostril.

catheter is required as the oral cavity is closed, airflow is stopped, and air pressure is relatively high and the same in all directions. As noted by Baken and Orlikoff (2000), perpendicular orientation of the catheter to the moving airstream is necessary for detection of air pressure associated with production of fricatives. Although the voiceless alveolar /t/ and velar /k/ can be targeted, placement of the catheter behind the tongue is difficult, especially for /k/. Typically, the catheter must be placed either along the buccal sulcus and angled around the posterior molar or passed through the nose and into the oropharynx to detect oral air pressure for /k/. Neither approach, however, is feasible with young children in a clinical setting. Warren and colleagues have also used the word *hamper* during pressure-flow studies (e.g., Warren, 1979; Warren, Dalston, Morr, & Hairfield, 1989). The rapid opening and closing gestures that occur during the nasal-plosive sequence are considered to stress the velopharyngeal mechanism and be more typical of closure obtained in connected speech.

Normal Velopharyngeal Function. Zajac (2000) provided norms for the pressure-flow method. He studied 181 children ranging in age from 6 to 16 years and 42 adults ranging in age from 18 to 37 years without cleft palate. The children were grouped into four age ranges: (a) 6 to 8 years (*n* = 47), (b) 9 to 10 years (*n* = 71), (c) 11 to 12 years (*n* = 41), and (d) 13 to 16 years (*n* = 22). All speakers produced the CV syllables /pi/, /pa/, and /mi/, the word *hamper*, and the sentence *peep into the hamper*. Peak oral air pressure, nasal airflow, and estimated velopharyngeal areas were determined for the /m/ and /p/ segments in syllables and *hamper*, both word and sentence levels.

Zajac (2000) reported that all children and adults achieved essentially complete velopharyngeal closure during production of /p/ in syllables and *hamper*. Mean nasal airflow during production of /p/ in *hamper* was less than 10 mL/s for the three youngest age groups and was only 14 mL/s for the 13- to 16-year-olds and 15 mL/s for adults. The single highest rate of nasal airflow during production of /p/ in *hamper* was 76 mL/s for an adult. This corresponded to a velopharyngeal opening of only 3.4 mm^2.

Zajac (2000) reported that nasal airflow and estimated velopharyngeal areas for /m/ in *hamper* typically increased across the speakers as a function of age. Mean nasal airflow was 87 mL/s for the 6- to 8-year-olds, 96 mL/s for the 9- to 10-year-olds, 122 mL/s for the 11- to 12-year-olds, 158 mL/s for the 13- to 16-year-olds, and 139 mL/s for the adults. Zajac attributed these findings to larger dimensions of the upper airways in the older children and adults. Conversely, oral air pressure during production of /p/ in *hamper* generally decreased as a function of age. Mean oral air pressure was 7.1 cm H$_2$O for the 6- to 8-year-olds, 7.2 cm H$_2$O for the 9- to 10-year-olds, 6.6 cm H$_2$O for the 11- to 12-year-olds, 5.6 cm H$_2$O for the 13- to 16-year-olds, and 5.3 cm H$_2$O for the adults. There was an approximate 2 cm of water pressure difference between the youngest children and adults. This occurred most likely because younger children simply tend to speak louder than adults.

Figures 9–13 and 9–14 illustrate pressure-flow recordings that show normal velopharyngeal function during production of the syllable /pa/ and the word *hamper*. Both speakers had repaired cleft palate but normal velopharyngeal function. The speaker in Figure 9–13 was a 13-year-old boy with repaired cleft lip and

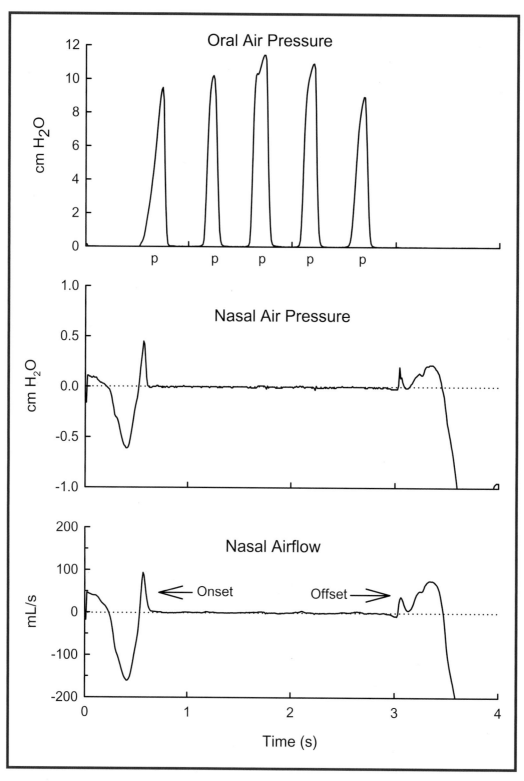

Figure 9–13. Pressure-flow recording showing complete velopharyngeal closure during repetition of /pa/ syllables. Note brief onset and offset nasal airflows.

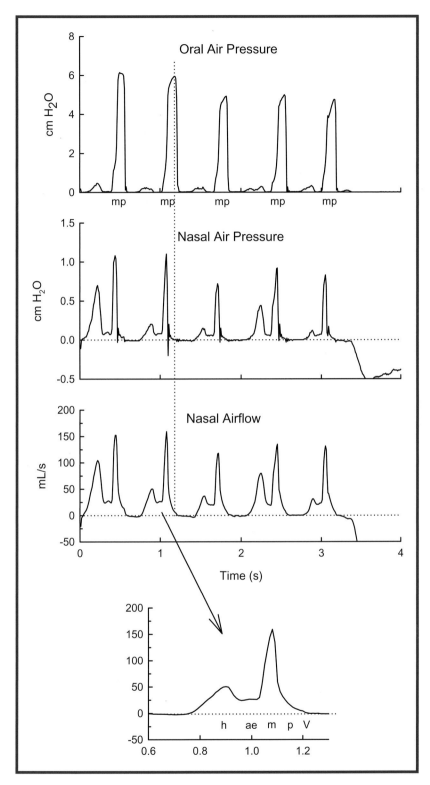

Figure 9–14. Pressure-flow recording showing normal velopharyngeal function during repetition of *hamper*. Expanded production at bottom shows anticipatory nasal airflow beginning with the /h/ segment.

palate who repeated the syllable /pa/ five times on a single breath. Peak oral air pressure associated with the stop segments of /p/ varied from approximately 9 to 12 cm of water pressure (top panel). Nasal air pressure (middle panel) and nasal airflow (bottom panel) indicated complete closure of the velopharyngeal port as reflected by zero or atmospheric values. There is normal onset nasal airflow at the beginning of the utterance and normal offset nasal airflow at the end. As indicated previously, these airflow events may be misinterpreted as velopharyngeal openings by low-tech devices (e.g., mirror testing).

The speaker in Figure 9–14 was a 14-year-old boy with repaired cleft palate who repeated the word *hamper* five times on a single breath. Peak oral air pressures associated with /p/ were rather consistent at approximately 5 to 6 centimeters of water for each word. The pattern of nasal airflow was also consistent during each word. Nasal airflow of the second production of *hamper* is expanded at the bottom of the figure. As shown, nasal airflow peaked at approximately 50 mL/s during the voiceless /h/ segment, dropped during the /ae/ segment, rose to over 150 mL/s during /m/, and rapidly shut down during the /p/ and final vowel segments. The nasal airflow that occurred during the /h/ and /ae/ segments was normal anticipatory airflow. As indicated by the vertical cursor in the main figure, the velopharyngeal port was essentially closed at the time of peak oral air pressure associated with /p/ as reflected by nasal airflow that was well below 20 mL/s.

As previously described, velar bounce is a slight up and down movement of the closed soft palate against the posterior pharyngeal wall during speech. It is normal movement that occurs due to levator veli palatini muscle contractions during syllable production. Velar bounce can cause some nasal airflow to occur even in the presence of complete velopharyngeal closure. Figure 9–15 illustrates an example of positive and negative nasal airflow due to velar bounce. The speaker was a 38-year-old male with repaired cleft lip and palate and a pharyngeal flap who produced the CV syllable /pa/ five times. The nasal airflow trace (bottom panel in the figure) shows consistent positive followed by negative nasal airflow associated with each syllable. The positive nasal airflow occurs when the soft palate (and/or pharyngeal flap) is rising and forces air out of the nose; the negative nasal airflow occurs when the soft palate (and/or pharyngeal flap) is falling and draws air into the nose. Whereas positive nasal airflow may be detected via mirror testing, only pressure-flow recordings can reveal negative nasal airflow as condensation will not occur on a mirror. The importance of using pressure-flow instrumentation is highlighted by this example as the speaker had a pharyngeal flap. The use of only low-tech devices may have detected the positive nasal airflow with the possibility of an unnecessary referral for imaging studies.

Velopharyngeal Dysfunction. Warren and colleagues (and others) have reported pressure-flow findings for speakers with cleft palate or VPI. As reviewed in Chapter 8, one common obligatory symptom of VPI is weak or reduced oral air pressure during production of obstruent consonants. The extent of the oral air pressure loss varies directly with the size of the velopharyngeal opening (Dalston, Warren, Morr, & Smith, 1988; Warren

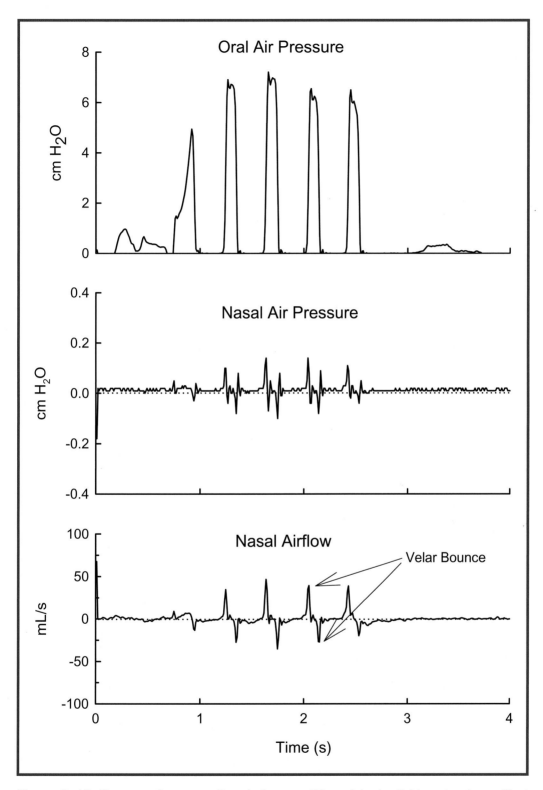

Figure 9–15. Pressure-flow recording during repetition of /pa/ syllables showing artifact nasal airflow as a function of velar bounce.

et al., 1989). Dalston et al. (1988) used the pressure-flow method to study 267 speakers with varying degrees of VPI ranging in age from 4 to 58 years. The speakers produced the word *hamper*, and estimates of velopharyngeal port size were calculated for the /p/ segment. Dalston et al. categorized the speakers into five groups based on velopharyngeal port size: (a) adequate—less than 5 mm², (b) adequate-borderline—5 to 9.9 mm², (c) borderline-inadequate—10 to 19.9 mm², (d) inadequate—20 to 80 mm², and (e) grossly inadequate—essentially equal oral and nasal air pressures that precluded accurate gap size estimates. Dalston et al. reported that peak oral air pressure associated with

the /p/ segment of *hamper* decreased systematically across the five groups of speakers: 6.7 ($SD = 2.4$), 4.5 ($SD = 1.9$), 4.1 ($SD = 1.7$), 3.5 ($SD = 2$), and 3.0 ($SD = 1.3$) centimeters of water, respectively.

Zajac (2003) reported interesting oral air pressure findings for speakers with repaired cleft palate. As noted in Chapter 8, he studied 176 speakers with repaired cleft palate and 223 controls who ranged in age from 5 to 51 years. Oral air pressure was determined during production of the syllable /pi/. Figure 9–16 shows peak oral air pressure levels of the speakers grouped by age, with three groups of children and the adults. Of interest, children with cleft palate used greater oral

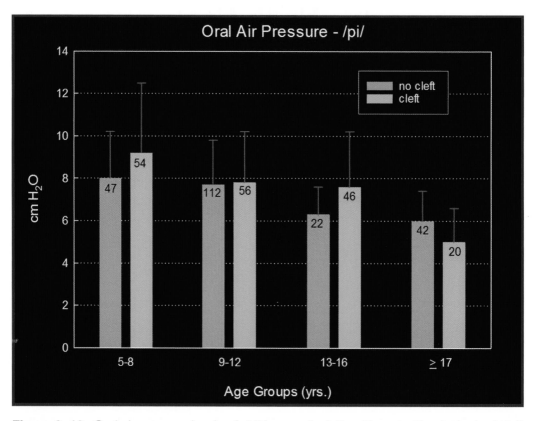

Figure 9–16. Oral air pressure levels of children and adults with and without repaired cleft palate during repetition of /pi/ syllables. Number of speakers per group are shown at tops of bars.

air pressure than the noncleft children. The differences between children with and without cleft palate in the youngest and oldest age groups were significant ($p < .05$). The adult speakers with cleft palate, however, used lower oral air pressure than the noncleft adults. It should be noted that most of the children with cleft palate (approximately 70%) had adequate velopharyngeal function, but most of the adults did not. Zajac suggested that the children with cleft palate might have used greater oral air pressure to achieve velopharyngeal closure. Fahey and Zajac (2013) reported similar findings of higher oral air pressure for children with repaired cleft palate who exhibited adequate velopharyngeal closure.

Warren et al. (1989) demonstrated that the magnitude of nasal airflow was also directly related to size of the velopharyngeal port. They used the pressure-flow method to study 107 speakers with repaired cleft palate ranging in age from approximately 5 to 58 years. All speakers produced the word *hamper* and were categorized into four groups based upon velopharyngeal port size associated with the /p/ segment. The velopharyngeal area categories and mean rates of nasal airflow were: (a) adequate (0–4.9 mm^2) – 32 mL/s ($SD = 25$), (b) borderline-adequate (5-9.9 mm^2) – 102 mL/s ($SD = 34$), (c) borderline-inadequate (10–19.9 mm^2) – 149 mL/s ($SD = 51$), and (d) inadequate (20+ mm^2) – 313 mL/s ($SD = 188$). It must be noted that while the relationship between velopharyngeal port size and nasal airflow is strong for areas up to 20 mm^2, it breaks down for larger areas (Laine, Warren, Dalston, & Morr, 1988). This occurs because at larger velopharyngeal areas (i.e., 40 mm^2 or greater), the smaller nasal valve region of the nose becomes the flow limiting structure.

Figures 9–17 to 9–19 illustrate pressure-flow recordings of marginal to inadequate velopharyngeal function. The term *marginal* is used to reflect Warren et al.'s (1989) categories of borderline-adequate and borderline-inadequate function characterized by velopharyngeal areas that range from 5 to 19.9 mm^2. Inadequate function refers to velopharyngeal areas that exceed 20 mm^2 or when oral and nasal air pressures are equal, reflecting complete oral-nasal coupling. Figure 9–17 shows a 12-year-old boy with repaired cleft palate who exhibited marginal function. The figure shows eight repetitions of the syllable /pi/. Although oral air pressure was adequate for production of /p/ (top panel), it was reduced from expected levels of 7 to 8 cm H$_2$O for 12-year-old children. Nasal airflow consistently occurred throughout the utterance (bottom panel), averaging 100 mL/s at peak oral air pressure of /p/ and approximately 20 to 50 mL/s during the vowel segments between the pressure peaks. Estimated velopharyngeal orifice area at peak oral air pressure of the fifth syllable was 6 to 7 mm^2. Perceptual symptoms exhibited by the boy included mild hypernasality and consistent visible nasal air emission.

Figure 9–18 shows the pressure-flow recordings from a 4-year-old boy who exhibited inadequate velopharyngeal function. He repeated the syllable /pi/ four times. Perceptually, the boy had severe hypernasality, reduced loudness, and audible nasal air emission. The figure shows that oral air pressure was significantly below expected age levels at only 2 cm H$_2$O. Nasal air pressure was the same magnitude as oral air pressure, indicating complete coupling of the oral and nasal cavities. Nasal airflow was consistent at approximately 200 mL/s during the /p/ segments. Valid velopharyngeal gap size

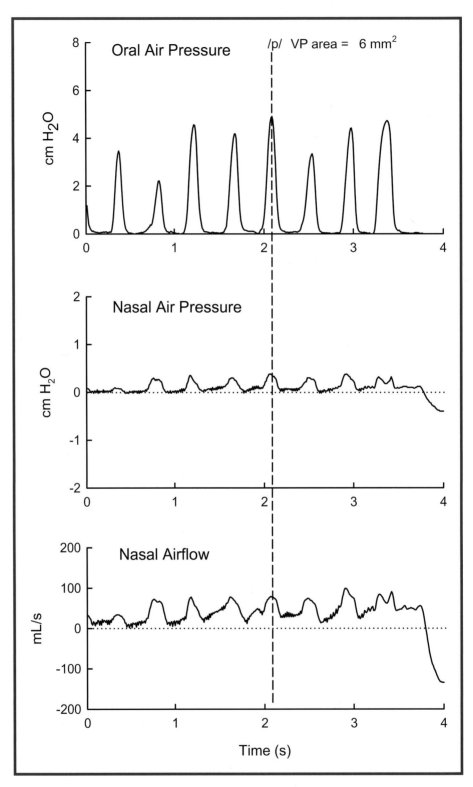

Figure 9–17. Pressure-flow recording during repetition of /pi/ syllables showing marginal velopharyngeal closure. Note consistent nasal airflow that approximates 100 mL/s during /p/ segments.

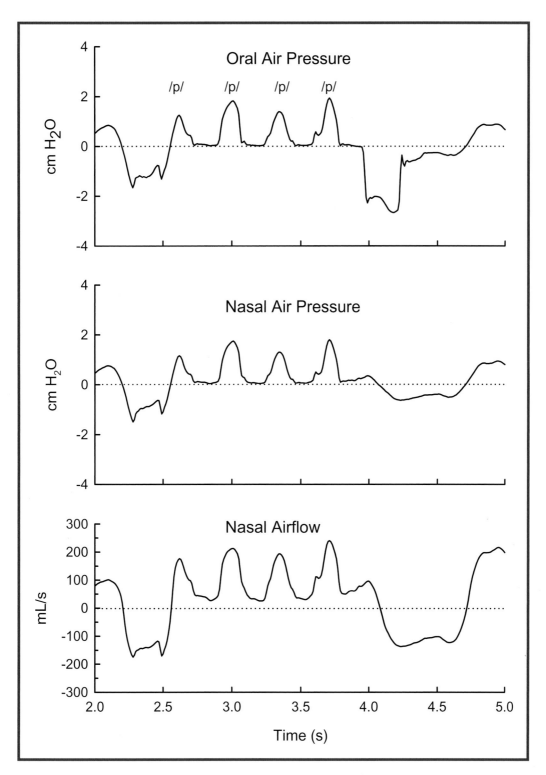

Figure 9–18. Pressure-flow recording during repetition of /pi/ syllables showing inadequate velopharyngeal closure. Note essentially equal oral and nasal air pressures during /p/ segments.

could not be estimated for the boy due to equal oral and nasal air pressures.

Last, Figure 9–19 shows the pressure-flow recordings from a 10-year-old girl with unrepaired submucous cleft palate who also exhibited inadequate velopharyngeal function. She repeated the word *hamper* four times. As shown in the figure, there is reduced oral air pressure and a complete overlap of the nasal airflow and oral air pressure pulses, indicating VPI. In essence, the girl was unable to aerodynamically separate the /m/ from the /p/ segments of *hamper*. Valid velopharyngeal areas could not be estimated due to equal oral and nasal air pressures. (Nasal air pressure is not shown in the figure.)

Advantages and Limitations. The pressure-flow method is minimally invasive, and most children readily tolerate the procedures. It provides objective information not only for velopharyngeal orifice size but also oral air pressure, nasal air pressure, and nasal airflow. Normative pressure-flow data have been reported by several studies (Searl & Knollhoff, 2013; Smith, Guyette, Patil, & Brannan, 2003; Zajac, 2000). Pressure flow is especially well suited to provide objective outcome data following secondary management (see Chapter 11), because it does not expose the child to additional radiation or physical discomfort associated with imaging procedures.

The primary limitation of the pressure-flow method is the uncertainty of the value for the *k* coefficient used in the equation to calculate port size. As indicated by Yates et al. (1990), velopharyngeal orifice size may be overestimated, perhaps by as

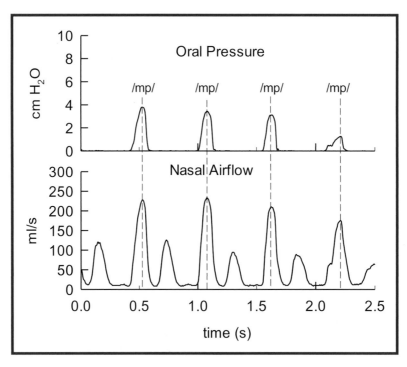

Figure 9–19. Pressure-flow recording during repetition of *hamper* showing inadequate velopharyngeal closure. Note complete temporal overlap of oral air pressure and nasal airflow pulses (nasal pressure not shown).

much as 30%, if a *k* value of 0.99 is more appropriate for the geometry of the port. Estimated velopharyngeal orifice areas, therefore, should be considered relative and not absolute. Interpreted in this way, area estimates still provide important diagnostic information across children.

As indicated in some of the examples above, area estimations are not possible when VPI is severe, and oral and nasal air pressures are equal. At times, nasal air pressure may even exceed oral air pressure. In such cases, clinicians may choose to report differential oral-nasal air pressure measures. Warren and colleagues have suggested that differential pressure that is less than 1 cm H_2O reflects inadequate velopharyngeal function, whereas differential pressure greater than 3 cm H_2O reflects adequate function. Differential pressures between these two values are considered to reflect marginal function. The use of differential pressure also circumvents the need to estimate area and the uncertainty of a *k* value.

Another limitation of the pressure-flow method is that it provides information primarily about voiceless stop consonants, not vowels. Therefore, estimates of velopharyngeal orifice size that are obtained during production of voiceless consonants do not correlate highly with perceived nasality, primarily a vowel phenomenon. Because of this, it is possible for a child who exhibits mild or even moderate hypernasality to have relatively small velopharyngeal areas during production of /p/, even in the adequate range (i.e., under 5 mm²). If this occurs, it should alert the clinician to carefully evaluate other aspects of speech production such as rate, segment duration, loudness, and/or oral opening that may be contributing to nasality.

Oral-Nasal Airflow. Separate oral and nasal airflows can be obtained by using a divided oral-nasal mask as previously shown in Figure 9–8. The inside of the mask has a partition that is placed against the upper lip to effectively separate the mouth from the nose. Pressure taps are inserted into each chamber of the mask and attached to calibrated, differential air pressure transducers. The screens of the mask act as pneumotachographs to create a pressure drop during speech that is converted to airflow. Speech is recorded with a microphone positioned outside of the oral chamber of the mask.

Figure 9–20 illustrates the audio, nasal airflow, and oral airflow signals obtained with a divided oral-nasal mask. The speaker was an 8-year-old girl without cleft palate who produced posterior nasal fricatives as substitutes for /s/ as part of phoneme-specific nasal air emission. The figure shows three productions of the syllable /si/. Oral airflow was absent during production of each /s/ segment due to occlusion of the oral cavity as part of the posterior nasal fricative. Because of oral stopping, all airflow was shunted through the nose to produce frication. As further shown in the figure, the vowels were produced with carryover nasal airflow resulting from the posterior nasal fricatives, causing the girl to exhibit assimilative nasality. This example highlights the occurrence of assimilative nasality that often accompanies phoneme-specific nasal air emission and should not be interpreted as velopharyngeal dysfunction.

Advantages and Limitations. The use of an oral-nasal airflow mask is noninvasive and minimally intrusive. It easily allows the assessment of continuous speech including vowel segments. Because oral airflow is obtained, information regarding oral articulations can be inferred. Available masks, however, are limited to child and adult sizes. This makes fitting

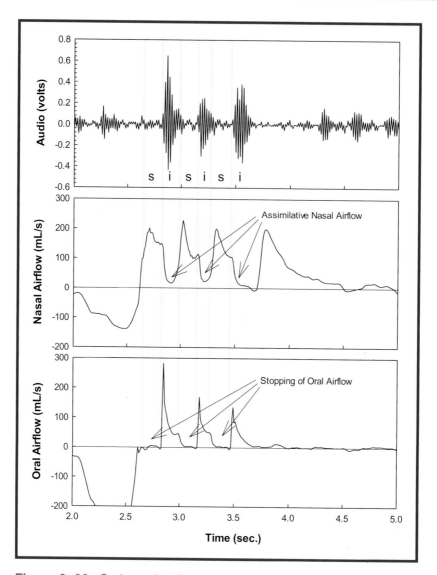

Figure 9–20. Oral-nasal airflow recording during production of active posterior nasal fricatives. Shown are audio signal (*top*), nasal airflow (middle), and oral airflow (*bottom*). Note assimilative nasal airflow during vowel segments and stopping of oral airflow during the nasal fricative segments.

and obtaining a good seal problematic for older children who may need an intermediate mask size.

Nasal Ram Pressure. Thom, Hoit, Hixon, and Smith (2006) described the use of nasal ram pressure (NRP) to assess velo-

pharyngeal function of infants without cleft palate. The procedure involves inserting the prongs of an oxygen-delivery cannula into the nostrils of an infant and attaching the other end to a differential pressure transducer (Figure 9–21A). The nasal cannula does not occlude the nose.

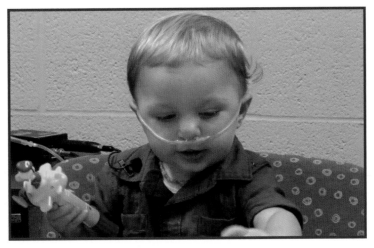

A

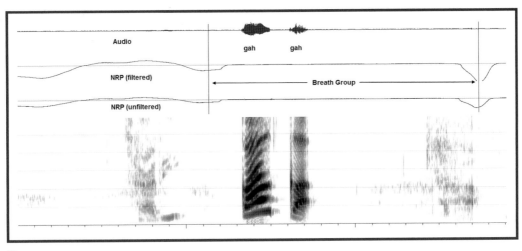

B

Figure 9–21. A. Nasal ram pressure (NRP) monitoring of an 18-month-old boy with repaired cleft lip and palate. **B.** NRP recordings from a 20-month-old girl without cleft palate showing velopharyngeal closure during production of "gah gah." Top of the figure shows audio, low-pass filtered NRP, and unfiltered NRP signals; bottom of figure shows a spectrogram of the audio signal.

A stagnation pressure, therefore, is not created as in the pressure-flow method. Rather, the prongs of the cannula act as a pitot tube to detect local changes in air velocity. A small microphone is used to record vocalizations of the infants. The procedure provides binary information on the status of the velopharyngeal port as being either open or closed. If positive NRP is detected during production of a stop consonant, for example, then the velopharyngeal port is inferred to be open. Zero (or atmospheric) NRP implies that the port is closed. Figure 9–21B shows NRP recordings from a 20-month-old girl without cleft palate who produced the syllable "gah" two times. NRP is zero throughout the breath group indicating complete velopharyngeal closure. Unlike the pressure-flow method, however, the procedure cannot provide an estimate of relative port size when positive NRP is detected.

Monitoring of NRP is a promising technique that may shed light on early velopharyngeal function of infants and toddlers with cleft palate following surgical repair. Zajac, van Aalst, Vallino, and Napoli (2011) attempted the procedure on 24 toddlers with repaired cleft palate (mean age = 23 months) and 5 toddlers without cleft palate (mean age = 24 months). The children were engaged in play activities designed to elicit production of stop consonants. Seventeen of the children with cleft palate tolerated wearing the nasal cannula and produced stop consonants (median number = 13, range of 2 to 53 stops). Four of the children without cleft palate also tolerated wearing the cannula and produced stop consonants (median number = 22, range of 10 to 48 stops). Zajac et al. reported that all four children without cleft palate achieved consistent VP closure as reflected by zero NRP on at least 90% of stops produced. Only 12 of the 17 children with cleft palate (70%), however, achieved VP closure on 90% or more of stops. One of the children with cleft palate achieved closure on only 50% of stops, and two achieved no closure. It should be noted that the percentage of children with cleft palate who achieved closure on 50% or less of stops (18%) is strikingly similar to the percentage of older children with cleft palate who are referred for secondary management procedures. To be sure, Krochmal, Zajac, Alhudaib, Emodi, and van Aalst (2013) reported evidence to show that early NRP testing may be predictive of later velo-pharyngeal function. They followed three children with 0% stop closure starting at 2 years of age and reported that two went on to receive secondary surgical procedures for VPI by 4 years of age.

Advantages and Limitations. NRP monitoring is a relatively easy procedure that most young children tolerate. Zajac et al. (2011) noted that approximately 80% of 2-year-old children tolerated wearing the nasal cannula. Disadvantages are that only binary information on velopharyngeal closure is provided and some children do not talk even if they tolerate wearing the cannula. Additional research is needed to further evaluate both the short- and long-term diagnostic significance of NRP findings.

Direct Methods: Radiographic Procedures

Lateral Still Cephalograms. Lateral cephalograms (radiographs) are standardized skull x-rays taken to show the occlusal relationship of the jaws and soft tissue dimensions of the face. Lateral cephalograms are a mainstay of orthodontic treatment and orthognathic surgery planning (see Chapter 13). Lateral cephalograms, for example, are used to document occlusal status, determine extent of orthodontic and surgical movement of structures (e.g., distance required to advance the maxilla), and evaluate treatment outcomes.

Subtelney and colleagues were among the first to use lateral cephalograms to study the speech of individuals with cleft palate (Aram & Subtelny, 1959; Subtelny, 1961). Typically, a speaker's head is stabilized during prolongation of a vowel such as /i/ or a continuant such as /s/. A radiograph is taken during production of the sound. Examination of the film allows assessment of the length of the velum, depth of the nasopharynx, and level and extent of velopharyngeal closure. Figure 9–22 shows a lateral cephalogram from a 5-year-old boy with unrepaired submucous cleft palate and cerebral palsy who prolonged the vowel /i/. A cephalostat and a locking nasal positioner stabilized his head. As seen in the figure, there is a 3- to 4-mm gap between the elevated velum and the posterior pharyngeal wall. The absolute gap size was calculated by comparing the measured distance on the cephalogram to the known distance marked in centimeters on the nasal positioner (see Williams, Henningsson, & Pegoraro-Krook, 1997).

Advantages and Limitations. Lateral cephalograms—also called *phonating cephs*—are relatively easy to obtain and interpret. Significant disadvantages are that information is obtained from a single, sustained speech sound and the child is exposed to radiation. As noted by Williams et al. (1997), velopharyngeal function during production of isolated, prolonged sounds may not be predictive of function during connected speech. Williams and Eisenbach (1981), for example, reported that use of lateral still cephalograms during production of sustained /i/ resulted in the misdiagnosis of 25% of speakers compared to lateral cinefluorography during continuous speech (described in the next section). Specifically, they reported that while 24 of 30 speakers failed to achieve closure during sustained /i/, only 18 demonstrated velopharyngeal inadequacy during connected speech.

Multiview Videofluoroscopy. Videofluoroscopy overcomes the disadvantage of single-exposure radiographs by recording the patient during connected speech. Initially, videofluoroscopy was restricted to the lateral view, due to limitations in technology (McWilliams & Girdany, 1964). Beginning in the late 1960s, Skolnick and colleagues described the use of multiview videofluoroscopy (MVVF) to assess patients (Skolnick, 1969, 1970, 1977; Skolnick & Cohn, 1989; Skolnick, McCall, & Barnes, 1973; Skolnick, Shprintzen, McCall, & Rakoff, 1975). As described by Skolnick and Cohn (1989), MVVF involves assessing the patient during a sequence of views and activities (Figure 9–23): (a) speaking in lateral view without barium contrast, (b) drinking barium in lateral view, (c) speaking and swallowing in base view after barium is instilled into the nostrils, (d) speaking and swallowing in frontal view after barium contrast, and (e) speaking and swallowing in lateral

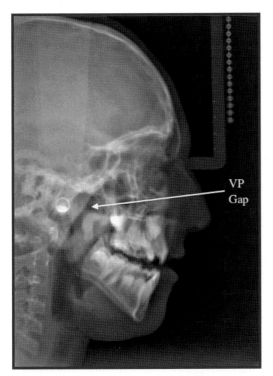

Figure 9–22. Lateral cephalogram during prolongation of /i/ showing inadequate velopharyngeal closure.

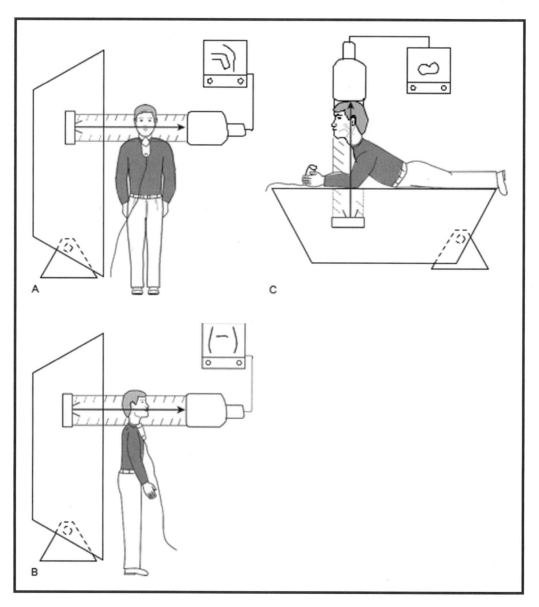

Figure 9–23. Multiview videofluoroscopy. **A.** Lateral view. **B.** Frontal view. **C.** Base view. (From Sloan, G., & Zajac, D. J., 2006. Velopharyngeal dysfunction. In S. Mathes [Ed.], *Plastic surgery. Volume 4: Pediatric plastic surgery* [2nd ed., pp. 311–337]. Philadelphia, PA: Saunders Elsevier. Used with permission.)

view after barium contrast. Typically, both an SLP and radiologist (or technician) perform MVVF examinations. The role of the SLP is to elicit speech samples and oversee the evaluation, and the role of the radiologist and technician is to obtain the radiographic images and ensure the safety of the patient.

Drinking barium in lateral view is designed to show the presence of a patent oronasal fistula in the hard or soft palates and reflux of barium into the nasopharynx during swallowing. Skolnick, Glaser, and McWilliams (1980) reported that MVVF assessment of 195 patients indicated that reflux of barium was always associated with either hypernasal speech or velopharyngeal gaps. The absence of reflux, however, was not reported to be diagnostic. That is, Skolnick et al. noted that more than 50% of patients who did not exhibit nasal reflux were nonetheless hypernasal or had velopharyngeal gaps during speech assessment. They attributed this finding to known differences in velopharyngeal mechanics during speech and nonspeech tasks (e.g., Bloomer, 1953; Moll, 1965).

Speaking in lateral view with barium contrast is designed to evaluate velopharyngeal structure and function. Velar length, depth of the nasopharynx, and dynamic movement of velopharyngeal structures, including formation of a Passavant's pad, are assessed. The speaker in

Figure 9–24 was a 4-year-old girl without cleft palate who developed mild nasality following adenoidectomy. As shown in the figure, there is almost touch closure of the soft palate against the posterior pharyngeal wall. This is evidenced by the presence of barium clearly outlining both the velum and the posterior pharyngeal wall, indicating a small gap (Figure 9–24A). The size of the gap is increased when the girl was instructed to extend the neck during speaking (Figure 9–24B). During head extension, there is reduced elevation of the velum as reflected by a diminished velar eminence and reduced forward extension of the posterior pharyngeal wall. Both of these physiological changes contribute to a larger velopharyngeal gap.

McWilliams, Musgrave, and Crozier (1968) recommended the use of head extension to enhance diagnostic interpretation of the lateral view. They studied 101 children with repaired cleft palate who were grouped according to the presence

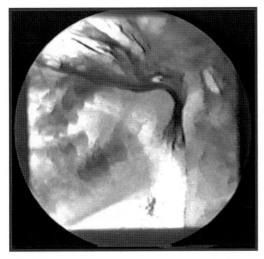
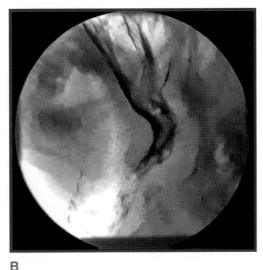

A   B

Figure 9–24. Lateral view videofluoroscopic images showing almost touch velopharyngeal closure during speech. **A.** Normal head position. **B.** Extended head position.

and absence of hypernasality. All children were assessed by lateral view videofluoroscopy in three head positions—upright, flexed, and extended. McWilliams et al. reported that of 22 hypernasal children who achieved closure in the upright position, 11 failed to maintain closure in the extended head position, presumably because of increased pharyngeal depth. McWilliams et al. suggested that use of head extension in the lateral view would facilitate obtaining complete diagnostic information.

The speaker in Figure 9–25 was a school-aged girl with repaired cleft who exhibited mild nasality. As shown in the figure, she exhibited a Passavant's pad that protruded from the posterior pharyngeal wall at the approximate level of the elevated velum. The formation of the Passavant's pad was consistent across different speech stimuli and head positions. The only time that the Passavant's pad

did not form was at the ends of utterances when the girl exhibited reduced loudness.

The base (or submentovertex) view is designed to assess movement and patterns of velopharyngeal closure during speech (Figure 9–26). A *circular* pattern of closure is due to relatively equal movement of the velum and lateral pharyngeal walls. *Coronal* closure is due primarily to movement of the velum while *sagittal* closure is due primarily to movement of the lateral pharyngeal walls. The base view is difficult to achieve at times, especially with young children. The speaker must be positioned in a sphinx-like position, often with the neck extended to obtain the view. As noted above, McWilliams et al. (1968) reported that head extension tended to promote velopharyngeal gaps in the lateral view. Because of this, Williams et al. (1997) advised that MVVF assessments in the base view should be interpreted with "caution."

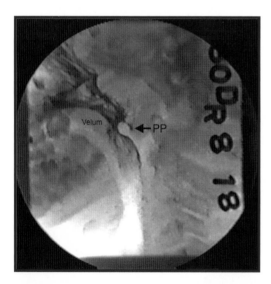

Figure 9–25. Lateral view videofluoroscopic image showing formation of a Passavant's pad (PP) during speech. Note that PP forms at the level of velar elevation but does not assist with closure.

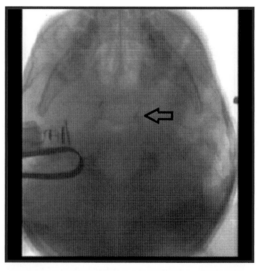

Figure 9–26. Base view videofluoroscopic image showing large coronal velopharyngeal gap during speech.

The frontal view is designed to assess multiple parameters during speech, including (a) lateral pharyngeal wall movement, (b) symmetry of lateral wall movement, (c) range of wall movement toward midline, and (d) location of maximum mesial wall movement relative to the level of velar-pharyngeal wall closure (Williams et al., 1997). Figure 9–27 illustrates the frontal view obtained from a child with repaired cleft palate and large tonsils. As seen in the figure, the tonsils touch in midline during speech well below the level of velopharyngeal closure. Of interest, this child exhibited a muffled, cul-de-sac resonance quality.

Advantages and Limitations. MVVF provides excellent imaging of velopharyngeal structure and function. It also provides information on tongue movement and place of articulation. Figures 8–3 and 8–4 in Chapter 8, for example, show pharyngeal articulations that were obtained during lateral view of MVVF.

All radiographic procedures expose the child to radiation. Although improvements in technology have reduced radiation exposure during MVVF to relatively low levels, it still exists. MVVF also requires cooperation from the child to drink barium, to instill barium into the nose, and for positioning in the base view. Young children may not cooperate or tolerate these procedures. Skolnick and Cohn (1989) recommended beginning MVVF procedures during speech without barium contrast in the lateral view. This is intended to provide some information even if the child does not comply with all procedures. As discussed in the next section on nasoendoscopy, a successful MVVF experience can be facilitated by adequately preparing the child and family in advance on the procedures.

Interpretation of videofluoroscopic images can be difficult. Although the base

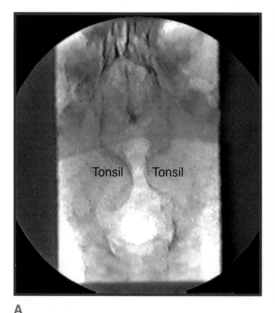
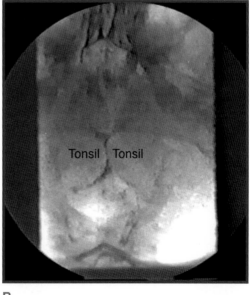

Figure 9–27. Frontal view videofluoroscopic images showing large tonsils. **A.** At rest. **B.** During speech. Note tonsils meet at midline.

view can provide important movement information, Shelton and Trier (1976) noted that it is often difficult to determine the level of movement. Last, videofluoroscopic images are subject to distortion due to movement of the child. As described by Williams et al. (1997), turning of the head in the lateral view may give the appearance of velar-pharyngeal wall contact even in the presence of a gap. Likewise, turning of the head in the frontal view may distort the image and give the impression of asymmetrical lateral pharyngeal wall movement.

Video Nasoendoscopy. Video nasoendoscopy involves insertion of a flexible fiberoptic endoscope through the nasal cavity to record movement of velopharyngeal structures during speech. The scope is connected to both a light source and a video camera (Figure 9–28). A microphone is used to record speech along with the video images. During a typical assessment, the patient is instructed to breathe quietly, swallow, and produce various speech samples.

Both an SLP and a physician, either an ENT or plastic surgeon, typically perform nasoendoscopic evaluations. Depending on the preferences of the physician, a topical anesthetic or nasal decongestant may be applied to the child's nasal passages. The scope is passed over the inferior turbinate and through the middle nasal meatus to obtain a view of the nasal velar surface. Passing the scope through the inferior nasal meatus, although somewhat easier than the middle, generally places the scope directly on top of the velum providing inadequate views of velopharyngeal closure (Karnell, 1994; Kummer, 2014).

Because of the physical insertion of a scope, many young children may be fearful of the procedure. Therefore, it is essential that young children be adequately prepared for the evaluation in advance. Many centers do this by having parents read booklets to the child that describe the procedures at an appropriate level of understanding, using "child terms." Some centers further attempt to reduce anxiety and facilitate cooperation of the child through active participation at the time of the procedure. That is, the child is encouraged to help pass the scope or control the video camera.

Figure 9–29A shows nasoendoscopy of a school-aged boy with repaired cleft pal-

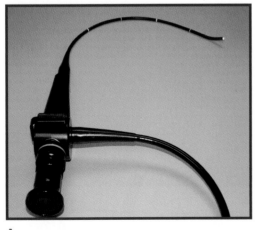
A

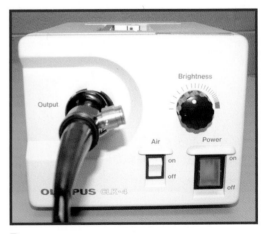
B

Figure 9–28. A. Flexible fiberoptic endoscope. **B.** Light source for scope.

ate who was diagnosed with VPI. There is a large velopharyngeal gap during production of oral pressure consonants. Figure 9–29B shows the boy during breathing approximately 3 months following surgical creation of a posterior pharyngeal flap (see Chapter 11). As seen in the figure, there is a wide flap of tissue from the posterior pharyngeal wall to the velum with open lateral ports on each side of the flap. During speech, resonance of the boy was hyponasal due to the wide width of the flap.

Advantages and Limitations. Although nasoendoscopy provides a clear view of the configuration of the velopharyngeal portal during attempted closure, the view is essentially limited to the nasal aspect of the velum and the superior aspect of the posterior and lateral pharyngeal walls. Thus, it may be difficult to discern overall activity level of the velum or if lateral pharyngeal wall movement occurs at a more inferior level. Related, Baken and Orlikoff (2000) point out that image

distortion occurs due to the wide-angle objective lens that is used. They note that this distortion, termed "barrel-type" or "convergence" effect, makes the center of the image appear larger than the periphery. Unlike MVVF, nasoendoscopy provides little, if any, information on lingual activity during articulation. Finally, similar to MVVF, reporting results from nasoendoscopy is largely subjective and not standardized. To overcome this limitation, a multidisciplinary group of clinicians formed a working group to develop standards for reporting results (Golding-Kushner et al., 1990). The group devised a rather complicated system of rating velopharyngeal closure based on the relative contributions of the velum and pharyngeal walls. It is not known if this reporting system has gained widespread acceptance.

Table 9–3 summaries the indirect and direct instrumental assessment techniques. The table indicates ease of use, quantifiable measures, and typical ages of patients that that can be assessed.

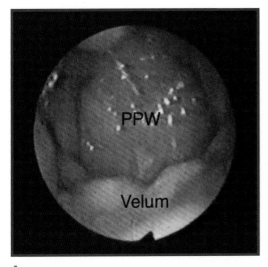
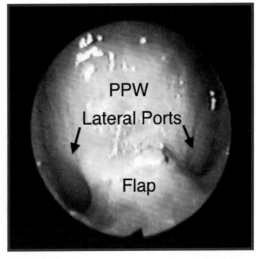

A

B

Figure 9–29. Nasoendoscopic images before and after pharyngeal flap surgery. **A.** Note large velopharyngeal gap during speech before surgery. **B.** Note wide pharyngeal flap during breathing following surgery.

Table 9–3. Summary of Instrumental Techniques to Assess Velopharyngeal (VP) Function

	Ease of Use	Quantifiable Measures	VP Port Estimates	Age Range of Patients
Indirect Techniques				
Nasometry	Easy; Noninvasive	Yes	No	Preschool to adults
Pressure-Flow	Relatively easy; Relatively noninvasive	Yes	Yes	Preschool to adults*
Oral-Nasal Airflow	Relatively easy; Noninvasive	Yes	No	Preschool to adults*
Nasal Ram Pressure	Relatively easy; Relatively noninvasive	Yes	No	Infants to toddlers
Direct Techniques				
Lateral Radiographs	Relatively easy; Noninvasive but radiation exposure	Yes**	Yes	School age to adults***
Videofluoroscopy	Moderately easy; Relatively noninvasive but radiation exposure	Yes**	Yes	School age to adults***
Video nasoendoscopy	Moderately easy; Invasive	Yes**	Yes	School age to adults***

Note. *Older children typically are more cooperative. **Relatively difficult to objectively quantify. ***Possible with cooperative younger children.

CHAPTER SUMMARY

The essential objective of the SLP when evaluating a child with repaired cleft palate is to determine the structural and functional integrity of the oral and velopharyngeal mechanisms for normal speech production. The SLP must carefully assess multiple speech parameters including resonance, nasal air emission, articulation, and phonation to make appropriate diagnostic decisions and treatment recommendations. Perceptual assessment procedures are the core of the diagnostic process and guide the need for objective instrumental assessments. Indirect instrumental procedures such as acoustics and aerodynamics are well suited to provide objective longitudinal information over time—to monitor effects of growth and adenoid involution—and following behavioral and physical interventions. The use of nasometric recordings to help clinicians differentiate passive from active nasal air emission is especially promising.

REFERENCES

Aram, A., & Subtelny, J. D. (1959). Velopharyngeal function and cleft palate prostheses. *Journal of Prosthetic Dentistry, 9,* 149–158.

Arkebauer, H. J., Hixon, T. J., & Hardy, J. C. (1967). Peak intraoral air pressures during speech. *Journal of Speech and Hearing Research, 10,* 196–208.

Baken, R. J., & Orlikoff, R. F. (2000). *Clinical measurement of speech and voice* (2nd ed.). San Diego, CA: Singular.

Baylis, A., Chapman, K., Whitehill, T. L., Group, T. A. (2014). Validity and reliability of visual analog scaling for assessment of hypernasality and audible nasal emission in children with repaired cleft palate. *Cleft Palate-Craniofacial Journal.* Advance online publication.

Bloomer, H. (1953). Observations on palatopharyngeal movements in speech and deglutition. *Journal of Speech and Hearing Disorders, 18,* 230–246.

Bundy, E., & Zajac, D. J. (2006). Estimation of transpalatal Nasalance during production of voiced stop consonants by non-cleft speakers using an oral-nasal mask. *Cleft Palate-Craniofacial Journal, 43*(6), 691–701.

Bzoch, K. R. (1979). Measurement and assessment of categorical aspects of cleft palate speech. In K. R. Bzoch (Ed.), *Communicative disorders related to cleft lip and palate* (2nd ed.). Boston, MA: Little, Brown.

Conture, E. G. (1997). Evaluating childhood stuttering. In R. F. Curlee & G. M. Siegel (Eds.), *Nature and treatment of stuttering: New directions* (2nd ed.). Boston, MA: Allyn & Bacon.

Dalston, R. M, Martinkosky, S. J, & Hinton, V. A. (1987). Stuttering prevalence among patients at risk for velopharyngeal inadequacy: A preliminary investigation. *Cleft Palate Journal, 24*(3), 233–239.

Dalston, R. M., Warren, D. W., & Dalston, E. T. (1991a). Use of nasometry as a diagnostic tool for identifying patients with velopharyngeal impairment. *Cleft Palate Journal, 28,* 184.

Dalston, R. M., Warren, D. W., & Dalston, E. T. (1991b). A preliminary investigation concerning the use of nasometry in identifying hyponasality and/or nasal airway impairment. *Journal of Speech and Hearing Research, 34,* 11.

Dalston, R. M., Warren, D. W., Morr, K. E., & Smith, L. R. (1988). Intraoral pressure and its relationship to velopharyngeal inadequacy. *Cleft Palate Journal, 25,* 210–219.

Fahey, R., & Zajac, D. (2013, November). *Oral air pressure during speech production in children with repaired cleft palate.* Paper presented at the Annual Convention of the American Speech-Language-Hearing Association, Chicago, IL.

Fletcher, S. G. (1970). Theory and instrumentation for quantitative measurement of nasality. *Cleft Palate Journal, 7,* 601.

Fletcher, S. G. (1976). "Nasalance" vs. listener judgments of nasality. *Cleft Palate Journal, 13,* 31.

Fletcher, S. G., Adams, L., & McCutcheon (1989). Cleft palate speech assessment through oral-nasal acoustic measures. In K. R. Bzoch (Ed.), *Communicative disorders related to cleft lip and palate.* Boston, MA: College-Hill Press.

Gildersleeve-Neumann, C. E., & Dalston, R. M. (2001). Nasalance scores in noncleft individuals: Why not zero? *Cleft Palate-Craniofacial Journal, 38*(2), 106–111.

Golding-Kushner, K., Argamaso, R. V., Cotton, R. T., Grames L. M., Henningsson, G., Jones, D. L., . . . Marsh, J. L. (1990). Standardization for the reporting of nasopharyngoscopy and multiview videofluoroscopy: A report from an international working group. *Cleft Palate Journal, 27,* 337.

Henningsson, G., Kuehn, D. P., Sell, D., Sweeney, T., Trost-Cardamone, J. E, Whitehill, T. L., & Speech Parameters Group. (2008). Universal parameters for reporting speech outcomes in individuals with cleft palate. *Cleft Palate-Craniofacial Journal, 45*(1), 1–17.

Karnell, M. P. (1994). *Videoendoscopy: From velopharynx to larynx.* San Diego, CA: Singular.

Kent, R. D., Weismer, G., Kent, J. F., & Rosenbek, J. C. (1989). Toward phonetic intelligibility testing in dysarthria. *Journal of Speech and Hearing Disorders, 54,* 482–499.

Krochmal, D. J., Zajac, D. J., Alhudaib, O. M., Emodi, O., & van Aalst, J. A. (2013). The assessment of velopharyngeal function using nasal ram pressure testing following palatoplasty. *Cleft Palate-Craniofacial Journal, 50*(5), 542–547.

Kuehn, D. P., Imrey, P. B., Tomes, L., Jones, D. L., O'Gara, M. M., Seaver, E. J., Smith, B. E., Van Demark, D. R., & Wachtel, J. M. (2002). Efficacy of continuous positive airway pressure for treatment of hypernasality. *Cleft Palate-Craniofacial Journal, 39*(3), 267–276.

Kuehn, D. P., & Moller, K. T. (2000). Speech and language issues in the cleft palate population: State of the art. *Cleft Palate-Craniofacial Journal, 37,* 348–383.

Kummer, A. W. (2014). *Cleft palate and craniofacial anomalies: Effects on speech and resonance* (3rd ed.). Clifton Park, NY: Cengage Learning.

Laine, T., Warren, D. W., Dalston, R. M., & Morr, K. E. (1988). Screening of velopharyngeal closure based on nasal airflow rate measurements. *Cleft Palate Journal, 25,* 220–225.

Lass, N. J., & Pannbacker, M. (2015). Low-tech assessment of resonance disorders. *Evidence-Based Communication Assessment and Intervention, 9*(1), 43–50.

Lohmander, A., Willadsen, E., Persson, C., Henningsson, G., Bowden, M., & Hutters, B. (2009). Methodology for speech assessment in the Scandcleft project—an international randomized clinical trial on palatal surgery: experiences from a pilot study. *Cleft Palate-Craniofacial Journal, 46*(4), 347–362.

Lubker, J. F., & Moll, K. L. (1965). Simultaneous oral-nasal air flow measurements and cinefluorographic observations during speech production. *Cleft Palate Journal, 2,* 257–272.

MacKay, I. R. A., & Kummer, A. W. (1994). Simplified nasometric assessment procedures. In Kay Elemetrics Corp. (Ed.), *Instruction manual: Nasometer model 6200-3* (pp. 123–142). Lincoln Park, NJ: Kay Elemetrics Corp.

McWilliams, B. J., & Girdany, B. (1964). The use of televex in cleft palate research. *Cleft Palate Journal, 1,* 398–401.

McWilliams, B. J., Musgrave, R. H., & Crozier, P. A. (1968). The influence of head position upon velopharyngeal closure. *Cleft Palate Journal, 5,* 117–124.

McWilliams, B. J., & Philips, B. J. (1979). *Velopharyngeal incompetence: audio seminars in speech pathology.* Philadelphia, PA: W. B. Saunders.

Milenkovic, P. (2000). Time-frequency for 32-bit Windows (software program). Madison, WI.

Moll, K. L. (1960). Cinefluorgraphic techniques in speech research. *Journal of Speech and Hearing Research, 3,* 227–241.

Moll, K. L. (1965). A cinefluorographic study of velopharyngeal function in normals during various activities. *Cleft Palate Journal, 2,* 112–122.

Morris, S. R., Wilcox, K. A., & Schooling, T. L. (1995). The preschool speech intelligibility measure. *American Journal of Speech-Language Pathology, 4*(4), 22–27.

Peterson-Falzone, S. J., Trost-Cardamone, J. E., Karnell, M. P., & Hardin-Jones, M. A. (2006). *The clinician's guide to treating cleft palate speech.* St Louis, MO: Mosby Elsevier.

Plante, C., Zajac, D. J., Queiros, F., & Vallino, L. (2011). *Comparison of nasalance scores obtained with the nasometer and the nasality visualization system: Prolonged vowels and low-pressure sentences.* Presented at the Annual Meeting of the American Cleft Palate-Craniofacial Association, San Juan, Puerto Rico, April.

Schiavetti, N. (1992). Scaling procedures for the measurement of speech intelligibility. In R.D. Kent (Ed.), *Intelligibility in speech* disorders: Theory, measurement and management (pp. 11–34). Philadelphia, PA: John Benjamins.

Schuster, M., Maier, A., Haderlein, T., Nkenke, E., Wohlleben, U., Rosanowski, F., . . . Nöth, E. (2006). Evaluation of speech intelligibility for children with cleft lip and palate by means of automatic speech recognition. *International Journal of Pediatric Otorhinolaryngology, 70*, 1741–1747.

Searl, J., & Knollhoff, S. (2013). Oral pressure and nasal flow on /m/ and /p/ in 3- to 5-year-old children without cleft palate. *Cleft Palate Craniofacial Journal, 50*, 40–50.

Shelton, R. L., & Trier, W. C. (1976). Issues involved in the evaluation of velopharyngeal closure. *Cleft Palate Journal, 13*, 127–137.

Shriberg, L. D., & Kent, R. D. (2003). *Clinical phonetics* (3rd ed.). Boston, MA: Allyn & Bacon.

Skolnick, M. L. (1969). Video velopharyngography in patients with nasal speech, with emphasis on lateral pharyngeal motion in velopharyngeal closure. *Radiology, 93*, 747–755.

Skolnick, M. L. (1970). Videofluoroscopic examination of the velopharyngeal portal during phonation in lateral and base projections—a new technique for studying the mechanics of closure. *Cleft Palate Journal, 7*, 803–816.

Skolnick, M. L. (1977). A plea of an interdisciplinary approach to the radiological study of the velopharyngeal port. *Cleft Palate Journal, 14*, 329–330.

Skolnick, M. L., & Cohn, E. R. (1989). *Videofluoroscopic studies of speech in patients with cleft palate.* New York, NY: Springer-Verlag.

Skolnick, M. L., Glaser, E. R., & McWilliams, B. J. (1980). The use and limitations of the barium pharyngogram in the detection of velopharyngeal insufficiency. *Radiology, 135*(2), 301–304.

Skolnick, M. L., McCall, G. N., & Barnes, M. (1973). The sphincteric mechanism of velopharyngeal closure. *Cleft Palate Journal, 10*, 286–305.

Skolnick, M. L., Shprintzen, R. J., McCall, G. N., & Rakoff, S. (1975). Patterns of velopharyngeal closure in subjects with repaired cleft palate and normal speech: A multiview videofluoroscopic analysis. *Cleft Palate Journal, 12*, 369–376.

Smith, B. E., Guyette, T. W., Patil, Y., & Brannan, T. S. (2003). Pressure-flow measurements for selected nasal sound segments produced by normal children and adolescents. *Cleft Palate-Craniofacial Journal, 40*(2), 158–164.

Stevens, S. S. (1974). Perceptual magnitude and its measurement. In E. C. Caterette & M. P. Friedman (Eds.), *Handbook of perception* (Vol. 2, pp. 22–40). New York, NY: Academic Press.

Stevens, S. S. (1975). *Psychophysics: Introduction to its perceptual, neural and social prospects.* New York, NY: Wiley.

Subtelny, J. D. (1961). Roentgenography applied to the study of speech. In S. Pruzansky (Ed.), *Congenital anomalies of the face and associated structures* (pp. 314–322). Springfield, IL: Thomas.

Subtelny, J. D., Worth, J. H., & Sakuda, M. (1966). Intraoral pressure and rate of flow during speech. *Journal of Speech and Hearing Research, 9*, 498–519.

Thom, S. A., Hoit, J. D., Hixon, T. J., & Smith, A. E. (2006). Velopharyngeal function during vocalization in infants, *Cleft Palate-Craniofacial Journal, 43*, 539.

Vallino-Napoli, L. D., & Montgomery, A. A. (1997). Examination of the standard deviation of mean nasalance scores in subjects with cleft palate: Implications for clinical use. *Cleft Palate-Craniofacial Journal, 34*(6), 512–519.

Warren, D. W. (1964a). Velopharyngeal orifice size and upper pharyngeal pressure-flow patterns in normal speech. *Plastic and Reconstructive Surgery, 33*, 148–162.

Warren, D. W. (1964b). Velopharyngeal orifice size and upper pharyngeal pressure-flow patterns in cleft palate speech: A preliminary study. *Plastic and Reconstructive Surgery, 34*, 5–26.

Warren, D. W. (1979). Perci: A method for rating palatal efficiency. *Cleft Palate Journal, 16*, 279–285.

Warren, D. W., Dalston, R. M., Morr, K. E., Hairfield, W. M., & Smith, L. R. (1989). The speech regulating system: Temporal and aerodynamic responses to velopharyngeal inadequacy. *Journal of Speech and Hearing Research, 32,* 566–575.

Warren, D. W., & DuBois, A. (1964). A pressure-flow technique for measuring velopharyngeal orifice area during continuous speech. *Cleft Palate Journal, 1,* 52–71.

Weinberg, B., Noll, J. D., & Donohue, M. (1979). TONAR calibration: A brief note. *Cleft Palate Journal, 16,* 158.

Whitehill, T. L. (2002). Assessing intelligibility in speakers with cleft palate: A critical review of the literature. *Cleft Palate-Craniofacial Journal, 39,* 50–58.

Whitehill, T. L., Lee, A. S., & Chun, J. C. (2002). Direct magnitude estimation and interval scaling of hypernasality. *Journal of Speech, Language, and Hearing Research, 45*(1), 80–88.

Williams, W. N., & Eisenbach, C. R. (1981). Assessing VP function: The lateral still technique vs. cinefluorography. *Cleft Palate Journal, 18,* 45–50.

Williams, W. N., Henningsson, G., & Pegoraro-Krook, M. I. (1997). Radiographic assessment of velopharyngeal function for speech. In K. R. Bzoch (Ed.), *Commuicative disorders related to cleft lip and palate* (4th ed., pp. 347–386). Austin, TX: Pro-Ed.

Yates, C. C, McWilliams, B. J., & Vallino, L. D. (1990). The pressure-flow method: Some fundamental concepts. *Cleft Palate Journal, 27,* 193–198.

Yorkston, K. M., & Beukelman, D. R. (1978). A comparison of techniques for measuring intelligibility of dysarthric speech. *Journal of Communication Disorders, 11,* 499–512.

Zajac, D. J. (2000). Pressure-flow characteristics of /m/ and /p/ production in speakers without cleft palate: Developmental findings. *Cleft Palate-Craniofacial Journal, 37,* 468–477.

Zajac, D. J. (2003). *Pressure-flow characteristics of speakers with repaired cleft palate.* Paper presented at the Annual Meeting of the American Cleft Palate-Craniofacial Association, Asheville, NC.

Zajac, D. J., Lutz, R., & Mayo, R (1996). Microphone sensitivity as a source of variation in nasalance scores. *Journal of Speech and Hearing Research, 39,* 1228.

Zajac, D. J., & Preisser, J. (2015). Age and phonetic influences on velar flutter as a component of nasal turbulence in children with repaired cleft palate. *Cleft Palate-Craniofacial Journal.* Advance online publication.

Zajac, D. J., van Aalst, J., Vallino, L, & Napoli, J. (2011). *Nasal ram pressure as an indicator of velopharyngeal closure during stop consonants in 2 year-olds following palate repair.* Paper presented at the Annual Meeting of the American Cleft Palate-Craniofacial Association, San Juan, PR.

Zraick, R. I., & Liss, J. M. (2000). A comparison of equal-appearing interval scaling and direct magnitude estimation of nasal voice quality. *Journal of Speech, Language, and Hearing Research, 43*(4), 979–988.

UNC Craniofacial Center Speech-Language Assessment: Child/Adolescent/Adult

UNC DENTISTRY   UNC Craniofacial Center Speech-Language Assessment: Child/Adolescent/Adult

Name_____ UNCH#_____ DOE_____
Dx_____ DOB_____
Date of last eval/Recs_____ Age_____
Background/Pt.Concerns_____
_____
_____
_____

SURGICAL Hx:	**ACADEMIC Hx:**
Lip repair_____	Grade/School_____
Palate repair_____	Special Services_____
Pharyngeal Flap/SP_____	Speech Tx: 0= Never/In Past
Fistula Repair_____	1=Articulation:_____
Bone Graft_____	2=Language:_____
PE Tubes_____	3=Voice_____
Lip/Nasal revision(s)_____	4=Other_____
Tonsillectomy/Adenoidectomy____	Frequency: _____ X per week/month
Other_____	Therapist:_____

ORAL-MOTOR:

Alveolar Ridge: Intact   Unrepaired   ONF_____
Hard Palate: Intact   Unrepaired   ONF_____
Soft Palate: Intact   Unrepaired   ONF_____
          bifid uvula   thin/V-shape   pal. notch
Velar Elevation: active   limited   none   CNT
          symmetrical   asymmetrical
LPW Motion: active   limited   none   CNT
     symmetrical   asymmetrical   Passavant's
Gag: hyperactive   active   limited   none   CNT
Tonsils: WNL   hypertrophied R/L   CNT
Adenoids: not visible   small/mod./large   CNT
Lip mobility: WNL   limited   CNT
Tongue mobility: WNL   limited ankylosed   CNT
Nasal regurgitation: none   occasional   frequent
          liquids   solids
Dental Occlusion: I   II   III
Cross/Open Bite: _____
Notes:

ARTICULATION:
0= CNT
1= WNL
2= Dev/Phonological
3= Obligatory/Dentition
4= Compensatory (for VPI)
Errors:_____
_____
_____

Intelligibility: 0= CNT
1=WNL
2= Mild
3= Moderate
4= Severe
Single Word _____%

COMPENSATIONS:
0= None
1= Glottal stop
2= Pharyngeal fricative
3= Pharyngeal stop
4= Pharyngeal affricate
5= Nasal fricative
6= Other_____

Additional Errors:
1=Mid-dorsum palatal stop
2=Posterior nasal fricative

LANGUAGE:
Receptive: 0= CNT   **Expressive:** 0= CNT
1= WNL   1= WNL
2= Mildly Delayed   2= Mildly Delayed
3= Moderately Delayed   3= Moderately Delayed
4= Severely Delayed   4= Severely Delayed
Test Scores:

VOICE Quality: O=CNT   **Intensity:** 0=CNT
WNL   WNL
Mildly Disordered   Reduced
Moderately Disordered   Excessive
Severely Disordered
Describe_____

FLUENCY: CNT   WNL   needs further testing

continues

HEARING: 0= CNT		
	Right ear	**Left ear**
Tympanometry	_____	_____
Pure Tone Screen	_____	_____
Fail R: 500 1K 2K 4K Hz		
Fail L: 500 1K 2K 4K Hz		

Hypernasality: 0= CNT	**Hyponasality:** 0= CNT
1= WNL	1=WNL
2= mild	2=mild
3= moderate	3= moderate
4= severe	4= severe
5= inconsistent	5= inconsistent
6= assimilative	6= cul-de-sac

VELOPHARYNGEAL ADEQUACY: 0= CNT
1= WNL/Adequate
2= marginal
3= inadequate

Nose pinch /i/: 1= no change 2= more oral 3= cul-de-sac

Notes/Comments:

Nasal Obstruction: 0= CNT

Right:	**Left:**
1= WNL right	1=WNL left
2= partial right	2= partial left
3= total right	3= total left

Potential source: _____

Nasal Air Emission: 0= CNT

Right:	**Left:**
1= WNL	1= WNL
2= visible p t k s	2= visible p t k s
3= audible p t k s	3= audible p t k s
4= inconsistent	4= inconsistent
5= compensatory	5= compensatory
6= nasal grimace	6= nasal grimace

PRESSURE FLOW:
Completed During Evaluation: Yes   No
VP Status: **Findings/Notes:**
1=WNL/Adequate
2=marginal
3=inadequate

NASOMETRY:
Completed During Evaluation: Yes   No
Zoo passage: _____ % (M/SD 15.5±4.8%)
Nasal sentences: _____% (M/SD 61.1%±6.6%)
LP sentences: _____ %
SNAP Oral Syllables: WNL   hypernasal
SNAP Nasal Syllables: WNL   hyponasal

Reduced nasalance with increased loudness? _____

ASSESSMENT SUMMARY/IMPRESSIONS:

___ VP dysfunction: marginal   inadequate
___ hypernasality
___ audible NE
___ compensatory artic
___ Articulation/phonological disorder
___ Other:

___ Language delay/impairment
___ Hearing impairment
___ Voice/fluency disorder
___ Resonance disorder unrelated to VPI
___ Dysarthria/apraxia

RECOMMENDATIONS:

___Complete speech/language evaluation
___Re-evaluation in ____months
___Initial palate repair
___Televex or Nasoendoscopy
___Secondary palate surgery/ONF repair
___ Audiological or ENT assessement
___Further evaluation for_____

___Continue/Enroll in speech/language therapy____times per week
___Suggested treatment goals include:
   1)_____
   2)_____
   3)_____
___See attached recommended speech therapy techniques
___Return for annual team evaluation in _____ year(s)/month(s)

_____
Speech/Language Pathologist

APPENDIX 9–B

Oral Examination Checklist

ORAL EXAMINATION CHECKLIST

Name: DOB: Age: Date of Exam:

Diagnosis:

Lip Structure   □ Normal   □ Abnormal   **Lip Function**   □ Normal   □ Abnormal
                    □ Scarred   □ Lips open at rest
                    □ Cleft   □ Asymmetrical at rest
                    □ Lip pits   □ Notched
                                                         □ Asymmetrical smile (L, R)

Comments:

Dentition   □ Normal   □ Abnormal
                    □ Maloclusion (Class I, Class II, Class III)
                    □ Open bite
                    □ Deep bite
                    □ Crossbite
                    □ Missing teeth
                    □ Interdental spaces

Comments:

Hard Palate   □ Normal   □ Abnormal
                    □ Cleft
                    □ Fistula (alveolus, hard palate, soft palate)
                    □ High
                    □ Narrow
                    □ Collapsed

Comments:

Uvula   □ Normal   □ Abnormal   **Soft Palate Elevation on "ah"**   □ Normal   □ Abnormal
                □ Bifid   □ Asymmetrial (L R)
                □ Absent   □ No elevation

Soft Palate   □ Normal   □ Submucous cleft palate (SMCP)

Pharyngeal Flap: □ None   □ Visualized

Comments:

Tonsils   □ Normal   □ Abnormal
                    □ Enlarged
                    □ Absent

Comments:

Tongue Structure   □ Normal   □ Abnormal   **Tongue Function**   □ Normal   □ Abnormal
                    □ Macroglossia   □ Protrudes at rest
                    □ Mircroglossia   □ Lateralizes to left
                    □ Deviates to one side at rest   □ Lateralizes to right
                    □ Asymmetrical at rest   □ Cannot elevate
                                                           □ Cannot depress

Comments:

10

School-Based Intervention

Dennis M. Ruscello

INTRODUCTION

Providing services to children with oral clefts can be a challenge for the school-based speech-language pathologist (SLP) for a variety of reasons. Most obvious is the fact that children with clefts constitute a low incidence population, and practitioners in the schools often report that their academic background and clinical experience are very limited in this area (Bedwinek, Kummer, Rice, & Grames, 2010). School SLPs indicate that in order to serve this population in an effective manner, there needs to be communication between the SLP and child's craniofacial team along with continuing education and professional development opportunities. The findings regarding lack of preparation in providing services to low incidence populations are consistent with other survey data reported by Vallino, Lass, Bunnell, and Pannbacker (2008). Such findings presented in the literature indicate the need to identify strategies for developing collaborations with a child's craniofacial team SLP and inservice educational opportunities for dealing with children

who present with low incidence communication disorders such as cleft palate. This chapter will deal with the issues identified by presenting the school SLP with collaborative strategies and assessment and treatment knowledge that may be utilized with this population. Prior to this discussion, information regarding developmental issues in this population will be discussed briefly, so that the SLP has a basis for understanding coexisting factors that may present in the population of school children with oral clefts.

NEUROPSYCHOLOGICAL, BEHAVIORAL, AND ACADEMIC VARIABLES

Richman, McCoy, Conrad, and Nopoulos (2012) provided a recent summary of the neuropsychological, behavioral, and academic outcomes research that has been conducted with children who were born with clefts across infancy, school age, and adolescence and young adulthood. In general, the school-age years are marked by children's development of self-concept and social skills that are necessary for interacting with authority figures and peers. In their review of the literature, the authors found that psychosocial and behavioral problems may be present in the child with cleft palate, if academic performance, relationships with peers, behavior, and disposition are at variance with a child's peer group. There can be a tendency for the problems to interact with the youngster's temperament and influence negatively behavior, self-concept, and socioemotional adjustment. The authors indicate that during this critical developmental period, adjustment is very important, as is a positive self-concept.

Recent brain imaging data suggest that there are differences in brain structure between children with clefts and matched controls. These findings have led researchers to propose that the neurological differences support a tentative hypothesis that genetic and biological factors may significantly influence cleft type, severity, and long-term outcomes in areas of cognitive development and performance. During the school years, cerebral maturation is occurring in children with associated changes in attention, concentration, and executive control. Studies of cognitive-linguistic performance typically show subtle language discrepancies in the cleft population. The results of different studies suggest that language impairment varies as a function of cleft type. Children with cleft lip and palate tend to exhibit expressive impairment in language skills such as verbal fluency and rapid information processing. Children with isolated cleft palate often show global deficits in both expressive and receptive language. Academic learning and reading disabilities have also been identified but not with a specific cleft type.

In summary, children with cleft palate are at risk for various problems across cognitive, linguistic, and social domains. It has also been identified in recent imaging data that neurological differences between children with clefts and control subjects exist. Language impairment and academic problems such as reading and learning disabilities are potential problems that may also be part of a child's clinical makeup. It is important that the school SLP be aware of the potential for coexisting problems, which are in addition to the speech and facial variations that are generally recognized as the stigmata of cleft lip and palate. The SLP needs to comprehend the potential totality of the cleft condition in order to work effectively with the child, craniofacial team, teachers, and parents.

ROLES OF THE SPEECH-LANGUAGE PATHOLOGIST

The SLP will function in different roles depending on the child in question. The most frequent role is that of treating the communication problems of a child who is managed by a craniofacial team (Karnell, Bailey, Johnson, Dragan, & Canady, 2005). General or explicit recommendations are made, and the school SLP is expected to carry out those recommendations, despite evidence cited previously that most school practitioners lack the knowledge and skills to provide appropriate assessment or treatment services. This is a practice dilemma, but there are strategies that can be employed to implement a successful collaboration and develop the requisite skills and knowledge base. Grames (2008) indicates that the child with a craniofacial anomaly requires a collaborative effort among all parties involved. The team SLP and school SLP must understand that the practice cultures of each are quite different, but both parties must agree to share control of the patient and power. It must be a coordinative relationship, not a subordinate relationship. In addition, each SLP must also be aware of his or her limitations and seek assistance and guidance, when necessary.

In sum, Grames is telling us that the overall goal of collaboration is to improve the communication skills of the child within the boundaries of one's knowledge and skills. In achieving this goal, we need to overcome any "turf issues" that may surface. For example, the therapeutic cultures of the hospital-based SLP and school-based SLP differ in terms of intervention. The hospital-based SLP is typically working from a medical reimbursement model and seeks to develop an inclusive intervention plan in conjunction with other professionals, while the school-based SLP is working on the child's communication skills within the context of its impact on school achievement and certain eligibility constraints that are legislatively mandated. In sum, collaboration means that one party is not subservient to the other, and there is a division of power with the child and parents, because each professional is responsible for different aspects of the child's care. Each demands respect and recognition for the skill set that each brings to the child's treatment plan.

COLLABORATIVE MODELS

Table 10–1 presents five different collaborative models described by Grames (2004). Note that each may be of use, but it will depend on the needs of the child, the parents, the purpose of the collaboration,

Table 10–1. Collaborative Models That May Be Employed in Treatment

Models of Collaboration	Key Components
1. Parallel Delivery	Each SLP is responsible for a certain aspect of the child's treatment. There is no overlap in service provision.
2. Informal Consultation	A consultant SLP provides guidance to the school SLP concerning the child's communication disorder. This is an informal arrangement with the consultant who relies on patient information provided by the school SLP.
3. Formal Consultation	The team SLP provides diagnostic services, which are communicated to the school SLP for implementation. It is a cooperative venture between the two entities.
4. Co-Provision of Care	The team SLP and school SLP share common treatment goals. They meet periodically to discuss progress and implement various agreed upon modifications in the treatment plan.
5. Collaborative Expansion	There is an expansion of the collaborative team to include other medical and educational specialists who may assist in achieving certain care goals. The child's parents may also be enlisted to help with the care plan.

and the recommendations of the SLPs. Keep in mind that successful implementation will depend in large part on shared power and understanding of each practitioner's work culture.

The first model is that of parallel delivery or distributed service delivery. The team SLP and school SLP provide individual services that differ in terms of the child's communication needs. For example, a child may present with compensatory speech sound errors and a coexisting language disorder. The team SLP may choose to work on the compensatory errors, because of his or her expertise in this area, while the school SLP will see the child for treatment of the language impairment. The school SLP is comfortable conducting language therapy and is able to work with the child's educators in implementing a curriculum-based language program. Each practitioner has agreed on a defined role that does not overlap but is designed to improve the overall communication skills of the client.

The second model is the informal consultation model and involves the employ of a consultant who provides resource information to the school SLP. Grames indicates that the client and family may or may not be informed about the use of a consultant. In the case of the latter, patient identification information would not be shared with the consultant. The consultant would rely on the patient data supplied by the school SLP, which must be accurate to insure that appropriate consultative services are delivered.

The third or formal consultative model defines explicitly the roles for the team and school SLPs. For instance, the team SLP conducts diagnostic services and communicates with the parents and school practitioner in terms of treatment recommendations. The school SLP carries out the treatment recommendations and shares progress notes with the team SLP. There is an open line of communication between the two entities, so that each is aware of what has been done and what needs to be done. This type of consultative model is probably the most frequently utilized, but it is typically implemented on an informal basis. As mentioned previously, shared power and understanding each practitioner's job culture are important to the success of such a consultative endeavor.

The fourth type of collaborative model is that of co-provision of care. Each of the professionals provides treatment in the context of their expertise. For instance, the team SLP may provide direct phonetic treatment of the youngster's compensatory errors through drill and practice, because he or she is well versed in techniques for modifying compensatory errors. The school SLP has expertise using a language-based approach to speech sound treatment and uses language facilitating techniques to incorporate the target sounds in discourse activities. The school practitioner also trains the child's teachers to use the facilitating techniques in the classroom. Both parties communicate periodically via e-mail, phone calls, and progress notes to ensure continuity of services. Parents also play an important role and need to be involved in information sharing and decision making.

The final model to be discussed is known as collaborative expansion. This is a cooperative variation, which consists of team members, the school SLP, and the family, if needed. There is a common goal or goals that need to be achieved, but an assisted effort from all involved is required. For example, a child with a significant VPI needs to undergo naso-endoscopy, but the child is apprehensive about the procedure. The team and school SLPs might work on the development of correct oral placements for the bilabial and alveolar plosives to facilitate an accurate assessment of the mechanism during speech. The team physician and psychologist may discuss the procedure in "child terms" and possibly display the scope, so that the child is familiar with the procedure. In addition, the parents may also play a supportive role in discussing what is planned and trying to minimize any apprehensiveness demonstrated by the child.

COLLABORATIVE STRATEGIES

Each of the models can be employed, but it will depend on the needs of the child and the constraints of the situation. Nevertheless, most children need coordinated services, unless all communication services are provided by the team. This is generally not the case, and SLPs in the schools need to include these children in their caseloads. Please refer to Table 10–2 for a summary of actions that the school and team SLPs can carry out to develop and enhance a collaborative interaction (Cohn,

Table 10–2. Actions That Should Be Considered in Developing and Maintaining a Successful Collaborative Interaction

School SLP	Team SLP
Provide contact information and preferred method of contact.	Provide contact information and preferred method of contact.
Obtain written parent consent to share information.	Obtain written parent consent to share information.
Maintain contact with the child's parents and make sure that you are apprised of the child's team appointments and other relevant medical issues.	Respond to queries that the parents and school SLP may have regarding current and future care.
Provide progress reports for the parents and team SLP.	Review progress reports and make recommendations.
Obtain reports from the team and modify treatment plan as needed.	Provide in-depth assessments including instrumental assessments when necessary for continued patient care.
Brief school colleagues on the child's status or needs when necessary.	Brief parents and school SLP regarding the child's communication status.
Monitor hearing status.	Monitor hearing status.
Attend team clinics with the child and parent.	
Obtain relevant medical data.	Maintain relevant medical data.
Maintain an open line of communication.	Maintain an open line of communication.
Be aware and sensitive to cultural differences of the family.	Be aware and sensitive to cultural differences of the family.

2013; LeDuc, 2008; Trost-Cardamone, 2013). Although many appear to be commonsense activities and are part of everyday practice, both parties have active caseloads, so conscious focus aids in establishing and maintaining a good collaborative relationship. For instance, contact between parties is very important, and determining the best method makes for the efficient flow of information. An e-mail contact for some is more effective than trying to reach someone via phone contact. Periodic reporting from the school SLP is another excellent strategy. In some cases, the team SLP sees a child for a brief clinic visit approximately two to three times a year, while the school SLP provides weekly treatment. Reports can alert the team SLP to certain problems that may require in-depth assessment, which include instrumental study generally not available in a local school system. For example, it may be necessary to conduct an aerodynamic study, so that air pressure and air flow may be measured for pressure sounds and inferences regarding the status of velopharyngeal closure for speech may be made and correlated with other instrumental techniques and perceptual indices.

Finally, the school and team SLPs need to be sensitive to cultural differences that may be present. The United States consists of a diverse group of people with different cultural beliefs and values (Torres, 2013). In the case of cleft palate, SLPs are dealing with a variety of communication disorders secondary to a birth defect that includes facial disfigurement. Even if one feels that a family in question is acculturated, Torres indicates that families very often retreat to entities that provide comfort and familiarity in emotionally charged situations. Understanding these differences and how they influence the dynamics of family relations is very important for the SLP to be cognizant of in service delivery. In summary communication, cooperation, and respect for each other are critical to providing the best possible collaborative services.

ASSESSMENT

Assessment activities require the SLP to apply clinical skills that are appropriate for children with cleft palate. The school SLP will generally collaborate with the team SLP in terms of implementing treatment recommendations via one of the models that was discussed. Consequently, it is important to have a protocol that enables the collection of assessment data in a consistent and reliable manner. Previously, a protocol for assessment of the child was presented in Chapter 9. Key components of this protocol are discussed below. If a child is in treatment, it is recommended that the protocol be administered at least twice per school year. Previously, the reader has been introduced to the concepts of compensatory, obligatory, and developmental errors in Chapter 8. Compensatory and obligatory errors differ significantly from the production errors of children, whose speech sound production deficits cannot be attributed to any type of structural deficit (Ruscello, 2008a). The school SLP must become familiar with these error types and their perceptual characteristics. Please refer to Table 10–3 for a brief review. There are several resources that include digital speech samples of various compensatory errors that may be used to acquaint the practitioner with the perceptual characteristics of cleft palate speech, and readers are strongly urged to review these (American Cleft Palate-Craniofacial Association; Peterson-Falzone, Trost-

Table 10–3. A Summary of the Different Speech Sound Categories and Related Information

Error Category	Developmental	Obligatory	Compensatory	Phoneme-Specific Nasal Emission
	Developmental errors observed in the speech of children with or without cleft palate. Errors may be outgrown or require treatment.	Speech sound errors that are related to some variation in oral structure. Errors are generally not responsive to speech therapy.	Speech sound errors that are a function of VPI. Treatment is necessary to develop correct oral placements.	Nasal articulation used in place of a fricative sounds(s) but not all fricative sounds.
Causal Factor	Mislearning	Oral structure variations	VPI	Mislearning
Surface Errors	Primarily, sound substitutions and deletions	Primarily, sound distortions due to place of articulation errors such as the dentalization of sounds	Primarily, sound substitutions of place of articulation and generally posterior to the VP valve such as glottal stops	Nasal substitution

Cardamone, Karnell, & Harden-Jones, 2006; Trost-Cardamone, 2013; Vallino & Ruscello, in preparation).

In addition, the protocol can be used to refer a client to a team when such cases are identified through screening programs or referrals from other educational specialists. Any child who presents with hypernasal speech or compensatory errors should be referred to a team for assessment. In addition, the SLP may identify a child with a repaired cleft who is not being followed by a team, and the child should be referred. Remember that the referral should first be discussed with the child's caregivers. Upon agreement, the team may be contacted and written permission from the parents given to forward relevant records and other information. If unsure where to refer, you may contact the American Cleft Palate-Craniofacial Association (http://www.acpa-cpf.org/team_care/) or the Cleft Palate Foundation (http://www.cleftline.org/parents-individuals/team-care/) for a listing of teams in your locale.

Protocol

The suggested protocol has four subsections that are summarized in Table 10–4, and the form is presented in Appendix 10–A. It has been adapted from the work of Henningsson et al. (2008) and Trost-Cardamone (2013).

Table 10-4. The Components of the Protocol and the Information That Is Collected

Protocol Subsections	Information
I. Identification and classification information	This is a brief section that consists of identifying information such as the name of the client, cleft type, additional anomalies, school treatment history, progress in treatment, and hearing status.

II. Assessment information	Components of the assessment
	1. Oral examination
	2. Speech assessment
	  A. Words
	  B. Sentences
	  C. Conversational speech
	  D. Resonance assessment
	  E. Voice assessment
	  F. Stimulability

III. Assessment findings	A summary of the findings.
IV. Summary and recommendations	A brief summary of the major findings is provided. Recommendations are made based on the findings of the assessment and the status of the child's treatment plan.

Identification and Classification Information

The first subsection is one of identifying information that is useful to both parties. It helps the school SLP focus on the child's presenting problems and assists the team SLP recall and focus on the child's presenting problems, know what is being treated, and the current outcome.

Oral Examination and Speech Assessment

This section includes the oral examination and a comprehensive speech evaluation. The oral examination is designed to examine the structure and function of the oral speech mechanism and identify any structural, sensory, or motor variations that my adversely affect speech production skills. Note that in most cases, significant motor or sensory problems would typically have been identified prior to the current testing. A major focus would be to identify structural variations. The SLP may use a standardized measure or self-developed instrument to obtain observations. Some of the standard observations in regard to structure (anatomy) and function (physiology) that pertain to children with cleft palate are presented in the protocol. For an in-depth review of oral anatomy and physiology, please refer to Chapter 1. Figure 10–1 shows a youngster with missing upper incisors and potential obligatory error.

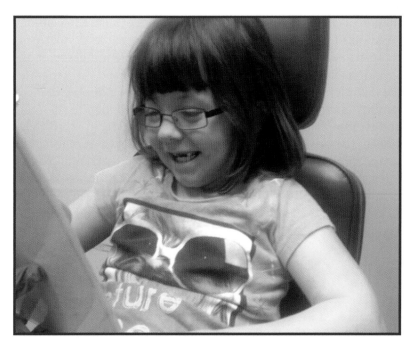

Figure 10–1. School-aged child with missing upper incisors and potential obligatory articulation error.

As previously reviewed in Chapter 8, dental, occlusal, and other oral anomalies are frequently found in the population of children with cleft palate, and they may be an obstacle to achieving correct speech sound production. They are generally obligatory errors and are not responsive to speech therapy. Dental, orthodontic, or surgical interventions are typically necessary to create an oral environment that is conducive to correct oral placement for obligatory errors. For example, a client with an open bite may exhibit distortion errors for sibilants such as the alveolars /s, z/. Intervention is necessary to create a dental environment that is conducive to precise sibilant production, rather than trying to modify tongue position. Other obligatory errors include hypernasality (resonance disorder), nasal emission, nasal turbulence, reduced intraoral pressure, and sound distortions due to the presence of oronasal fistulae (Golding-Kushner, 2001). Appropriate targets for treatment are compensatory and residual developmental errors. Compensatory errors include such speech sound substitutions as glottal stops, velar fricatives, pharyngeal fricatives, and pharyngeal stops. Please note that the compensatory errors are used by the child as substitutions for oral pressure sounds or coproduced with an oral placement (Trost-Cardamone, 2009). That is, some children will articulate an oral sound simultaneous with a posterior production. For example, a youngster might articulate /t/ and simultaneously valve a glottal stop, so that there is a coproduction. Perceptually, the SLP needs to have the auditory skills to identify such productions.

The speech assessment section needs to be comprehensive, because of the possible coexistence of other speech disorders in this population of children. In addition, it enables the school SLP to identify speech sound error types (compensatory, obligatory, and developmental), determine the impact of the disorder(s) on other listeners (intelligibility and severity), examine stimulability, establish eligibility for receiving services, determine progress or lack thereof, and provide current performance data for school status reports, the child's parents, and team SLP.

Word-Level Assessment

A standardized test(s) can be administered such as the *Goldman-Fristoe Test of Articulation* (2nd ed.) (2000), *Arizona Articulation Proficiency Scale* (3rd ed.) (2000), or *Templin-Darley Tests of Articulation* (1960). The *Templin-Darley Tests of Articulation* include the *Iowa Pressure Articulation Test*, which may be used to assess the production of speech sounds that require the generation of oral pressure. General regulations for school eligibility require standardized testing and multiple measures of speech sound production. In addition, the application of developmental normative data are considered. However, it should be noted that obligatory and compensatory errors are nondevelopmental sound variations. Obligatory errors are not responsive to treatment due to structural causal problems, whereas compensatory errors are the sequelae of VPI and the targets of treatment.

The protocol also includes clinician-devised word sets that can also be pictured. Remember that in terms of speech sound production, the pressure consonants (plosives, fricatives, and affricates) are most problematic for children with clefts and VPI. Vowel and oral sonorant speech sounds provide information on the child's resonance. Guidelines for the de-

velopment of such clinician-devised materials are available from Trost-Cardamone (2013) and Henningsson et al. (2008) and have been used to generate the word items. A listing of potential word items is included in Appendix 10–A.

In addition to word items, it is also recommended that at least 20 to 25 short sentences be used imitatively (Henningsson et al., 2008) to assess the production of pressure sounds in context. The criteria for construction of the stimuli are similar to that of the word list with the exception that five of the sentence items should contain nasals without pressure consonants, but oral sonorants may be included. Examples taken from Trost-Cardamone (2013) are

/p/ Puppy will pull a rope.

/s/ Sissy saw Sally race.

/g/ Give Aggie a hug.

/n/ Anna knew no one.

A complete list prepared by Trost-Cardamone is included in Appendix 10–A.

A 3- to 5-min sample of conversational speech will allow for judgment of spontaneous connected speech and its impact on a listener. Various procedures such as storytelling, story retelling, interactive play, interaction with a caregiver, or interaction with peers may be used to elicit the sample.

Resonance Assessment

Resonance disorders coexist and are assessed by the examiner during the production of vowels, oral sonorants, and nasals (see Chapter 9). The SLP needs to determine if the child is hypernasal, hyponasal, or presents with mixed nasality. The speech materials described previously can be used for this purpose along with some other measures. The cul-de-sac testing procedure (see Chapter 9) is a low-technology technique that is utilized. The testing is as follows:

Cul-de-sac testing:

The child is instructed to produce the high vowels /i/ and /u/ in a prolonged manner, while the SLP or child alternately opens and closes the nostrils with digital pressure. A change in resonance under the two conditions is indicative of hypernasal resonance.

Another assessment measure requires the child to read or produce imitatively the Zoo passage (Fletcher, 1972). This is a reading passage that contains no nasal consonants and provides information on the presence of hypernasal resonance. Finally, the child's production of nasal consonants in word, sentence, and conversational testing material allows for judgment of hyponasality or the lack of nasal resonance during the production of nasal speech sounds.

Intelligibility

A rating of intelligibility is based on the SLP's overall assessment of the client's communication across the different levels of evaluation. Intelligibility is defined by Yorkston, Beukelman, Strand, and Hakel (2010) as the degree to which a listener understands another speaker. According to the authors, intelligibility is a composite of the communication disorder and any compensatory strategies that are utilized by the speaker. Whitehill (2002) carried out a review of cleft palate literature and identified several issues related to the employ of intelligibility measures

including the type of procedure used to estimate intelligibility. For this proposed assessment tool, a 5-point interval rating scale is proposed.

Stimulability

Stimulability for speech sound errors is the final component of the assessment (Golding-Kushner & Shprintzen, 2011). Speech sounds in error are selected and presented to the child. The child is asked to *watch the SLP and imitate a model produced by the SLP*. Depending on the child and circumstances, he or she may be asked to produce the speech sound errors at the isolation, syllable, and word levels, whichever is appropriate. If the child can imitate the models successfully, he or she is stimulable, and the prognosis for future phonetic treatment is positive. Please note that stimulability testing is not only designed to examine oral placement, but we are also interested in the impact of stimulability on oral pressure generation and resonance. That is, is there also a change in VPI when a child is stimulable for error productions? This would be a very positive finding for a child who presents with VPI in terms of intervention.

Assessment Findings

This portion of the protocol allows the SLP to record the assessment findings. There are separate subsections for reporting speech sound production errors, resonance balance, and phonatory observations (D'Antonio, Muntz, Providence, & Marsh, 1988; Kummer, 2001a). There is also a section for rating overall communicative intelligibility and severity. In addition, there is a portion to report the results of stimulability testing.

Summary and Recommendations

The final section of the protocol is a brief summary of the assessment and recommendations based on the assessment. The SLP writes a brief summary of the findings and can also provide specific status, referral, and other recommendations. For example, the school SLP may recommend that certain instrumental testing be conducted such as endoscopy or that a referral be made for some specific problem that was identified during the testing.

TREATMENT

As discussed in the assessment section, treatment also entails the application of unique clinical skills. Remember that clinical expertise in this low incidence population is a composite of acquiring the necessary knowledge base through study and interaction with colleagues, developing the auditory perceptual skills requisite to identifying cleft palate speech production errors, and applying clinical concepts in assessment and treatment. Initially, general treatment concepts will be discussed, followed by treatment recommendations that will be geared to specific sound classes and individual speech sounds.

General Treatment Concepts

1. There is disagreement regarding the theoretical characterization of cleft palate speech errors. Some authors have proposed that the sound system errors are phonologically based (Chapman, 1993; Pamplona & Ysunza, 1999), while others have proposed a phonetic explanation for the errors. For example, Golding-Kushner (2001)

has stated that a glottal stop is a physiologically based error, not a phonologically based error. This explanation assumes an error in motor output, and not an error at the linguistic output level. It is important to note that a physiological cause underlies many of the errors. Others (Trost-Cardamone & Bernthal, 1993) have also taken this position, and treatment concepts in this chapter will be based on a phonetic rationale.

2. Children with cleft lip and palate are typically followed by a cleft palate craniofacial team, but treatment is frequently carried out by community-based SLPs through some type of formal or informal collaboration. There are different collaborative models that may be employed and have been discussed previously. Regardless of the model utilized, shared power and understanding of each practitioner's work culture are important in developing and maintaining a productive collaboration. It is also important to note that one of the key factors in maintaining a successful collaboration is keeping an open line of communication.

3. Generally, cleft lip repair is done between the ages of 2 and 3 months, and palate repair is carried out between 8 and 14 months of age. If the alveolus, which is that portion of the maxilla providing support for the dentition, is cleft, closure via bone graft is typically delayed until there is eruption of the primary dentition and establishment that the permanent teeth are developing in the area of the cleft. In terms of age, this can range between 7 and 12 years of age (Swift, 2009). SLPs need to be mindful of the fact that prior to repair of the alveolus, there is typically an oral-nasal fistula in that

anatomical location due to the lack of fusion of bony and soft tissue (gum).

4. Children who have undergone successful palatal surgery prior to 12 to 14 months of age will generally develop normal speech. According to Morris (1992), approximately 75% of children undergoing palatal repair develop normal speech.

5. Most children who present with VPI after their initial surgery will need additional management. Generally, treatment options may include a secondary surgical repair(s) or the use of a speech appliance (see Chapter 11).

6. Treatment should be directed to the modification of compensatory errors. If the child presents with VPI, treatment of compensatory errors should not be delayed until secondary surgery or prosthetic intervention is undertaken. The type of therapy will vary as a function of the child's chronological age and level of development. There is evidence that the elimination of compensatory errors has a positive effect on velopharyngeal movement for speech (Henningsson & Isberg, 1986). Compensatory errors include glottal stops, nasal fricatives, velar fricatives, pharyngeal fricatives, pharyngeal stops, and mid-dorsum palatal stops. Correct place of articulation can stimulate velopharyngeal movement; however, hypernasality and nasal emission may continue to some degree. Note that hypernasality is a resonance disorder and nasal emission is an articulatory disorder, and both are obligatory because of VPI.

7. Children enrolled in speech treatment and undergoing secondary surgical repair may recommence treatment with a doctor's clearance. Speech treatment does not need to be delayed for a long period of time (Golding-Kushner, 2001).

8. Middle ear infections and fluctuating hearing loss are very common in this population, and the SLP should be cognizant of the problem (McWilliams, Morris, & Shelton, 1990). The SLP needs to alert the child's parents, teachers, and other caregivers about the potential negative effects of hearing loss on speech and language development.

9. Many children with cleft palate are at risk for language delay and academic learning problems; consequently, interventions may be needed for language and academic learning issues (Peterson-Falzone, Hardin-Jones, & Karnell, 2010).

10. The SLP should be alert to the fact that there is a small subset of children who will present with phoneme-specific nasal emission. As reviewed in Chapter 8, this is a sound substitution of mislearning and should not be confused with structural-based VPI. It involves channeling air and acoustic sound energy through the nose during the production of a fricative sound or sounds but not all fricative sounds. The cause is attributed to phonological mislearning during the developmental period (see Chapter 8). Phoneme-specific nasal emission is often used in substitution of /s, z/, and the problem is amenable to speech treatment; there is no structural problem with the velopharyngeal mechanism.

11. Most children with cleft palate do not have oral muscle weakness. Nonspeech oral motor treatment procedures (NSOMEs) such as blowing, sucking, or specific resistance exercises to improve lip or tongue strength

are not appropriate for treatment. In addition, such oral motor strengthening techniques have not been successful in improving velopharyngeal movement for speech (Ruscello, 2008b; Skahan, Watson, & Lof, 2007).

Evidence Base

Prior to discussing treatment techniques, the SLP needs to be aware that the evidence base for different treatments is not supported by substantial research. There is some evidence from randomized studies, cohort studies, case studies, descriptive studies, and expert opinion (Bessell, Sell, Whiting, Roulstone, Albery, & Persson, 2013; Golding-Kushner, 2001; Vallino-Napoli, 2012), but the level of evidence would be classified as fair evidence for the support of treatment in this clinical population (Justice & Fey, 2004). The treatment concepts that will be summarized are based primarily on the work of Golding-Kushner (2001) and Trost-Cardamone (2009, 2013) and can be modified depending on the needs of the child.

Selection of Speech Sounds for Treatment

The actual selection of a speech sound or sounds will depend on the testing that has been conducted and the incorporation of any recommendations from the team SLP. Sound system errors are classified as developmental, obligatory, or compensatory. The SLP needs to note that developmental errors may or may not be potential treatment targets depending on the age of the client. For instance, treatment for the /r/ speech sound would be appropriate for a child who is approximately 7 years

of age or older and has not spontaneously corrected the error. Please note that /r/ is not a pressure sound and not subject to being produced in a compensatory manner. Obligatory errors are not targets, because the errors are a function of a structural problem. Sometimes SLPs will attempt to teach placements for sounds that are not achievable because of structural differences that exist, but referral to appropriate medical or dental specialists are necessary for correction of structural problems, which are the causal factors of obligatory errors. After dental or medical treatment, speech-language pathology follow-up is routinely carried out; however, correct function is frequently achieved and speech treatment is not needed (Moller, 1994; Ruscello, Tekieli, & Van Sickels, 1985).

Compensatory errors are targeted for treatment and have been discussed in this section. Because the goal is correct production of speech sounds currently being substituted by more posterior articulations, concentrated practice is important for success. The SLP needs to keep in mind that compensatory errors have distinct perceptual features and familiarity with these errors is paramount. Sources for audio samples of these errors have been identified for the reader.

Phonetic Sound Teaching

If the child is not stimulable for a specific compensatory error, phonetic teaching techniques will need to be used to obtain correct oral placements. Each teaching technique will be discussed individually, but children using compensatory errors frequently need a combination of prompts, cues, and differing types of stimulation to acquire initial production of a target sound. To that end, phonetic teaching techniques will be summarized and followed by other types of stimulation and feedback procedures that can be used in combination with the former.

Williams (2003) classifies phonetic teaching techniques under the categories of sound awareness and direct instructional activities. The sound awareness techniques consist of metaphoric reference, describing and demonstrating placements, and the use of tactile cues. Specific examples are presented in Table 10–5. These are teaching methods that most SLPs use, and they can be useful for this population. The use of metaphors assists the child in forming a mental image or contrast between a specific target sound and a posterior articulation such as a glottal stop. Generally, the SLP is trying to contrast a posterior point of articulation with an anterior/oral place of articulation. The description and demonstration of a target sound is designed to furnish additional information to the child, so that an awareness of correct production is achievement. For example, the oral explosion of air during plosive production can be illustrated for the child and that feedback made directly available during isolation trials. Touch cues are also used for providing supplemental feedback, and one that can be very effective is the nostrils occlusion or cul-de-sac technique.

Table 10–5. Examples of Sound Awareness Activities

Phonetic Sound Establishment	
Sound Awareness Activities	**Examples**
Metaphoric reference	The purpose is to create an image in the child's mind of a desired sound feature through contrast.
	For example, glottal stop contrast with oral pressure sound placement.
	"throaty" versus "tippie" (tongue tip)
	"coughing sound" versus "mouthie sounds"
Description and demonstration	The purpose is to create an awareness of the production features of a sound.
	For instance, having the child produce an oral pressure sound and place a tissue in front of the child's mouth to show oral airflow is an example.
	Another example is placing a straw near the lips and directing the oral articulated airstream into the straw (e.g., tuh,tuh,tuh).
Tactile cueing	The purpose is to facilitate oral productions by occluding the child's nostrils or having the child do it. This technique allows the youngster to generate sufficient oral pressure, while making an oral point of articulation.

There are other cueing procedures such as using tongue blades and commercial devices to provide tactile placement cues for the child.

Direct instructional activities include the use of phonetic placement and different shaping cues to effect correct articulatory placements. One of the most frequently used of the isolated sound activities is that of phonetic placement. The SLP provides simple verbal cues regarding the movement and placement of a target sound. The instructions need to be simple and concise for the child to follow. Verbal placement cues can also be supplemented with a mirror, so that the child can observe his or her productions, or simple diagrams or models that demonstrate correct placement of a sound. Shaping can take a number of different forms, but the rationale behind the method is to break down the desired behavior into steps that lead to the correct production of the target sound. The steps can encompass transition from one sound to the desired target sound, or the use of nonphonetic oral gestures that lead to correct target articulation. In the latter, the SLP might teach the individual placements for a target sound such as lip rounding and tongue placement individually and then blend the movements requisite to the desired target sound. Shaping or transitioning from a sound produced correctly to a target sound that is currently misarticulated is also frequently employed by many SLPs. Please see Table 10–6 for specific examples.

Other Feedback and Stimulation Techniques

In addition to the different phonetic teaching methods, there are other ways

Table 10–6. Examples of Direct Instructional Activities

Phonetic Sound Establishment	
Direct Instructional Activities	**Examples**
Phonetic placement	The purpose is to achieve correct sound production through the use of instructional cues regarding the positioning and movement of the articulators.
	"Put your lips together, hold your lips together and then blow out the air (e.g., puh). Watch in the mirror as you make the sound.
	Look at this picture of the lips and your teeth. See the upper teeth touching the lower lip. Now, I want you to touch your front teeth with your lower lip like this (visual demonstration) and then blow air (e.g., fuh)."
Shaping cues	The purpose is to achieve correct sound production through facilitation of a sound produced correctly.
	The child is asked to produce the /t/ sound rapidly in a repetitive manner and then transition to producing the fricative /s/ (e.g., tttttt-s).

of providing the child with feedback and stimulation in achieving and maintaining oral place of articulation. One method that has been discussed is nostrils occlusion or the cul-de-sac technique. Occluding the nostrils, for example, will prevent active nasal air emission as part of nasal fricatives or passive nasal air emission as part of pharyngeal fricatives during trial productions of these oral pressure sounds and allow feedback of unwanted air or acoustic energy passing into the nose.

The See-Scape (Pro-Ed, Austin, Texas) is a commercial product that will also sense nasal airflow (see Chapter 9, Figure 9–5). It consists of tubing that is connected to a glass piston. The glass piston contains a small piece of Styrofoam that is sensitive to airflow. A nasal olive connected to the tubing is placed in contact with one naris, and any unwanted nasal air pressure will be sensed by displacement of a Styrofoam cylinder within the piston. The device can also be used to furnish visual feedback of oral pressure for anterior pressure sounds such as /p, b/. The nasal olive is positioned between the lips, and the release of the oral air pressure is visually available for the client. A simple drinking straw may also be used for feedback purposes. When placed between the lips, the oral release of air into the straw will create an auditory percept of an oral production. The SLP should keep in mind that there is also sophisticated instrumentation that can be used for feedback purposes such as the nasometer and pressure/flow equipment (reviewed in the previous chapter), but many school-based practitioners do not have access to such equipment, because of cost and the fact that cleft palate is a low incidence population.

In some cases, a child will not acquire correct production of a target sound immediately and require the presentation of a combination of cues and prompts. One must keep in mind that the child has been substituting the compensatory error(s) for an extended period of time. To that end, the sound elicitation techniques can be used in combination. For example, it may be necessary to use metaphoric reference, diagrams of articulator placement, and occluding the nostrils and a mirror in combination to achieve correct target sound production. Once the sound is acquired, the child should be taught to self-monitor productions, so that an awareness of the correct target versus the compensatory error substitution is created. The use of multiple elicitation cues and auditory self-monitoring cannot be overemphasized with this population of children with speech sound disorders. Correct production of target sounds is the primary goal and the SLP should not introduce any type of contextual practice, until the target sound is perceptually identified as being articulated correctly.

The Sequence and Treatment of Target Sounds

The decision as to the sequence of speech sounds to be taught will depend on the severity of the child's speech sound disorder. If there is significant use of compensatory errors, it is often useful to introduce /h/ initially. The reason is that /h/ is articulated with the vocal folds in the open position; consequently, the articulation is not compatible with a glottal stop. Once acquired, the speech sound /h/ will also serve as a facilitating sound for other oral pressure sounds. When introducing /h/, it is generally helpful to have the child imitate the SLP's modeling of the target. The models can be sustained to approximate a whispered production.

Whisper is also a treatment method that physiologically acts to minimize the triggering of glottal stops. When correct production is achieved, /h/ should be practiced in various contextual levels such as syllables (pre- and intervocalic positions), words, phrases, and sentences. Treatment is designed so that the youngster first acquires correct target sound production and then transfers the skill to different contextual levels.

An additional reason for beginning with /h/ is that it can be used to draw attention to the open/closed activity of the vocal folds. The SLP can contrast /h/ ("open sound or breathy sound") versus the glottal stop ("coughing sound") (Golding-Kushner, 2001) using metaphoric reference. The vocal fold distinction can also be used when targeting oral pressure sounds. The contrast might consist of the "coughing sound" versus "the lip popping sound" such as /p/. These contrasts help the child to form a correct percept of oral target sound placements. For example, if the child substitutes a glottal stop during a training trial, the SLP may respond: "No you made the coughing sound. I need you to make the /puh/ lip popping sound! Let's try it again."

After /h/ has been acquired, oral compensatory errors are targeted for treatment. Golding-Kushner (2001) suggests that an anterior to posterior progression of sound treatment be employed. For instance, bilabial pressure sounds /p,b/ are treated before alveolar pressure sounds /s,z,t,d/; however, the order can be modified in cases where a sound or sounds are found to be stimulable. In the case of treating cognate pairs, Trost-Cardamone (2009) recommends that the voiceless cognate be taught prior to the voiced. Treatment recommendations for the acquisition of oral pressure sounds by place and manner

are discussed below, and different teaching techniques recommended by various authors are also included.

The first set of sounds are the bilabials, and they include the plosives /p, b/ and the nasal /m/. Typically, a youngster with a cleft can produce the /m/ correctly; however, it will need to be targeted, if in error. Golding-Kushner (2001) recommends a shaping method wherein the child is directed to close the lips and "hum" a song. This elicitation procedure will often facilitate correct production of /m/. Correct production of the bilabial pressure sounds requires the generation of satisfactory intraoral air pressure, and a glottal stop is a frequent substitution for the bilabial plosives. Golding-Kushner (2001) recommends that the SLP use a shaping technique by having the child sustain /h/ and then close and open the lips to produce the /p/ sound. The nostrils occlusion technique can be used in combination with the shaping technique to achieve correct production, when nasal emission is a problem for the child. The aim is to create the explosion or release of air for the plosive with the air impounded behind the lips. When providing models, it is important to use normal loudness levels as increased loudness may create a coproduced articulation by the child. That is, the target sound may be produced correctly but coproduced with a glottal stop. Correct placement of the cognate /b/ may be obtained by informing the child to "make a sound just like /p/ but use your voice engine." Another elicitation method is to have the client produce an /m/ and then occlude both nostrils to achieve articulation of /b/. Once production is obtained, contextual practice is introduced.

The labiodental fricatives /f, v/ are targeted following acquisition of the bilabial plosives. Children will often substitute a pharyngeal fricative in place of the target sounds. It is suggested that the child be instructed to prolong the /h/ and then bring the lower lip and upper teeth together to produce the target sound. Golding-Kushner (2001) advises against using the verbal cue "bite the lip," because it may limit range of motion and result in a restricted constriction of the lip and teeth. When practicing the sound, the SLP should occlude the client's nares with digital occlusion, because air is often directed through the nasal tract during the initial stages of treatment. When the child is capable of controlling the airstream orally and uses the correct place of articulation, digital occlusion may be stopped. The voiced cognate /v/ is taught by having the client overlay the voicing signal with the labiodental production. Verbal imagery prompts such as "buzz like a bee" or "make a humming sound" may be employed to facilitate voicing. Occlusion of the nostrils is also used with the voiced cognate, if necessary.

The next suggested group of sounds to be taught are those at the lingua-dental and alveolar places of articulation. The fricative pair /θ, ð/ are visible sounds that are taught in the same way as the labiodental fricatives. The difference is that the placement cues will differ. The child is usually taught to "place the tongue tip between the teeth and make the air come out your mouth." Occluding the nostrils may be needed during the initial teaching of the target sounds. Golding-Kushner (2001) recommends that /θ, ð/ be used as shaping agents for the fricatives /s, z/, so correct placement can be very important when the alveolar fricatives are introduced in treatment. For example, the child is instructed to articulate /θ/ and then gradually "Pull the tongue back just behind the teeth. The /s, z/ speech

sounds can be very difficult for the child with cleft palate to produce, and occlusion of the nostrils may be necessary to assist in generation of oral air pressure. Riski (2003) has proposed a number of teaching strategies for eliciting the alveolar fricatives. For instance, one strategy is to have the child articulate /t/ and then release the tongue tip to produce /s/ or generate repetitions of /t/ and transition to an /s/ production /t t t t t sssss/. Golding-Kushner (2001) recommends utilizing phonetic context by selecting a word with /t/ in the postvocalic position. The child is instructed to produce a word such as /pit/ and instructed to prolong the /t/ at the end of the word. This elicitation method frequently results in the target production of /s/ in a cluster /pits/. The /z/ can be produced by prompting the child to produce a sustained /s/ and then "turning on the speech motor," so that the voiced /z/ is made /sssssszzzzzz/. Correct placement of the alveolar fricatives is a significant achievement for the youngster with cleft palate.

The lingua-alveolar sounds /n, t, d/ are then taught if they are not in the child's phonetic inventory. The nasal /n/ is taught first and then the plosives /t, d/. The child is directed to "Open your mouth a little and touch your tongue behind your upper teeth. Once you touch, you need to let your tongue go." In addition to the phonetic placement instructions, the child should also be informed that /n/ is made like /m/; consequently, there will be sound energy channeled through the nose. Golding-Kushner (2001) suggests that the same shaping technique used for /p, b/ also be used for /t, d/, since they are also plosive sounds. The child sustains the /h/ and alternately contacts and releases the tongue tip as it forms a constriction with the alveolar ridge.

The shaping procedure can be modeled for the child, so that the requisite auditory and visual information is clearly presented (/hhhhhhhtuh/). Following introduction of the alveolar sounds, Golding-Kushner (1995) recommends that attention be directed to the velar sounds rather than the palatal sounds. She feels that many children experience problems in developing correct production of the velar plosives /k, g/, because placement is most posterior of the oral pressure sounds, and intended productions often initiate pharyngeal or glottal stop substitutions. The nasal /ŋ/, which occurs in the inter- and postvocalic word positions is first taught. A coarticulation technique for achieving correct placement of /ŋ/ is to have the client produce the sound in the intervocalic position using the high front vowel /i/ in the sequence of VCV (/i ŋ i/). Golding-Kushner (2001) indicates that the contextual arrangement decreases the likelihood of eliciting a more posterior articulation, since the vowel is a high front vowel. After production of /ŋ/ is accomplished, the nasal can be used as a facilitating agent for the voiced velar plosive /g/. The child is instructed to "make the sound with the back of the tongue and make it a longer sound while I hold your nose." The clinician can then provide an imitative model of the sequence /i ŋ gi-i ŋ gi-i ŋ gi/ for the child to practice. This stimulus is then imitated with the nostrils occluded. With occlusion, the production is a transition to the desired stimulus /guh/. Once the /g/ productions are achieved, the target sound can be practiced in context such as in syllable or word items without occluding the nostrils. The /k/ speech sound follows with the child instructed to make the /guh/ sound but "don't turn on your voice motor, just let the air come out when you make the sound." The voiced velar plosive was taught first, which is a departure from the typical voiceless/voiced sequence that has been presented. The rationale for this change is the clinical premise that children with cleft palate have less of a problem acquiring /g/ than /k/, and /ŋ/ is a facilitating agent for teaching /g/.

The final set of sounds in the teaching sequence are the palatal fricatives /ʃ, ʒ/ and affricates /tʃ, dʒ/. These sounds are also frequently misarticulated by children with clefts, because of their significant pressure requirement. Some placement methods for eliciting /ʃ/ are discussed and include shaping procedures such as instructing the child to "pull the tongue back a little bit when you make /sssss/, so that you make /ʃ/." The lingual movement from /s/ to /ʃ/ frequently results in the desired placement for the sound (Riski, 2003). If necessary, the child's nostrils can be occluded to assist with oral air pressure buildup. Kummer (2001b) suggests that the child be taught to generate a "big sigh" with the teeth closed and lips rounded. The child can employ the technique, while prompted to "move the tongue until you make the whisper sound /ʃ/. Voicing cues such as "turn on your motor and make the sound /ʒ/" can be used after correct placement of /ʃ/ is achieved.

The affricates are speech sounds that combine the production features of both stops and fricatives. There is a complete blockage of the vocal tract, which is followed by a sustained release. A recommended placement technique has the youngster repeat /t/ such as /tuh,tuh, tuh,tuh/ and then shift the tongue tip to the palatal point of articulation and make

/tʃ/. An additional placement strategy is to teach the child to "sneeze" by starting with the mouth closed and then producing the /tʃ/ (Kummer, 2001b). The voiced cognate /dʒ/ can be elicited in the same way as discussed with /ʒ/ by " Turning on your speech motor."

Additional Speech Sound Errors

The primary goal of speech treatment is the modification of compensatory speech errors, but it has been noted by some that many children with cleft palate often lateralize production of the lingual fricatives and affricates. Trost-Cardamone (1990a) has observed that some children with cleft lip and palate who present with a lateral crossbite may exhibit lateralization. Lateralization is a nondevelopmental distortion error that is articulated by directing the airstream off the sides of the tongue, rather than using a central airstream. Because it has been observed in a subgroup of children with a dental problem, an SLP might conceptualize the error as an obligatory error (see discussion in Chapter 8); however, this error type is also found in the speech of children without VPI and should be corrected.

The oral semivowels /w, j, l, r/ were included in the discussion of specific placement techniques, because they are voiced sounds and do not require the generation of oral pressure.

They may, however, be produced with hypernasal resonance. Trost-Cardamone (1990b) wrote that the /l, r/ speech sounds are occasionally produced with a velar point of articulation by some children with cleft palate. The /l/ → /L/ and the /r/ → /R/. The SLP should be alert to the possibility that these error types may be observed and should be treated, if identified.

Target Sound Practice

Practice is an important component in the treatment of compensatory errors, because they can be very ingrained in the motor output of children with clefts. Although motivational games and activities are important for maintaining attention and interest, purposeful and varied types of practice cannot be overemphasized and should be carried out by the SLP and the child's caregivers. Because treating compensatory errors is the goal of phonetic-based therapy, the SLP is interested in replacing a pattern of movement (compensatory error) with a new movement pattern (correct oral placement). Ruscello (2008a) has conceptualized phonetic treatment as consisting of various learning stages. During the initial stages of treatment, basic instructions, different feedback procedures, and modeling are key components in helping the learner to acquire correct placement of the target sound. Practice of the target via drill activities is a key component as is feedback regarding the performance of the child. Drill is just not repetition of the target sound; it is the formation of conscious control of the muscular movements requisite to the sound. It also includes introspection and judgment of correct versus error productions. At the introductory stage of treatment, the goal is to develop correct placement and make sure that the child can reliably discriminate between the target sound and the former error.

After the child has acquired correct production of the target sound, practice continues to extend the production of the target in context. The practice hierarchy of isolation, syllables, words, phrases, sentences, and conversation is used to facilitate transfer of the target sound. Different forms of practice are introduced, because the goal is refinement and retention of the target sound. Performance feedback remains important but is gradually faded as the child improves. The final stage is a time of automating the target sound and is characterized by effortless and accurate practice (Ruscello, 2008a). The child is not focused on conscious control of the target sound but incorporating the target in more spontaneous production tasks. Similar to the previous stage, different types of practice can be a very effective for transfer or generalization. One such practice variation is that of mental practice or mentally rehearsing the target. It is a task that can help the child automate the target sound and facilitate generalization, so that the new oral sound is incorporated in his or her phonetic system. Some examples of lesson plans, which utilize different variations of practice, are summarized in Appendix 10–B.

Adolescent Clients

Even though most clients seen by the SLP are in the elementary grades, adolescents with repaired clefts may also be part of the caseload. Riski (1995) points out that physical growth changes, hormonal alterations, and increased physiologic learning characterize the adolescent period. He also indicated that speech and resonance outcomes continue to improve as a function of improved care; however, he also stated that there are adolescents who present with speech impairment and need treatment. Peterson-Falzone (1995) essentially stated the same, indicating that

there is a subset of adolescent clients who still present with communication problems. Generally, these are clients who had minimal or no care due to such factors as geographic locale, or for whatever reason have regularly missed appointments. She surveyed the speech records of 110 adolescent clients, and the results indicated that approximately 46% presented with communication problems related to the cleft condition. Peterson-Falzone expressed the opinion that poor speech outcomes were a function of many factors, such as a lack of regular team care, which prevented the appropriate and timely implementation of necessary interventions.

Table 10–7 summarizes three different client scenarios that may possibly be seen by the school SLP. They are by no means inclusive; however, they constitute some frequently seen patient scenarios.

The first are clients who are regularly seen by their craniofacial team, and there is a collaborative relationship with the school SLP and the craniofacial SLP. In most cases, there may be some minor communication issues that are in the process of being resolved. For example, it could be that the school SLP is working with the client on the generalization of certain compensatory errors that are corrected but require transfer to spontaneous use. It is more of "fine tuning" the youngster's communication skills.

The second scenario is a situation wherein the school SLP identifies a client who needs the services of a craniofacial team but has not consistently received needed services. There are many potential problems that face some families such as travel distance and lack of transportation, which are barriers to obtaining service. In this situation, it is recommended that the school SLP contact the family and discuss the importance of team care and the tim-

Table 10–7. Possible Clinical Scenarios That May Seen By the School SLP

Status of Care	Role of the School SLP
1. The client is receiving services from a team on a regularly scheduled basis.	Provide services as per collaboration with the team SLP and other team members as needed. This may include direct and/or indirect services.
2. The client is not receiving services from a team due to certain constraints such as travel distance, lack of family resources, etc.	Initiate contact with family to discuss the importance of team care and seek permission for referral to a team. If granted permission, refer and work collaboratively with the team SLP and other team members as needed.
3. The client is scheduled to receive services from a team, but appointments are not consistently maintained.	Initiate contact with family to discuss the importance of team care and seek permission to contact the team coordinator. If granted permission, monitor team appointments and work collaboratively with the team SLP and other team members as needed.

ing of services. If the family is willing, the SLP should contact the craniofacial team coordinator, so that there is a resumption of service. This may require interacting with the school counselor and local social service agencies to arrange travel and other needs. In some cases, it is extremely helpful if the school SLP assists the family and accompanies them to scheduled appointments. It can be comforting for the family, and it also allows the school direct contact with team members.

The third and final situation is failure to keep scheduled appointments with the craniofacial team due to lack of parental motivation. The client is part of a team's caseload, but the family fails to keep scheduled appointments. In this scenario, it is recommended that the school SLP make contact with the family and discuss the importance and timing of team care. It is not a contact for putting the caregivers on the defensive but to emphasize the need for services. One should always

"keep the door open" in these situations. If the family agrees, the school SLP should contact the team coordinator and convey the family's willingness to recommence visits and proposed care. It is also recommended that the school SLP be informed of team visits, so that he or she can monitor visits, accompany the family, provide gentle reminders, and discuss the results of individual team meetings with the family. The school SLP would also carry out collaborative treatment efforts, if necessary.

The above scenarios and recommended strategies are based on the clinical experience of the author and are not based on a strong level of evidence. An additional factor in working with adolescent clients that needs to be considered is the client's level of motivation. The adolescent years come with significant challenges, and many clients have received years of speech treatment. Peterson-Falzone (1995) writes that some adolescents with clefts may be resigned to fact that they have communication problems or simply deny that a problem exists. These cases are extremely difficult to treat, and they may elect to terminate services with the approval of their parents. In these cases, the SLP can point out that speakers often react negatively to individuals with speech problems (Ruscello, 2008a) and inform the client that treatment is available, if there is a change in attitude. The team SLP should be informed of the client's decision to withdraw from treatment due to a lack of motivation.

CHAPTER SUMMARY

Working with children who have oral clefts can be a very fulfilling experience. In many cases, school SLPs report a lack of knowledge and clinical skills to provide appropriate services, but there are ways to overcome such obstacles and prepare oneself to work effectively with this population. First, the SLP must become knowledgeable of the cognitive, social, motor, and communicative problems that are associated with this population. Children with cleft palate may present with a variety of problems, and the SLP must be prepared to understand those problems and provide appropriate service and referrals. In addition, the SLP must develop the auditory perceptual skills requisite to the assessment of the speech, resonance, and voice characteristics of children with clefts. Because most children are receiving services from a team, the school SLP needs to work collaboratively with the team SLP. There are a number of different collaborative models, and the implementation of a specific model will depend on the type of collaboration; however, professionals must keep in mind that success depends

on shared power and cooperation. Each SLP plays a key role in the overall treatment process; there is no subordinate relationship in the delivery of services.

The evaluation of communication disorders in this population requires the use of some specialized assessment materials, which have been discussed in length. It is important to examine the speech, resonance, voice, and language skills of these children, so that an appropriate course of action may be taken. In addition, the school SLP must be alert to the fact that middle ear infection is common and can have a negative influence in the acquisition and development of speech and language. Speech production errors are very prevalent and need to be categorized as developmental, obligatory, and compensatory, which is a departure for those SLPs who typically treat children without cleft palate. Compensatory errors are legitimate targets for treatment prior to and after secondary surgical repair, if done. Treatment for compensatory errors was characterized as a phonetic teaching endeavor that requires different forms of practice as the child first acquires and then automates the target sound(s). Cooperation and competence among professionals are extremely important and are the key to successful interactions with the child and his or her caregivers.

REFERENCES

American Cleft Palate-Craniofacial Association. (n.d.). *Speech samples.* Retrieved from http://www.acpa-cpf.org/education/edu cational_resources/speech_samples/

Bedwinek, A. P., Kummer, A. W., Rice, G. B., & Grames, L. M. (2010). Current training and continuing education needs of preschool and school-based speech-language pathologists regarding children with cleft lip/palate. *Language, Speech, and Hearing Services in Schools, 41,* 405–414.

Bessell, A., Sell, D., Whiting, P., Roulstone, S., Albery, L., & Persson, M. (2013). Speech and language therapy interventions for children with cleft palate: A systematic review. *Cleft Palate-Craniofacial Journal, 50,* e1–e17.

Chapman, K. (1993). Phonologic processes in children with cleft palate. *Cleft Palate-Craniofacial Journal, 30,* 64–71.

Cleft Palate Foundation. (n. d.). *U.S. Team listing.* Retrieved from http://www.cleftline.org/parents-individuals/team-care/

Cohn, E. (2013, June 6). On the pulse: Combining strengths in craniofacial treatment: Cleft palate and craniofacial teams provide a long-established model of interprofessional care. *The ASHA Leader, 18,* 30–31.

D'Antonio, L. L., Muntz, H., Providence, M., & Marsh, J. (1988). Laryngeal/voice findings in patients with velopharyngeal dysfunction. *Laryngoscope, 98,* 432–438.

Fletcher, S. G. (1972). Contingencies for bioelectric modification of nasality. *Journal of Speech and Hearing Disorders, 37,* 329–346.

Fudala, J. B., & Reynolds, W. M. (2000). *Arizona Articulation Proficiency Scale* (3rd ed.). Austin, TX: Pro-Ed.

Golding-Kushner, K. J. (1995). Treatment of articulation and resonance disorders associated with cleft palate and VPI. In R. J. Shprintzen and J. Bardach (Eds.), *Cleft palate speech management: A multidisciplinary approach* (pp. 327–351). St. Louis, MO: Mosby.

Golding-Kushner, K. J. (2001) *Therapy techniques for cleft palate speech and related disorders.* San Diego, CA: Singular.

Golding-Kushner, K. J., & Shprintzen, R. J. (2011). *Velo-cardio-facial syndrome: Volume II. Treatment of communication disorders.* San Diego, CA: Plural.

Goldman, R., & Fristoe, M. (2000). *Goldman-Fristoe Test of Articulation* (2nd ed.). San Antonio, TX: Pearson.

Grames, L. M. (2004). Implementing treatment recommendations: Role of the craniofacial team speech-language pathologist in working with the client's speech-language pathologist. *SIG 5 Perspectives on Speech Science and Orofacial Disorders, 14,* 6–9.

Grames, L. M. (2008, May 6). Advancing into the 21st century: Care for individuals with cleft palate or craniofacial differences. *The ASHA Leader, 13,* 10–13.

Henningsson, G. E., & Isberg, A. M. (1986). Velopharyngeal movements in patients alternating between oral and glottal articulation: A clinical and cineradiographical study. *Cleft Palate Journal, 23,* 1–9.

Henningsson, G., Kuehn, D. P., Sell, D., Sweeny, T., Trost-Cardamone, J. E., & Whitehill, T. L. (2008). Universal parameters for reporting speech outcomes in individuals with cleft palate. *Cleft Palate-Craniofacial Journal, 45*(1), 1–17.

Justice, L. M., & Fey, M. E. (2004, September 9). Evidence-based practice in schools: Integrating craft and theory with science and data. *ASHA Leader, 9,* 4–32.

Karnell, M. P., Bailey, P., Johnson, L., Dragan, A., & Canady, J. W. (2005). Facilitating communication among speech pathologists treating children with cleft palate. *Cleft Palate-Craniofacial Journal, 42,* 585–588.

Kummer, A. W. (2001a). Perceptual assessment. In A. W. Kummer (Ed.), *Cleft palate and craniofacial anomalies: The effects of speech and resonance* (pp. 265–292). San Diego, CA: Singular.

Kummer, A. W. (2001b). Speech therapy for effects of velopharyngeal dysfunction. In A. W. Kummer (Ed.), *Cleft palate and craniofacial anomalies: The effects of speech and resonance* (pp. 459–482). San Diego, CA: Singular.

LeDuc, J. A. (2008). Cleft palate and/or velopharyngeal dysfunction: Assessment and treatment. *SIG 16 Perspectives on School-Based Issues, 9,* 155–161.

McWilliams, B. J., Morris, H. L., & Shelton, R. L. (1990). *Cleft palate speech* (2nd ed.). Philadelphia, PA: B.C. Decker.

Moller, K. T. (1994). Dental-occlusal and other oral conditions and speech. In J. Bernthal & N. Bankson (Eds.), *Child phonology: Characteristics, assessment, and intervention with special populations* (pp. 3–28). New York, NY: Thieme Medical.

Morris, H. L. (1992). Some questions and answers about velopharyngeal dysfunction during speech. *American Journal of Speech-Language Pathology, 1*, 26–28.

Pamplona, M., & Ysunza, A. (1999). A comparative trial of two modalities of speech intervention for cleft palate children: Phonologic vs. articulatory approach. *International Journal of Pediatric Otorhinolaryngology, 49*, 2–27.

Peterson-Falzone, S. J. (1995). Speech outcomes in adolescents with cleft lip and palate. *Cleft Palate-Craniofacial Journal, 32*, 125–128.

Peterson-Falzone, S. J., Hardin-Jones, M. A., & Karnell, M. (2010). *Cleft palate speech* (4th ed.). St. Louis, MO: Mosby.

Peterson-Falzone, S. J., Trost-Cardamone, J. E., Karnell, M., & Hardin-Jones, M. A. (2006). *Treating cleft palate speech.* St. Louis, MO: Mosby.

Richman, L. C., McCoy, T. E., Conrad, A. L., & Nopoulos, P. C. (2012). Neuropsychological, behavioral, and academic sequelae of cleft: Early developmental, school age, and adolescent/young adult outcomes. *Cleft Palate-Craniofacial Journal, 49*(4), 387–396.

Riski, J. E. (1995). Speech assessment of adolescents. *Cleft Palate-Craniofacial Journal, 32*, 109–113.

Riski, J. E. (2003). *Improving your clinical competence with unique articulation disorders.* Retrieved from Craniofacial Services: Speech Pathology Laboratory website: http//www .choa.org./craniofacial/speech-3.shtml

Ruscello, D. M. (2008a). *Treating articulation and phonological disorders in children.* St. Louis, MO: Mosby Elsevier.

Ruscello, D. M. (2008b). An examination of non-speech oral motor exercises for children with VPI. *Seminars in Speech and Language, 29*, 294–303.

Ruscello, D. M., Tekieli, M. E., & Van Sickels, J. E. (1985). Speech production before and after orthognathic surgery: A review. *Oral Surgery, Oral Medicine, and Oral Pathology, 59*, 10–14.

See-Scape. Austin, TX: Pro-Ed.

Skahan, S. M., Watson, M., & Lof, G. L. (2007). Speech-language pathologists' assessment practices for children with suspected speech sound disorders: Results of a national survey. *American Journal of Speech-Language Pathology, 16*, 246–259.

Swift, J. Q. (2009). Oral and maxillofacial surgery: Management of the alveolar cleft and jaw discrepancies. In K. T. Moller & L. E. Glaze (Eds.), *Cleft lip and palate: Interdisciplinary issues and treatment* (2nd ed., pp. 573–600). Austin, TX: Pro-Ed.

Templin, M. C., & Darley, F. L. (1960). *The Templin-Darley Tests of Articulation.* Iowa City, IA: University of Iowa Bureau of Educational Research and Service.

Torres, I. G. (2013, February 1). Know what you don't know. *The ASHA Leader, 18*, 38–41.

Trost-Cardamone, J. E. (1990a). The development of speech: Assessing cleft palate misarticulations. In D. A. Kernahan & S. W. Rosenstein (Eds.), *Cleft lip and palate* (pp. 225–235). Baltimore, MD: Williams & Wilkins.

Trost-Cardamone, J. E. (1990b). Speech: Anatomy, physiology, and pathology. In D. A. Kernahan & S. W. Rosenstein (Eds.), *Cleft lip and palate* (pp. 91–103). Baltimore, MD: Williams & Wilkins.

Trost-Cardamone, J. E. (2009). Articulation and phonologic assessment procedures and treatment decisions (2nd ed.). In K. T. Moller & L. E. Glaze (Eds.), *Cleft lip and palate: Interdisciplinary issues and treatment* (pp. 377–414). Austin, TX: Pro-Ed.

Trost-Cardamone, J. E. (2013). *Cleft palate speech.* Rockville, MD: ASHA Product Sales.

Trost-Cardamone, J. E., & Bernthal, J. E. (1993). Articulation assessment procedures and treatment decisions. In K. T. Moller & C. D. Starr (Eds.), *Cleft palate: Interdisciplinary issues and treatment* (pp. 307–336). Austin, TX: Pro-Ed.

Vallino, L. D., Lass, N. J., Bunnell, H. T., & Pannbacker, M. (2008). Academic and clinical training in cleft palate for speech-language pathologists. *Cleft Palate-Craniofacial Journal, 45*, 371–380.

Vallino, L. D., & Ruscello, D. M. (In preparation). *Primer on cleft lip and palate.*

Vallino-Napoli, L. D. (2012). Evaluation and evidence-based practice. In A. Lohmander & S. Howard (Eds.), *Cleft palate speech: Assessment and intervention* (pp. 317–358). West Sussex, UK: Wiley.

Whitehill, T. L. (2002). Assessing intelligibility in speakers with cleft palate: A critical review of the literature. *Cleft Palate-Craniofacial Journal, 39,* 50–58.

Williams, A. L. (2003). *Speech disorders resource guide for preschool children.* Clifton Park, NY: Thomson Delmar Learning.

Yorkston, K. M., Beukelman, D. R., Strand, E. A., & Hakel, M. (2010). *Mangement of motor speech disorders in children and adults.* Austin, TX: Pro-Ed.

APPENDIX 10–A

A Suggested Assessment Protocol

IDENTIFICATION AND CLASSIFICATION INFORMATION

Date of Assessment:

Patient:

Birthdate: ____/____/____   Gender: M___   F___

Cleft Type: UNCLP   BLCLP   Cleft of Hard & Soft Palate

Cleft of Soft Palate   Other:

Other Anomalies: YES   NO   Describe:

Syndrome: YES   NO   Describe:

Patient's Team: Team SLP:

Contact Information:

School SLP:

Contact Information:

School Treatment History:

Current Treatment Goals:

Progress to Date:

Hearing Status:

ASSESSMENT INFORMATION

Date: Age of Client:

Assessment: Live judgment ___   Audio recording ___   Video recording ___

1. Oral Examination

Purpose: Examine the structure and function of the oral speech mechanism to identify any structural, sensory, or motor variations that may adversely affect speech production skills. The SLP may use a standardized measure or self-developed instrument to obtain observations.

Oral posture of mouth/lips at rest

Appearance and mobility of the lips

    Scarring

    Lip pits or mounds on lower lip

    Dentition

    Missing teeth

    Ectopic teeth

    Supernumerary teeth

    Rotated teeth

Occlusion of the maxilla and mandible

    Overjet

    Underjet

    Open bite

    Crossbite

Tongue size, appearance, and mobility

Configuration of the hard palate

Appearance and mobility of soft palate

    Zona pellucida

    Bony notch in the posterior nasal spine

Appearance of uvula

    Bifid

Size and position of the palatine tonsils

continues

Presence and location of oronasal fistula

Presence of an oral appliance

Dental braces

Breathing at rest

Oral

Nasal

Speech motor control (Diadochokinesis)

2. Speech Assessment

Purpose: Assess the child's speech sound skills, resonance, and voice in the contexts of words, sentences, and conversation. Testing enables the school SLP to identify error types (compensatory, obligatory, and developmental), determine the impact of the speech sound disorder on other listeners (intelligibility and severity), establish eligibility for receiving services in the schools, determine progress or lack thereof, and provide current performance data for the child's parents and craniofacial team.

2A. Word-Level Assessment. A standardized test(s) can be administered such as the *Goldman-Fristoe Test of Articulation* (2nd ed.) (2000), *Arizona Articulation Proficiency Scale* (3rd ed.) (2000), or *Templin-Darley Tests of Articulation* (1960). The SLP should also supplement observations with a clinician-devised set of words that can also be pictured. Guidelines for the development of such materials are available from Trost-Cardamone (2013) and Henningsson et al. (2008), and a listing of word items is as follows:

Oral Pressure Sounds

1. /p/ pea, peel, pear, rip, lap, leap
2. /b/ bee, bye, boo, rub, rib, lube
3. /t/ tea, two, toe, rat, light, root
4. /d/ dew, D, doll, read, lid, rod
5. /k/ key, cow, car, ache, rake, leak
6. /g/ go, goal, gay, rig, wig, leg
7. /f/ fee, fear, fell, leaf, reef, roof
8. /v/ veil, V, veal, weave, wave, Eve
9. /θ/ three, Thor, thigh, wreath, math, Ruth
10. /ð/ thee, there, they, lathe, loathe, wreathe
11. /s/ see, Sue, sew, race, lice, rice
12. /z/ zoo, zero, Zoe, rose, hose, wheeze
13. /ʃ/ she, shoe, shy, leash, wash, rash
14. /ʒ/ beige, luge, rouge
15. /h/ high, hill, who, he
16. /tʃ/ chew, chill, chair, leech, reach, wrench
17. /dʒ/ joy, Joe, Jill, age, ridge, huge

Nasals

18. /m/   me, moo, mail, lamb, ram, room
19. /n/   nail, new, no, run, one, lawn
20. /ŋ/   ring, long, lung

2B. Sentence-Level Assessment. Use at least 20 to 25 short phrases or sentences imitatively (Henningsson et al., 2008) to include pressure sounds, oral sonorants, and nasals. These materials are taken from Trost-Cardamone (2013) and are as follows:

1. /p/   Puppy will pull a rope.
2. /b/   Buy baby a bib.
3. /f/   A fly fell off a leaf.
4. /v/   I love every view.
5. /θ/   Thirty-two teeth.
6. /ð/   The other feather.
7. /t/   Your turtle ate a hat.
8. /d/   Do it today for Dad.
9. /l/   Laura will wear a lily.
10. /s/   Sissy saw Sally race.
11. /z/   Zoey has roses.
12. /ʃ/   She washed a dish.
13. /tʃ/   Watch a choo-choo.
14. /dʒ/   George saw Gigi.
15. /k/   A cookie or a cake.
16. /g/   Give Aggie a hug.
17. /h/   Hurry ahead, Harry.
18. /r/   Ray will arrive early.
19. /w/   We were away.
20. /m/   Mom and Amy are home.
21. /n/   Anna knew no more.
22. /ŋ/   We are hanging on.
23. /m,n,ŋ/ We ran a long mile.
24. *nasals, high-pressure, low-pressure targets—*
       Summer is sunny, winter is windy and cold.

From *Cleft Palate Speech: Causes, Identification, and Assessment* (Part 1, p. 219), by Judith E. Trost-Cardamone, 2013, Rockville, MD: American Speech-Language-Hearing Association. Copyright 2013 by the American Speech-Language-Hearing Association. Adapted with permission.

2C. Contextual Speech Assessment. A 3- to 5-minute sample of conversational speech will allow for judgment of contextual speech and its impact on a listener. Various procedures such as storytelling, story retelling, interactive play, interaction with a caregiver, or interaction with peers may be used to elicit the sample.

2D. Resonance Assessment. The SLP needs to assess resonance to determine if the child is hypernasal, hyponasal, or has mixed nasality.

continues

Cul-de-sac testing

The child is instructed to produce the high vowels /i/ and /u/ in a prolonged manner, while the SLP or child alternately opens and closes the nostrils with digital pressure. A change in resonance under the two conditions is indicative of hypernasal resonance.

Production of nasal consonants

The child's production of nasal consonants in word, sentence, and conversational testing materials allows for judgments of hyponasality.

The Zoo Passage

The child can read or recite the Zoo passage. This is a reading passage that contains no nasal consonants and provides information on the presence of hypernasal resonance:

Look at this book with us. It's a story about a zoo. That is where bears go. Today it's very cold out of doors, but we see a cloud overhead that's a pretty white fluffy shape. We hear that straw covers the floor of cages to keep the chill away; yet a deer walks through the trees with her head high. They feed seeds to birds so they're able to fly.

Source: Fletcher, S. G. (1972). Contingencies for bioelectric modification of nasality. *Journal of Speech and Hearing Disorders, 37,* 329–346.

2E. Voice Assessment. The different assessment tasks permit perceptual judgments of vocal pitch, loudness, and quality.

2F. Stimulability. Speech sounds in error are selected and presented to the child. The child is asked to watch the SLP and imitate a model produced by the SLP. Depending on the child and circumstances, he or she may be asked to produce the speech sound errors at the isolation, syllable, or word levels, whatever is appropriate. If the child can imitate the models successfully, we say that he or she is stimulable, and the prognosis for future phonetic treatment is positive. Conversely, the SLP may choose not to treat the speech sound error, because the child may develop the correct production without intervention (Ruscello, 2008a). Keep in mind that our stimulability testing is not only designed to examine oral placement, but we are also interested in the impact of stimulability on oral pressure generation and resonance. That is, is there also a change in VPI when a child is stimulable for error productions? This would be a very positive finding for a child who presents with VPI in terms of intervention.

ASSESSMENT FINDINGS

3. *Summary of Assessment Results*

The results of the assessment are summarized according to speech sound production, resonance, and voice.

3A. Summarize findings of the oral mechanism examination: _____

_____

_____

3B. Speech production skills as modified from Henningsson et al. (2008):

WNL   Compensatory Errors   Obligatory Errors   Developmental Errors

Compensatory Error Categories:

1. Audible nasal emission
2. Backing of oral pressure sounds to postvelar point of articulation.
3. Oral backing to mid-dorsum velar or uvular point of articulation.
4. Nasal fricative that is or is not phoneme specific.
5. Nasal consonant is in substitution of oral consonant.
6. Weak pressure sounds.

3C. Resonance Balance

Judgment of Hypernasality

WNL	Mild	Moderate	Severe
0	1	2	3

Judgment of Hyponasality

WNL	Present
0	1

3D. Voice

Pitch   Loudness
WNL   High   Low   WNL   High   Low

Quality
WNL   Hoarse   Harsh   Breathy

continues

3E. Overall Intelligibility and Severity. Based on the collected evidence, the SLP needs to rate the child's intelligibility or ability to be understood by others and severity or the impact of the speech disorder on a listener.

Intelligibility

0 Intelligible   1 Intelligible with some limitations   2 Intelligibility difficult

3 Intelligibility very difficult   4 Cannot understand

Severity

0 normal 1 mild 2 moderate 3 severe 4 profound

3F. Stimulability

Stimulable: _____

_____

Not Stimulable: _____

SUMMARY AND RECOMMENDATIONS

Summary of the current findings: _____

_____

_____

_____

☐ Current Communication Status:

☐ Recommendations for communication treatment:

☐ Referral for further assessment:

☐ Other recommendations:

APPENDIX 10–B

Therapy Approach for a School-Aged Child

HYPOTHETICAL CASE

C. R. is a 7-year-old female with a complete unilateral cleft of the primary and secondary palates. The lip was repaired at 3 months of age, and the palate was closed at 11 months. She presents with hypernasality (obligatory resonance disorder), nasal emission (obligatory phonetic error), weak pressure generation (obligatory phonetic error), pharyngeal fricatives (compensatory speech error), and glottal stops (compensatory speech error). The client will undergo a pharyngoplasty in 6 months to improve velopharyngeal closure for speech. She is currently enrolled in speech treatment.

Phonetic Inventory

Nasals: /m, n, ŋ / Produced with correct placement.

Glides and Liquids: /j, w, l, r/ Produced with correct placement but perceived as hypernasal.

Affricates: /tʃ, dʒ/ Produced with correct placement but with weak pressure.

Fricatives: /h/ is produced correctly. /f, v, θ, ð/ Produced with correct placement but with weak pressure. /s, z, ʃ, ʒ/ are produced as pharyngeal fricatives.

Stops: /p, b/ Produced with correct placement but with weak pressure. /t, d, k, g/ are produced as glottal stops.

Treatment Targets

The goal of treatment is to eliminate the pharyngeal fricatives and glottal stops currently used by the client. They are both compensatory errors and subject to treatment. Individual target sounds to be introduced initially in treatment are /s/ and /t/.

INITIAL THERAPY SESSION

Therapy Goals

Correct oral placement of /s/ and /t/ in isolation* and CV syllables.

*Note that the plosive /t/ is not a continuant sound and cannot be produced in isolation.

Ten-Minute Introductory Period

The purpose of therapy is discussed, because the chronological age of the client indicates that she is capable of comprehending information regarding her speech problem and what will be done to treat the compensatory errors. Following the short explanation, contrasts of incorrect placement versus correct placement are modeled for the client. A metaphoric reference of "throaty" versus "tongue tippy" sounds is introduced, so that the child can connect conceptually to the different points of articulation and develop an internal auditory percept of correct versus incorrect.

Rationale

The child is given simple instructions and a frame of reference for what is to be done to treat the compensatory speech sound errors. It also serves as an introductory activity for error identification, because the imagery contrast is employed to help the youngster discriminate between correct and incorrect production.

Twenty-Minute Placement Activity

Oral placement for /s/ is introduced through simple phonetic placement instructions and having the client occlude her nostrils during training trials.

Rationale

Beginning practice should incorporate very basic skills (sound in isolation), use simple instructions (e.g., "Place your tongue just behind your front teeth and blow out some air. Make the sound _____."), and heighten sensory awareness (nostrils occlusion). Practice trials deal exclusively with the target sound, and verbal performance feedback is used. The speech-language pathologist (SLP) needs to cue and prompt the child to make adjustments in tongue position and airflow that will result in correct target production. After production in isolation is achieved, practice is carried with the target sound in five different CV syllables.

Twenty-Minute Placement Activity

The same procedures used above are employed for /t/.

INTERMEDIATE THERAPY SESSION

Therapy Goals

Correct oral placement of /s/ and /t/ in all word positions including cluster combinations in single words.

THERAPY SESSION TREATMENT ACTIVITIES

Ten-Minute Introductory Period

Progress in treatment is discussed with the client. Examples of words produced as "throaty" and "tongue tippie" by the SLP are identified by the client using the imagery concepts.

Rationale

The introductory period is a review of progress and also serves as an error detection activity.

Ten-Minute Drill Period

Ten target words containing /s/ in different contextual arrangements are practiced by the client.

Rationale

Current practice should involve more advanced contextual material (sound in different contexts), and use different instructional cues to elicit responses (e.g., "Say _____."; "Say this picture."). Practice trials are varied, because the child practices different contextual configurations of the target sound. Feedback consists primarily of correct/incorrect verification, but it is used on a variable basis, because target sound production is improving.

Ten-Minute Drill Period

The 10 target words used above are randomly presented with 10 other words that do not contain the target /s/ speech sound.

Rationale

Current practice should involve more advanced contextual material (sound in different contexts), and use different instructional cues to elicit responses (e.g., "Say _____."; "Say this picture."). Practice trials are varied additionally, because the child practices different contextual configurations of the target sound, and the practice items are interspersed with items that do not contain the target sound. Feedback consists primarily of correct/incorrect verification, but it is used on a variable basis, because target sound production is improving.

Twenty-Minute Drill Period

The same procedures used above are employed for /t/.

ADVANCED THERAPY SESSION

Ten-Minute Introductory Period

Therapy progress is reviewed with the child. The SLP also furnishes two examples each of words, phrases, and sentences containing each of the two target sounds.

The SLP produces each practice item and prompts the child to "think about how the sound is made in your mouth, and then make the sound in your brain and then say _____."

Rationale

The introductory period is used to review progress and introduce a mental rehearsal activity for the child to carry out.

Fifteen-Minute Drill Period

Twenty sentences containing the two targets each in a single word are used for practice. The child produces the target sentences, and the SLP has the child alter speaking rate in each presentation of the sentence stimuli set. The aim of the "speed drills" is to increase speech rate, while sustaining high levels of response accuracy. This drill activity is designed to automate the use of the target sounds. A stopwatch is used for timing purposes, and the SLP collects response accuracy data.

Rationale

Practice trials provide varied context and alterations in speaking rate in this automation drill. After each trial set, the time and accuracy rate are calculated and reviewed with the client.

Fifteen-Minute Drill Period

The SLP and child participate in scripted conversational interchanges. A topic is introduced, and the child is instructed that "one topic at a time" will be discussed in therapy. The SLP informs the child that he or she needs to use the "new sounds" correctly, when talking. The child is queried regarding a word or words that include the target sound. The child needs to identify words containing the target sounds and assess the accuracy of his or her productions.

Rationale

This is a spontaneous speaking task that is designed to automate the target sounds. The child must employ error detection skills (self-monitoring), and the SLP gives variable verbal feedback regarding performance.

11

Secondary Management of Velopharyngeal Inadequacy

INTRODUCTION

The goal of team management for the child born with cleft palate is normal speech by the time he or she enters school. The overall success in obtaining this goal, however, is difficult to assess due to the varied approaches to management and the lack of standardized procedures to assess outcomes across centers. Peterson-Falzone, Hardin-Jones, and Karnell (2001) estimated that at least 50% of children with repaired cleft palate will receive speech therapy at some time in their lives, most for articulation issues. In addition, approximately 20% to 30% of children will exhibit obligatory symptoms of velopharyngeal inadequacy (VPI) following initial palatal surgery (Morris, 1973; Peterson-Falzone, 1990; Riski, 1979). This estimate is similar to the percentage of 2-year-old children with repaired cleft palate who lacked consistent velopharyngeal closure as reported by Zajac, van Aalst, Vallino, and Napoli (2011).

The primary symptoms of VPI in school-aged children with repaired cleft palate are hypernasality and audible nasal air emission, including nasal turbulence.

Fortunately, because cleft palate is a low-incidence anomaly, the absolute number of children who experience VPI is relatively small. Nevertheless, the presence of obligatory symptoms such as hypernasality can significantly impact a child's intelligibility and social acceptance, especially if severe. The purpose of this chapter is to describe some behavioral, surgical, and prosthetic management options for children with repaired cleft palate who persist in exhibiting obligatory symptoms of VPI.

BEHAVIORAL APPROACHES

As reviewed in the previous chapter, non-speech oral motor exercises designed to increase muscle strength have not been shown to be effective relative to improving velopharyngeal function for speech (Ruscello, 2008; Skahan, Watson, & Lof, 2007). The most frequent cause of VPI in children with repaired cleft palate is not muscle weakness, but rather inadequate length or movement of the soft palate and limited movement of the lateral pharyngeal walls (see discussion of posterior pharyngeal flaps later in the chapter). The reason that nonspeech oral motor exercises are ineffective is because patterns of muscle activation and velopharyngeal closure are different between speech and nonspeech tasks (McWilliams & Bradley, 1965; Moll, 1965). Moll (1965) used cinefluoroscopy to describe velopharyngeal movements during speech, blowing, swallowing, sucking, and cheek puffing of adults with and without repaired cleft palate. The adults with cleft palate all exhibited VPI. Moll reported patterns of velopharyngeal closure that were different for speech, blowing, and swallowing compared to sucking and cheek puffing. For the former tasks, there was always velum to posterior pharyngeal wall contact, with the greatest contact occurring during blowing. McWilliams and Bradley (1965) reported similar findings and concluded that closure during blowing was "gross and purposeful," while closure during speech was "precise and automatic." Moll additionally reported two findings that have direct implications for the use of nonspeech oral motor exercises. First, he found that velar-pharyngeal wall contact did not occur during sucking and cheek puffing for many of the adults without cleft palate. Rather, they used tongue to palate contact during the tasks. Second, Moll reported that although all of the adults with cleft palate achieved velopharyngeal closure during swallowing, they did so in part by lifting the velum with the back of the tongue, a maneuver that is not possible during normal speech production.

Although there is a clear lack of evidence, some speech-language pathologists (SLPs) still persist in recommending nonspeech oral motor activities such as sucking in the hope of strengthening velar muscles and eliminating hypernasality. Organizations such as the American Speech-Language-Hearing Association and the American Cleft Palate-Craniofacial Association have recently stepped up efforts to educate SLPs that such activities are ineffective. In fact, time spent doing these activities will use up resources and deprive patients of valuable, cost effective evidence-based treatment.

It is our opinion that behavioral approaches to treating VPI must include speaking and should be directed primarily to reducing severity of symptoms rather than attempting to improve velopharyngeal function per se. As reviewed in Chapter 8, there are multiple speech parameters that may affect hypernasality—and perhaps nasal turbulence—including pitch, loudness, and rate. SLPs can manipulate these parameters during "diagnostic" therapy to assess the effects on hypernasality. As defined by Owens, Metz, and Haas (2003), diagnostic therapy is ongoing assessment as intervention takes place.

Selection of candidates is an important factor when considering behavioral approaches. A young child who exhibits severe hypernasality with instrumental findings showing frank VPI is obviously not a candidate for behavioral therapy. Rather, a child who has mild to moderate symptoms, especially when inconsistent in nature, and who is old enough to understand the therapeutic approach is a candidate for behavioral therapy. The following review of behavioral approaches is limited to those that cite some supporting evidence relative to efficacy. The reader is referred to Peterson-Falzone et al. (2001) for coverage of additional approaches that they consider as largely experimental.

Biofeedback

Behavioral therapy can be facilitated via biofeedback provided by various instruments. One obvious choice of instruments is the nasometer. Although originally intended by Fletcher to be used as a therapeutic device (e.g., Fletcher, 1972, 1978), there have been surprisingly few studies that used the nasometer for therapy since its introduction. Starr (1993) cited an unpublished study (Burrell, 1989) that included one adult speaker with repaired cleft palate. Starr reported that hypernasality was reduced in the speaker following biofeedback with the nasometer. Starr further noted, however, that imagining studies showed no evidence of improved velopharyngeal function. As suggested by Peterson-Falzone et al. (2001), successful reduction in nasalance via feedback with the nasometer may occur due to "oral articulatory adjustments that decrease oral resistance" (p. 309).

Given the widespread availability of the nasometer and similar devices, we believe that clinicians should consider nasometric feedback more frequently.

One option that might be considered is feedback of "oralance" versus nasalance (Figure 11–1). That is, both the nasometer (model 6450 at least) and the Nasalance Visualization System include display options that reverse the nasalance trace. This means that a rising signal indicates more oral acoustic energy relative to total (i.e., oral plus nasal) acoustic energy. Obviously, it may be easier for a child to improve oral resonance via clear instructions to increase mouth opening than to decrease nasal resonance by vague instructions to be less nasal.

The use of video nasoendoscopy has also been reported to be a successful biofeedback tool. Hoch, Golding-Kushner, Siegel-Sadewitz, and Shprintzen (1986) provided biofeedback to nine patients ranging in age from 6 to 29 years who had various types of VPI. Four patients had Type 3 VPI, described as "inconsistent VPI of structural origin." Two patients had Type 5 VPI, described as "inconsistent VPI

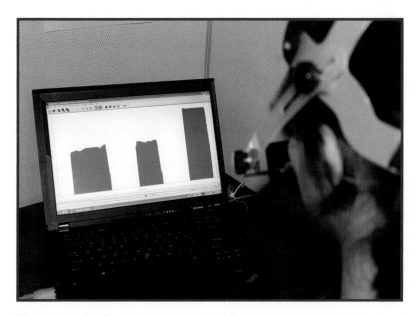

Figure 11–1. Oralance feedback using the nasometer. Increased mouth opening and oral resonance results in higher display bars.

in otherwise normal individuals." These patients were further described as having phoneme-specific VPI. Three patients had Type 6 VPI, described as "arrhythmic valving." Hoch et al. noted that Type 6 VPI is characterized by several closing and opening gestures within a non-nasal production. Hoch et al. provided weekly video nasoendoscopy sessions to the patients that consisted of feedback showing speech attempts with maximal closure contrasted to attempts with minimal closure. After the patients understood the mechanics involved in maximal closure, they were given feedback during all speech attempts. Hoch et al. reported that eight of nine patients showed improved valving after four to nine sessions. Although two of these patients subsequently underwent surgery (pharyngeal flaps), six showed complete resolution of VPI with follow-ups that ranged from 1 to 3 years. It should be noted that two of the patients who showed complete resolution had Type 5 or phoneme-specific VPI. Even with these two patients excluded, Hoch et al. reported impressive results in that four of seven patients (greater than 50%) achieved complete resolution of symptoms and avoided the need for surgery.

Continuous Positive Airway Pressure Therapy

Kuehn and colleagues described a novel behavioral therapy that uses continuous positive airway pressure (CPAP) during speech (Kuehn, 1991; Kuehn et al., 2002). The therapy program consists of an 8-week schedule of speech exercises that use CPAP applied to the nasal cavity. Both speaking time and magnitude of CPAP are systematically increased over the 8-week period. The goal of the program is to strengthen the velopharyngeal muscles

during speech in the face of increasing levels of aerodynamic resistance provided by CPAP. Kuehn, Moon, and Folkins (1993), for example, have shown that levator veli palatini muscle increases activity when intranasal air pressure is applied. Kuehn and colleagues developed multiple lists of disyllables to be used during the therapy. The disyllables contain nasal-obstruent (stop, fricative, and affricate) sequences that are assumed to maximize aerodynamic resistance during the transition from the nasal to the oral obstruent segment. Participants are instructed to stress the second syllable that contains the oral obstruent segment.

Kuehn et al. (2002) investigated the effectiveness of CPAP therapy in reducing hypernasality in children and young adults with repaired cleft palate. They studied 43 speakers ranging in age from approximately 4 to 24 years. All were diagnosed with various levels of hypernasality. The speakers participated in 8 weeks of 6 days-per-week home therapy that systematically increased speaking time from 10 to 24 minutes and CPAP from 4 to 8.5 cm H_2O. Trained listeners who were blinded to the conditions rated pre- and post-therapy recordings of the speakers for hypernasality. Kuehn et al. reported that the therapy was "substantially" effective in reducing hypernasality for some participants.

Although CPAP therapy is based on sound scientific principles, it is not clear that aerodynamic resistance is actually maximized during the closing phase of some of the nasal-obstruent sequences that are used as speech stimuli. Weaver (2003), for example, showed that both intraoral and nasal mask pressures were essentially the same during the /mp/ sequence of nonsense syllables when CPAP was applied. This occurs because during a nasal-plosive sequence, the mouth is closed and pressure equalizes through-out the nasal and oral cavities. Weaver showed that nasal pressure increased only after velopharyngeal closure had occurred. It is also possible that CPAP therapy might trigger an increase in respiratory and vocal effort in speak-ers. Increased vocal effort may occur in response to increasing CPAP levels or due to therapy instructions to stress the sec-ond syllable of the disyllabic stimuli. We observed a boy with marginal VPI who underwent CPAP therapy with a private SLP. Although post-therapy pressure-flow testing showed almost complete velopha-ryngeal closure, the boy also exhibited moderate to severe hoarseness that was not present before therapy. Last, it must be noted that CPAP is a medical device used to treat sleep apnea and requires a physician's prescription. Obtaining a CPAP device, therefore, may require co-management with the patient's primary care provider or other medical specialist.

SECONDARY SURGICAL MANAGEMENT

When symptoms of VPI are consistent and severe enough to reduce intelligibil-ity or create social stigmata, surgical inter-vention is usually recommended. The SLP on the craniofacial team is primarily responsible for making recommendations for surgery to improve velopharyngeal function for speech. The SLP, therefore, must have a thorough understanding of the cause of the speech symptoms, the child's current developmental status, future plans for treatment, and the sur-gical procedures available. As discussed in Chapter 8, obligatory nasal turbulence due to VPI may be perceptually indistin-guishable from posterior nasal fricatives that are learned in the presence of an adequate mechanism. Even experienced

SLPs may be hard pressed to make a dif-ferential diagnosis based solely on per-ceptual assessment. The SLP must be con-fident of a diagnosis and that surgery will resolve symptoms with a high degree of probability. At times, a child may exhibit both learned nasal fricatives and mild to moderate obligatory symptoms of VPI. In these cases, it is our opinion that speech therapy should always be recommended before surgery. Successful elimination of perceptually salient nasal fricatives may shift the diagnostic threshold for the need of secondary surgery.

The SLP also needs to be aware of the child's current developmental status and future treatment plans. At times, older children may develop hypernasality or audible nasal air emission due to invo-lution of adenoids during the pubertal growth spurt (Mason & Warren, 1980). Although obligatory symptoms may reach a threshold for a surgical recom-mendation, it may be in the best interest of the child to wait if he or she is likely to need maxillary advancement surgery in the near future (see Chapter 13). Maxillary advancement may increase the extent of VPI and exacerbate obligatory symptoms. If so, then careful assessment of the child following maxillary advancement with a recommendation for surgery or prosthet-ics at that time may be the best approach.

Posterior Pharyngeal Flaps

Because of its long history, surgical cre-ation of a posterior pharyngeal flap is perhaps the most common procedure to correct VPI. Essentially, a pharyngeal flap obturates the velopharyngeal space (Fig-ure 11–2). The German physician Passa-vant in 1865 first described the adhesion of the posterior border of the soft palate to the posterior pharyngeal wall in an

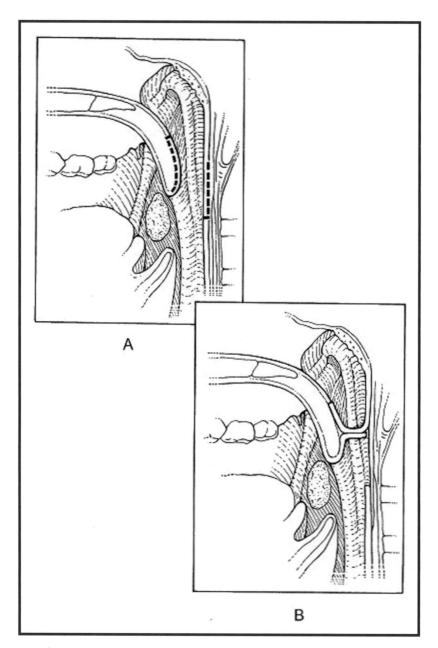

Figure 11–2. Superior-base posterior pharyngeal flap. (From Sloan, G., & Zajac, D. J. [2006]. Velopharyngeal dysfunction. In S. Mathes [Ed.], *Plastic surgery. Volume 4: Pediatric plastic surgery* [2nd ed., pp. 311– 337]. Philadelphia, PA: Saunders Elsevier. Used with permission.)

attempt to correct VPI (Sloan & Zajac, 2006). This was followed by the true attachment of a posterior pharyngeal flap to the palate by Schoenborn, another German physician, in 1875. Schoenborn first created flaps with inferior attachments but switched to superior attachments over time (discussed below). Padgett (1930) promoted the use of the superior-based pharyngeal flap in the United States as a procedure to treat VPI.

As illustrated in Figure 11–2, a superior-based pharyngeal flap is created by making incisions in the posterior pharyngeal wall, releasing a myomucosal flap of tissue, and inserting the flap into the soft palate. Because the base of the flap that remains attached to the pharyngeal wall is higher than the part inserted into the soft palate, it is called a superior-based flap. Early attempts to create inferior-based flaps were largely abandoned due to difficulty in creating flaps that were of adequate length. If an inferior-based flap is too short or too low, it may restrict elevation of the velum (Padgett, 1930).

Surgeons vary in their methods of creating pharyngeal flaps, especially regarding attachment to the soft palate. Sloan and Zajac (2006) described a method of splitting the soft palate in the midline and elevating flaps from the nasal surface of the soft palate to line the pharyngeal flap (see Figure 11–2B). Lining the flap may help prevent tissue shrinkage during postsurgical healing. Sloan and Zajac also recommended closing the donor site on the posterior pharyngeal wall, if possible.

Pharyngeal flaps are essentially static structures. Success of the operation in eliminating or reducing obligatory speech symptoms, therefore, is primarily dependent on the position and width of the flap relative to the location of attempted velopharyngeal closure. Mesial movement of the lateral pharyngeal walls to meet the flap and close the lateral ports is critical to achieving success. Flaps that are placed too low in the pharynx may miss the level of attempted closure. Even if positioned at the appropriate level, the lateral pha-

ryngeal walls may fail to meet a flap that is too narrow. Shprintzen et al. (1979) recommended that flaps be "tailor-made." That is, they recommended that surgeons plan the width of flaps by estimating the relative degree of lateral pharyngeal wall movement during preoperative imaging procedures such as multiview videofluoroscopy and nasoendoscopy.

Peterson-Falzone et al. (2001) noted a wide range of reported success rates for pharyngeal flap surgery from 60% to 100% across studies. They emphasized, however, that too many studies used only vague categories of speech outcomes such as "normal" or "improved" and that many studies did not consider overcorrection (i.e., hyponasality) as a negative outcome. Hogan (1973) reported an overall success rate of 98% (91 of 93 patients) for the "total elimination" of hypernasality following pharyngeal flap surgery; he reported three cases that resulted in hyponasality. Hogan also reported "negligible" increases in nasal resistance during breathing for all patients. Hogan attributed his impressive results to lateral port control during surgery. Specifically, Hogan inserted two 4 mm–diameter catheters into each lateral port and sutured the marginal edges of the pharyngeal flap around the catheters to create a known port size. The combined area of the resulting two flap ports was approximately 25 mm^2. Hogan stated that this port size was targeted because speech studies—including aerodynamic studies by Warren and colleagues—showed that definite symptoms of VPI occurred when velopharyngeal port size exceeded 20 mm^2. Hogan reported that pressure-flow studies performed on the 91 successfully treated patients indicated an average velopharyngeal port area during speech of 5.8 mm^2. He attributed the reduction in area from the targeted 25 mm^2 of the portals at rest to mesial movement of the lateral pharyngeal walls. It is not known, however, to what degree, if any, shrinkage of the ports due to postsurgical healing contributed to the findings.

Argamaso (1990) reported impressive results when preoperative movement of the lateral pharyngeal walls was used to determine flap width. He reported on 356 consecutive patients operated on between 1980 and 1986. The patients received either narrow, moderately wide, very wide, or "obstructing" pharyngeal flaps depending on the extent of medial pharyngeal wall movement. Obstructing flaps were limited to patients who showed "gross" VPI reflected by poor or absent lateral pharyngeal wall movement. Argamaso reported correction of hypernasality in 97.8% of cases, including 9.5% of patients who developed hyponasality. He concluded that success of pharyngeal flap surgery is based on adequate movement of the lateral pharyngeal walls. He further commented that a pressing problem was the treatment of patients who showed limited lateral pharyngeal wall movement. He noted that these patients were "destined either for very wide flaps that may induce hyponasality or for short or subobstructing flaps" that did not resolve symptoms (p. 268).

Zajac et al. (2015) suggested that successful pharyngeal flap surgery should include adequate function for (a) oral speech segments, (b) nasal speech segments, and (c) nasal breathing. They used aerodynamic criteria to evaluate speech following pharyngeal flap surgery by a single surgeon in 14 children. Adequate function for oral speech segments was defined as estimated velopharyngeal orifice areas under 5 mm^2 during production of /p/ in syllables and words. Adequate function for nasal speech segments was defined as velopharyngeal orifice areas greater than 5 mm^2 during production of /m/ in words. The latter criterion was rather liberal as typical velopharyngeal areas for the nasal consonant /m/ have been reported to be at least 10 mm^2 depending upon age of the speaker (Zajac, 2000). Zajac et al. (2015) reported that 10 of 14 children (71%) were adequate on oral speech segments following surgery, while 8 of 12 children (67%) were adequate on the nasal speech segment (data were not available for two children). Only 4 of 12 children (33%), however, were categorized as adequate on *both* oral and nasal speech segments. These results suggest that success rates of pharyngeal flap surgery may not be high when objective aerodynamic criteria are used to evaluate outcomes regarding both oral and nasal speech segments. Zajac et al. cautioned, however, that they did not consider perceptual outcomes of the children. It is not known, therefore, if significant hyponasality was associated with any of the children who exhibited small velopharyngeal areas during nasal consonants.

The most serious negative consequence of pharyngeal flap surgery is obstructive sleep apnea (OSA). Some studies have estimated that 20% to 30% of individuals may experience persistent OSA following pharyngeal flap surgery (Orr, Levine, & Buchanan, 1987; Sirios, Caouette-Laberge, Spier, Larocque, & Egerszegi, 1994). A recent study, however, indicated that OSA was not significantly more prevalent in middle-aged adults with pharyngeal flaps than in those without pharyngeal flaps (Campos et al., 2015). If OSA is confirmed via sleep studies, then CPAP may be tried to prevent airway collapse and alleviate symptoms. In most cases, however, successful resolution of OSA will require surgical revision or division of the flap (Agarwal et al., 2003; Katzel et al., 2015). Agarwal et al. (2003) performed surgical division of pharyngeal flaps in 12 patients diagnosed with OSA. Of interest, they reported that significant symptoms of VPI returned in only one of the patients. Agarwal et al. suggested that speech did not deteriorate in most patients due to a combination of the bulk of the flap remaining on the posterior pharyngeal wall and a general narrowing of the velopharyngeal port due to scarring. In essence, division of the flap may have resulted in posterior pharyngeal wall augmentation (discussed later in the chapter). It is also possible that the presence of the pharyngeal flap may have stimulated lateral pharyngeal wall movement—perhaps due to increased aerodynamic resistance—that continued or even increased following division of the flap.

Sphincter Pharyngoplasty

Beginning in the 1950s, surgeons began to devise other procedures to correct VPI. Hynes (1950) described pharyngoplasty by means of muscle transplantation, or more commonly referred to as sphincter pharyngoplasty (Figure 11–3). Hynes initially performed a two-stage surgical procedure. In the first stage, he divided the soft palate to gain access to the nasopharynx, raised bilateral muscle flaps from salpingopharyngeus, and attached the flaps in a side-by-side fashion to the posterior pharyngeal wall. In a second surgery, Hynes would repair the soft palate. Later, Hynes (1953) began using bulkier flaps taken from the salpingopharyngeus, palatopharyngeus, and part of the superior constrictor muscles and abandoned a two-stage approach. The flaps were attached to the posterior pha-

ryngeal wall in an end-to-end fashion with some overlap to tighten the sphincter. Orticochea (1968) advocated a *dynamic* sphincter pharyngoplasty. This procedure differed from Hynes in two ways. First, Orticochea placed the bilateral flaps at a lower position than Hynes, substantially below the level of velopharyngeal closure. Second, Orticochea also raised a separate, inferior flap from the posterior pharyngeal wall and sutured the two lateral flaps to this flap. Of interest, Orticochea performed sphincter palatoplasty routinely on all patients 6 months after initial palate surgery, regardless of velopharyngeal status. A third variant of sphincter pharyngoplasty was described by Jackson and Silverton (1977). Their procedure was similar to that of Orticochea except they raised superior-based posterior pharyngeal flaps. This was done to create a higher sphincter than that of Orticochea.

Unlike posterior pharyngeal flaps, sphincter pharyngoplasty was thought to produce a dynamic mechanism to correct VPI. As suggested by Pigott (1993), the sphincter pharyngoplasty may work by (a) passively augmenting the posterior pharyngeal wall (the initial intent of Hynes), (b) passively reducing the transverse dimension of the nasopharynx, or (c) actually producing dynamic sphincter-like closure by means of palatopharyngeus muscle activity. Although evidence is sparse, at least one study has shown that dynamic muscle activity does not occur. Ysunza et al. (1999) studied 25 patients who had undergone the Jackson and Silverton method of sphincter pharyngoplasty. All patients were simultaneously examined by video nasoendoscopy and electromyography (EMG). Hook-wire electrodes were inserted into the levator veli palatini, superior constrictor, and palatopharyngeus muscles. Ysunza et al.

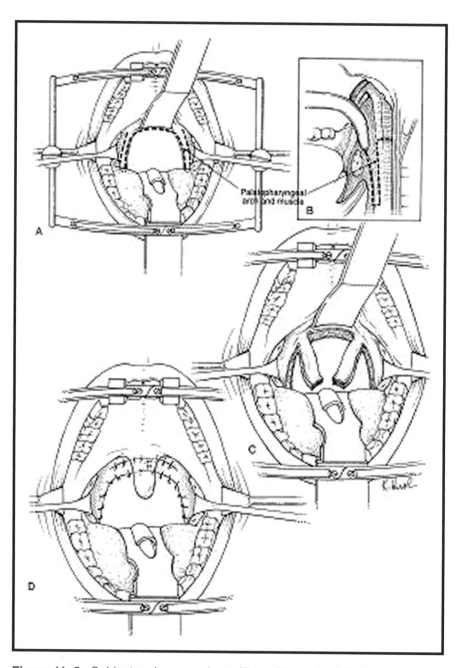

Figure 11–3. Sphincter pharyngoplasty. (From Sloan, G., & Zajac, D.J. [2006]. Velopharyngeal dysfunction. In S. Mathes [Ed.], *Plastic surgery. Volume 4: Pediatric plastic surgery* [2nd ed., pp. 311–337]. Philadelphia, PA: Saunders Elsevier. Used with permission.)

reported that 23 of 25 patients showed complete, sphincter-like velopharyngeal closure. EMG activity, however, was observed only from levator and superior constrictor muscles. They concluded that sphincter-like activity of the port was passive and caused by contraction of the superior constrictor muscle, not palatopharyngeus. Figure 11–4 shows a sphincter pharyngoplasty in a teenage patient. The patient's speech was characterized by excessive hypernasality. There was little movement of the sphincter during phonation, which appears to be placed too low to assist with closure.

Sphincter pharyngoplasties have been considered less disruptive to sleep breathing than pharyngeal flaps. There is little empirical evidence, however, to support this claim. Abyholm et al. (2005) reported no long-term difference in the incidence of OSA between patients who were randomized to receive either pharyngeal flap or sphincter pharyngoplasty. Although they stated that OSA is rare with either pro-

cedure, this conclusion is not consistent with other studies. It should also be noted that Abyholm et al. did not describe the relative widths of the pharyngeal flaps in their patients.

Palatal Lengthening

Furlow (1986) described the double-opposing Z-plasty (DOZ) as a surgical technique for primary repair of palatal clefts. As reviewed in Chapter 5, this technique retropositions the levator sling while lengthening the soft palate. Because of its lengthening potential, DOZ has been used as a surgical procedure (either primary or secondary) for older children with VPI (Figure 11–5). Chen, Wu, Chen, and Noordhoff (1994) performed DOZ on 18 speakers with repaired cleft palate and VPI. They carefully selected the patients based on presurgical assessment of velopharyngeal closure patterns and size of the gap. Chen et al. reported that

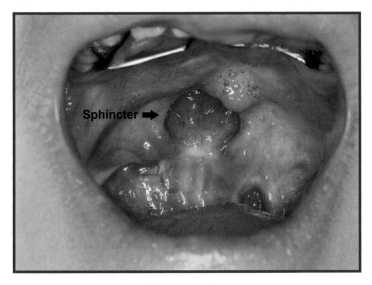

Figure 11–4. Teenager with a sphincter pharyngoplasty. Also note palatal expander (see Chapter 12).

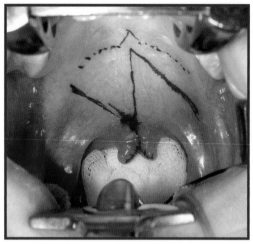 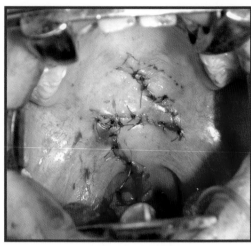

A   B

Figure 11–5. A. Surgical markings for double-opposing Z-plasty in a child with submucous cleft palate. **B.** Same child following surgery. (Courtesy of Joseph A. Napoli, MD, DDS, Plastic, Maxillofacial, and Craniofacial Surgery, Alfred I. duPont Hospital for Children, Wilmington, DE.)

"complete" velopharyngeal closure was achieved in 16 speakers. Fifteen of the speakers had presurgical gaps between the velum and posterior pharyngeal wall that were less than 5 mm as determined by lateral view fluoroscopy. A linear distance of 5 mm between the velum and posterior pharyngeal wall would be approximately 20 mm^2 assuming a circular pattern of closure. The two speakers who did not improve both had presurgical gaps that were greater than 10 mm. This linear gap distance would be greater than 70 mm^2, again assuming a circular pattern of closure. Chen et al. concluded that DOZ is a promising secondary surgical procedure to correct VPI, especially for relatively small velopharyngeal gaps.

Posterior Pharyngeal Wall Augmentation

Various procedures have been used to augment the posterior pharyngeal wall to eliminate VPI. Blocksma (1964) reviewed early attempts to inject materials such as Vaseline and paraffin, at times with disastrous results. Later procedures have ranged from insertion of autogenous cartilage to fat injections to implants of alloplastic materials such as silicone, Teflon, and Proplast. Significant disadvantages of these procedures, especially alloplastic implants, include infection, extrusion, and migration of the materials. Although some recent reports have noted success with autogenous fat injections, these procedures may have to be repeated due to absorption of the fat (Leuchter, Schweizer, Hohlfeld, & Pasche, 2010).

An Algorithm for Selecting Secondary Procedures

Gart and Gosain (2014) described an algorithmic approach to assessing and surgically treating the patient with VPI. The approach is briefly described here not because we believe that it is necessarily the best, but because it exemplifies the use of careful presurgical assessment and, for the most part, evidence-based selection of procedures.

Gart and Gosain (2014) recommended surgical procedures based on the pattern of attempted velopharyngeal closure and size of the residual gap. They suggested that a sagittal closure pattern occurs due to a deficiency in either length or movement of the velum. For small sagittal gaps less than 9 mm, they recommended DOZ; for sagittal gaps greater than 9 mm, they recommended pharyngeal flap. Gart and Gosain's recommendation of pharyngeal flaps for large sagittal gaps is consistent with the need to obturate in the absence of adequate velar length or movement. The recommendation of DOZ for smaller sagittal gaps, however, is more difficult to understand, at least for certain scenarios. For patients who lack velar movement, it is not clear if increased length of a non-moving velum will facilitate closure.

Gart and Gosain noted that coronal patterns of attempted velopharyngeal closure indicate the lack of lateral pharyngeal wall movement. Accordingly, they recommended sphincter pharyngoplasty when gaps are less than 9 mm and a combination of DOZ and sphincter pharyngoplasty when gaps are greater than 9 mm. Relative to the latter, they reported an 85% success rate in eliminating VPI in 13 patients.

For circular gaps, Gart and Gosain recommended DOZ when the gap is less than 9 mm and narrow pharyngeal flaps when gaps are larger. They based these recommendations on the observation that circular closure indicates movement of both the velum and lateral pharyngeal walls. They believe, therefore, that length-ening the palate can effectively eliminate small gaps whereas narrow pharyngeal flaps can be successful for larger gaps. Finally, Gart and Gosain noted that children with 22q deletion syndrome present with challenging surgical management decisions due to frequently encountered hypodynamic velopharyngeal mechanisms. They recommended wide obstructing pharyngeal flaps for these children.

PROSTHETIC MANAGEMENT

The American Dental Association defines prosthodontics as "The dental specialty pertaining to the diagnosis, treatment planning, rehabilitation and maintenance of the oral function, comfort, appearance and health of patients with clinical conditions associated with missing or deficient teeth and/or oral and maxillofacial tissues using biocompatible substitutes." Because individuals with cleft lip and palate often have dental anomalies, prosthodontists have long been vital members of the craniofacial team. As noted in Chapter 5, the Academy of Cleft Palate Prosthesis was the forerunner of the current American Cleft Palate-Craniofacial Association. The craniofacial prosthodontist has expertise not only in restoring missing teeth via dentures and implants, but also in restoring maxillary and velopharyngeal function via various types of obturators and speech appliances. At times, other dental specialists, such as the orthodontist or pediatric dentist, may have expertise in fabricating prosthetic appliances.

Typically, two types of removable speech appliances are used to manage VPI: speech bulb obturators and palatal lifts. Speech bulb appliances are generally used when a speaker has some velopharyngeal movement but the soft palate is short or the nasopharynx is excessively deep. Palatal lift appliances are generally used when a speaker has limited velar movement.

Speech Bulbs

A speech bulb appliance consists of an anterior maxillary section that is held in place by clasps attached to the teeth and a tail section that extends into the nasopharynx as an obturating bulb (Figure 11–6). The bulb extension must be carefully formed to fit snuggly in the nasopharyngeal space without exerting undue pressure on the posterior pharyngeal wall. The anterior portion should not be bulky to interfere with articulation. The velum and lateral pharyngeal walls must be mobile to elevate and close around the bulb during speech. The bulb must not be too large as to interfere with breathing and production of nasal consonants.

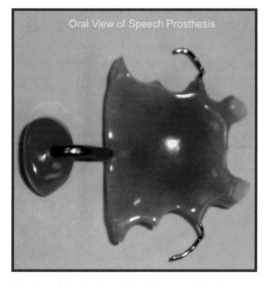

Figure 11–6. Combination partial denture to replace missing anterior teeth and speech bulb appliance. (Courtesy of Dennis Ruscello, PhD, University of West Virginia.)

A speech bulb appliance is typically indicated when the velum is short or the nasopharynx is deep. Candidates for speech bulbs must have adequate dentition to hold the appliance, practice good oral hygiene, not have an excessive gag reflex, and be motivated to comply with procedures. Typically, speech bulbs are recommended for individuals who are not good surgical candidates due to coexisting medical problems such as OSA or who have already exhausted surgical options without success. Generally, young children are not good candidates due to the need for cooperation when fabricating the appliance and the need for frequent modifications due to growth.

Golding-Kushner, Cisneros, and Le-Blanc (1995) described three primary uses of speech appliances, including bulbs. First, the appliance is used as a permanent solution for VPI. This typically occurs when the individual is either not a surgical candidate or chooses not to have surgery. Second, the appliance is used for a temporary period of time prior to surgery. This may occur if there are other pressing medical needs that might delay surgery. Third, the appliance is used as part of bulb-reduction therapy (Blakely, 1964; Golding-Kushner et al., 1995). This therapy is designed to stimulate velar and lateral pharyngeal wall movement over time by gradually reducing the size of the bulb. Typically, the speaker wears the bulb appliance for 1 to 3 months. If nasoendoscopy shows complete velopharyngeal closure, then the bulb is reduced in size. The speaker wears the reduced bulb appliance for another 1 to 3 months, and the bulb is reduced in size again. This cycle is repeated until the speaker (a) shows complete velopharyngeal closure without the bulb, or (b) reaches some optimal level of closure. In the latter case, the speaker either continues to use the bulb as a permanent appliance or seeks surgical management.

Golding-Kushner et al. (1995) reported interesting results of speech-bulb reduction therapy. They enrolled 31 patients ranging in age from 3½ to 50 years who presented with VPI due to nonsyndromic and syndromic cleft palate, neurological problems, and idiopathic reasons. Of 17 patients who completed the program, they reported that symptoms of VPI were "completely eliminated" with the appliance in place and that some reduction in bulb size was possible for each. Golding-Kushner et al. reported that two patients appeared to achieve complete velopharyngeal closure—one required 13 visits over a period of 21 months, and the other required 10 visits over 13 months—and did not need surgery. Finally, although they reported that 10 of 17 patients went on to receive pharyngeal flaps, six needed less obstructive flaps following bulb-reduction therapy due to increased lateral pharyngeal wall movement.

Although Golding-Kushner et al. (1995) reported impressive results, they noted several disadvantages of speech bulbs. These included the potential to interfere with needed orthodontic treatment and cause excessive wear of the teeth. They also noted that because most of the patients had also received simultaneous speech therapy for compensatory articulations, it was difficult to separate the effects of the bulb-reduction therapy from possible improvement in velar function due to the elimination of compensatory errors.

Palatal Lifts

A palatal lift appliance differs from a speech bulb in that its primary purpose is to physically lift and position the soft palate against the posterior pharyngeal wall versus obturating the nasopharyngeal space (Figure 11–7). Palatal lifts are often recommended for patients who have adequate velar length and mass but who lack movement due to congenital neuromuscular disorders or acquired head trauma.

Similar to speech bulb appliances, candidates for palatal lifts must have adequate dentition, practice good oral hygiene, not have an excessive gag reflex, and be highly motivated. The patient's

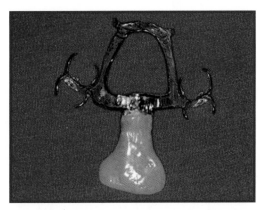

A

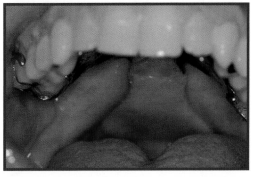

B

Figure 11–7. A. Palatal lift appliance. **B.** Patient wearing appliance. (Courtesy of Luiz Andre Pimenta, DDS, MS, PhD, Craniofacial Center, University of North Carolina at Chapel Hill.)

ability to tolerate and benefit from a palatal lift can be determined by an SLP. While instructing the patient to prolong a low vowel, the SLP can use a tongue depressor to manually lift the soft palate up and against the posterior pharyngeal wall. If there is a definite shift in resonance—and the patient does not exhibit a severe gag reflex—then he or she may be a good candidate for a palatal lift.

Nasal Valve Appliances

There have been several reports of construction of nasal valve appliances to eliminate or reduce nasal air loss during speech due to VPI (Hakel, Buekelman, Fager, Green, & Marshall, 2004; Suwaki, Nanba, Ito, Kumakura, & Minagi, 2008). These devices operate as one-way valves that are inserted into the nostrils (Figure 11–8). The valves open during inspiration and close during expiration or speech when a positive pressure is applied. Candidates for such devices are typically adult patients with head trauma who cannot tolerate palatal lifts. Hakel et al. (2004) constructed one-way nasal valves using commercially available nose filters fitted with rubber flaps and O-rings. They reported that the nasal valves reduced air escape and increased oral air pressure in two speakers with severe dysarthria and VPI.

CHAPTER SUMMARY

Obligatory symptoms of VPI such as hypernasality, weak oral air pressure, and nasal air emission persist in some children

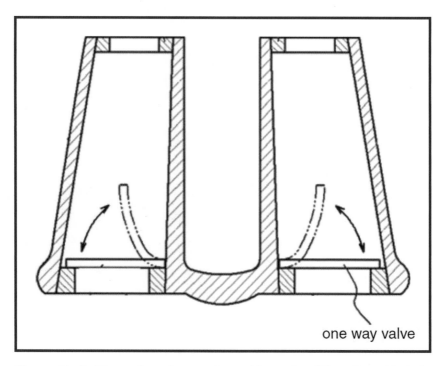

one way valve

Figure 11–8. Plane view of a nasal speaking valve. (From Suwaki et al., 2008). Nasal speaking valve: A device for managing velopharyngeal incompetence. *Journal of Oral Rehabilitation, 35,* 73–78. Used with permission.)

with repaired cleft palate. In some cases, behavioral approaches such as instrumental biofeedback during speech may be effective in reducing or eliminating symptoms. In most cases, however, physical management of the velopharyngeal mechanism via surgery or prosthetics will be required to eliminate symptoms.

REFERENCES

Abyholm, F., D'Antonio, L., Davidson Ward, S. L., Kjøll, L., Saeed, M., Shaw, W., . . . VPI Surgical Group. (2005). Pharyngeal flap and sphincterplasty for velopharyngeal insufficiency have equal outcome at 1 year postoperatively: Results of a randomized trial. *Cleft Palate-Craniofacial Journal, 42*(5), 501–511.

Agarwal, T., Sloan, G. M., Zajac, D. J., Uhrich, K. S., Meadows, W., & Lewchalermwong, J. A. (2003). Speech benefits of posterior pharyngeal flap are preserved after surgical flap division for obstructive sleep apnea. *Journal of Craniofacial Surgery, 14*, 630–636.

Argamaso, R. V. (1990). The pharyngeal flap. In D. A. Kernahan & S. W. Rosenstein (Eds.), *Cleft lip and palate: A system of management* (pp. 263–269). Baltimore, MD: Williams & Wilkins.

Blakely, R. W. (1964). The complimentary use of speech prostheses and pharyngeal flaps in palatal insufficiency. *Cleft Palate Journal, 1*(2), 194–198.

Blocksma, R. (1964). Silicone implants for velopharyngeal incompetence: A progress report. *Cleft Palate Journal, 1*(1), 72–81.

Burrell, K. (1989). *The modification of nasality using Nasometer feedback* (Unpublished master's thesis). University of Minnesota, Minneapolis.

Campos, L. D., Trindade-Suedam, I. K., Sampaio-Teixeira, A. C., Yamashita, R. P., Lauris, J. R., Lorenzi-Filho, G., & Trindade, I. E. (2015). Obstructive sleep apnea following pharyngeal flap surgery for velopharyngeal insufficiency: A prospective polysomnographic and aerodynamic study in middle-aged adults. *Cleft Palate-Craniofacial Journal.* Advance online publication.

Chen, P. K., Wu, J. T., Chen, Y. R., & Noordhoff, M. S. (1994). Correction of secondary velopharyngeal insufficiency in cleft palate patients with the Furlow palatoplasty. *Plastic and Reconstructive Surgery, 94*(7), 933–941.

Fletcher, S. G. (1972). Contingencies for bioelectronic modification of nasality. *Journal of Speech and Hearing Disorders, 37*, 329–346.

Fletcher, S. G. (1978). *Diagnosing speech disorders from cleft palate.* New York, NY: Grune & Stratton.

Furlow, L. T. (1986). Cleft palate repair by double opposing Z-plasty. *Plastic and Reconstructive Surgery, 78*, 724–736.

Gart, M. S., & Gosain, A. K. (2014). Surgical management of velopharyngeal insufficiency. *Clinics in Plastic Surgery, 41*(2), 253–270.

Golding-Kushner, K. J., Cisneros, G., & LeBlanc, E. (1995). Speech bulbs. In R. J. Shprintzen & J. Bardach (Eds.), *Cleft palate speech management: A multidisciplinary approach* (pp. 352–363). St. Louis, MO: Mosby.

Hakel, M., Buekelman, D. R., Fager, S., Green, J. R., & Marshall, J. (2004). Nasal obturator for velopharyngeal dysfunction in dysarthria: Technical report on a one-way valve. *Journal of Medical Speech Language Pathology, 12*(4), 155–159.

Hynes, W. (1950). Pharyngoplasty by muscle transplantation. *British Journal of Plastic Surgery, 3*, 128–135.

Hynes, W. (1953). The results of pharyngoplasty by muscle transplantation in "failed cleft palate" cases, with special reference to the influence of the pharynx on voice production. *Annals of the Royal College of Surgeons of England, 13*, 17–35.

Hoch, L., Golding-Kushner, K., Siegel-Sadewitz, V. L., & Shprintzen, R. J. (1986). Speech therapy. *Seminars in Speech and Language, 7*(3), 313–326.

Hogan, V. M. (1973). A clarification of the goals in cleft palate speech and the introduction of the lateral port control (L.P.C.) pharyngeal flap. *Cleft Palate Journal, 10*, 331–345.

Jackson, I. T., & Silverton, J. S. (1977). The sphincter pharyngoplasty as a secondary procedure in cleft palates. *Plastic and Reconstructive Surgery, 59*, 518–524.

Katzel, E., Naran, S., MacIsaac, Z., Camison, L., Goldstein, J., Grunwaldt, L., . . . Losee, J. (2015, April). *Speech outcomes following clinically indicated posterior pharyngeal flap takedown.* Paper presented at the Annual Meeting of the American Cleft Palate-Craniofacial Association, Palm Springs, CA.

Kuehn, D. P. (1991). New therapy for treating hypernasal speech using continuous positive airway pressure (CPAP). *Plastic and Reconstructive Surgery, 88*, 959.

Kuehn, D. P., Imrey, P. B., Tomes, L., Jones, D. L., O'Gara, M. M., Seaver, E. J., . . . Wachtel, J. M. (2002). Efficacy of continuous positive airway pressure for treatment of hypernasality, *Cleft Palate-Craniofacial Journal, 39*, 267.

Kuehn, D. P., Moon, J. B., & Folkins, J. W. (1993). Levator veli palatini muscle activity in relation to intranasal air pressure variation. *Cleft Palate Craniofacial Journal, 30*, 361.

Leuchter, I., Schweizer, V., Hohlfeld , J., & Pasche, P. (2010). Treatment of velopharyngeal insufficiency by autologous fat injection. *European Archives of Otorhinolaryngology, 267*(6), 977–983.

Mason, R. M., & Warren, D. W. (1980). Adenoid involution and developing hypernasality in cleft palate. *Journal of Speech and Hearing Disorders, 45*(4), 469–480.

McWilliams, B. J., & Bradley, D. P. (1965). Ratings of velopharyngeal closure during blowing and speech. *Cleft Palate Journal, 45*, 46–55.

Moll, K. L. (1965). A cinefluorographic study of velopharyngeal function in normal during various activities. *Cleft Palate Journal, 31*, 112–122.

Morris, H. L. (1973). Velopharyngeal competence and primary cleft palate surgery, 1960–1971: A critical review. *Cleft Palate Journal, 10*, 62–71.

Orr, W. C., Levine, N. S., & Buchanan, R. T. (1987). Effects of cleft palate repair and pharyngeal flap surgery on upper airway obstruction during sleep. *Plastic and Reconstructive Surgery, 80*, 226–230.

Orticochea, M. (1968). Construction of a dynamic muscle sphincter in cleft palates. *Plastic and Reconstructive Surgery, 41*, 323–327.

Owens, R. E., Metz, D. E., & Haas, A. (2003). *Introduction to communication disorders: A life span perspective* (2nd ed.). Boston, MA: Pearson Education.

Padgett, E. C. (1930). The repair of cleft palates after unsuccessful operations, with special reference to cases with an extensive loss of palatal tissue. *Archives of Surgery, 20*, 453–472.

Peterson-Falzone, S. J. (1990). A cross-sectional analysis of speech results following palatal closure. In J. Bardach & H. L. Morris (Eds.), *Multidisciplinary management of cleft lip and palate* (pp. 750–756). Philadelphia, PA: W.B. Saunders.

Peterson-Falzone, S. J., Hardin-Jones, M. A., & Karnell, M. P. (2001). *Cleft palate speech* (3rd ed.). St. Louis, MO: Mosby.

Pigott, R. W. (1993). The results of pharyngoplasty by muscle transplantation by Wilfred Hynes, *British Journal of Plastic Surgery, 46*, 440–442.

Riski, J. E. (1979). Articulation skills and oral-nasal resonance in children with pharyngeal flaps. *Cleft Palate Journal, 16*, 421–428.

Ruscello, D. M. (2008). An examination of non-speech oral motor exercises for children with VPI. *Seminars in Speech and Language, 29*, 294–303.

Shprintzen, R. J., Lewin, M. L., Croft, C. B., Daniller, A. I., Argamaso, R. V., Ship, A. G., & Strauch, B. (1979). A comprehensive study of pharyngeal flap surgery: Tailor-made flaps. *Cleft Palate Journal, 16*, 46–55.

Sirois, M., Caouette-Laberge, L., Spier, S., Larocque, Y., & Egerszegi, E. P. (1994). Sleep apnea following a pharyngeal flap: A feared complication. *Plastic and Reconstructive Surgery, 93*(5), 943–947.

Skahan, S. M., Watson, M., & Lof, G. L. (2007). Speech-language pathologists' assessment practices for children with suspected speech sound disorders: Results of a national survey. *American Journal of Speech-Language Pathology, 16,* 246–259.

Sloan, G., & Zajac, D. J. (2006). Velopharyngeal dysfunction. In S. Mathes (Ed.), *Plastic surgery. Volume 4: Pediatric plastic surgery* (2nd ed., pp. 311–337). Philadelphia, PA: Saunders Elsevier.

Starr, C. D. (1993). Behavioral approaches to treating velopharyngeal closure and nasality. In K. T. Moller & C. D. Starr (Eds.), *Cleft palate interdisciplinary issues and treatment: For clinicians by clinicians* (pp. 337–356). Austin, TX: Pro-Ed.

Suwaki, M., Nanba, K., Ito, E., Kumakura, I., & Minagi, S. (2008). Nasal speaking valve: A device for managing velopharyngeal incompetence. *Journal of Oral Rehabilitation, 35,* 73–78.

Weaver, L. A. (2003). *Respiratory and velar EMG responses to nasal CPAP variations during speech* (Unpublished master's thesis). University of North Carolina at Chapel Hill, Chapel Hill, NC.

Ysunza, A., Pamplona, M. C., Molina, F., Chacón, E., & Collado, M. (1999). Velopha-ryngeal motion after sphincter pharyngoplasty: A videonasopharyngoscopic and electromyographic study. *Plastic and Reconstructive Surgery, 104*(4), 905–910.

Zajac, D. J. (2000). Pressure-flow characteristics of /m/ and /p/ production in speakers without cleft palate: Developmental findings. *Cleft Palate-Craniofacial Journal, 37,* 468–477.

Zajac, D. J., van Aalst, J., Vallino, L., & Napoli, J. (2011, April). *Nasal ram pressure as an indicator of velopharyngeal closure during stop consonants in 2 year-olds following palate repair.* Paper presented at the Annual Meeting of the American Cleft Palate-Craniofacial Association, San Juan, PR.

Zajac, D. J., Vivaldi, D., Drake, A., van Aalst, J. A., Warren, T., Eshghi, M., & Feldbaum, M. (2015, April). *Pharyngeal flap outcomes based upon aerodynamic assessment of oral and nasal speech segments: Preliminary findings.* Paper presented at the Annual Meeting of the American Cleft Palate-Craniofacial Association, Palm Springs, CA.

12

Alveolar Cleft Repair

Joseph A. Napoli

INTRODUCTION

The need for a multidisciplinary team approach to cleft care is well established, and nicely demonstrated during management of the alveolar process cleft. During this aspect of cleft treatment, there is need for close communication and coordination of care, especially among the surgeon, dental specialists, and speech-language pathologist (SLP).

For children born with complete cleft lip and palate, the reconstruction for repair of the cleft is most commonly done in three stages with each stage addressing a different anatomic zone (Figure 12–1).

The first two stages, cleft lip repair and cleft palate repair, have already been discussed in Chapter 5. With the lip and palate repairs completed during infancy, the zone between the lip and palate, which include the alveolar process of the maxilla, usually remains unrepaired during this early stage of life. Although some reconstructive approaches include repair of the alveolar process during infancy, either with bone graft ("primary alveolar bone graft") or without bone graft (gin-

givoperiosteoplasty or GPP), each with its advantages and disadvantages (and proponents and detractors), this chapter will cover alveolar process cleft repair

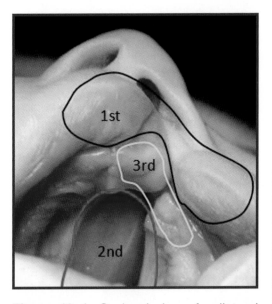

Figure 12–1. Occlusal view of unilateral cleft lip and palate showing the three general zones of the cleft requiring repair: lip outlined in blue, palate outlined in red, and alveolar process region outlined in yellow.

as it is done during the mixed dentition stage. This is the most common approach, and there is a great body of evidence over several decades supporting it. We will describe each specialist's role, including the orthodontic preparation usually required before surgical repair, the effect on speech, the interaction among the specialists, and the expected outcome of treatment. In this chapter, the terms "alveolar process" and "alveolar ridge" will be used interchangeably.

ANATOMY AND FUNCTION OF THE ALVEOLAR PROCESS

Knowledge of the normal and pathologic anatomy of the entire vocal tract, including the alveolar process, enhances an understanding of the etiology and differential diagnosis of speech errors. The alveolar ridge is the part of the maxilla that protrudes into the oral cavity and contains the developing and erupted teeth and their supporting bone (Figure 12–2).

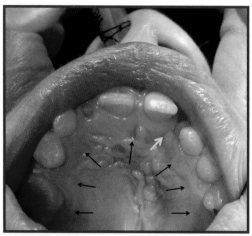

A

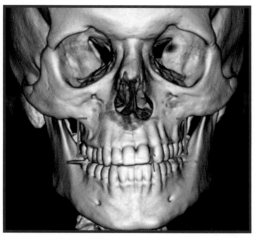

B

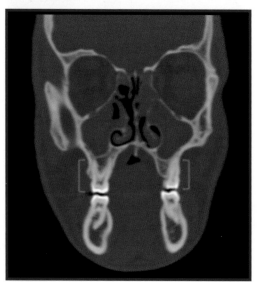

C

Figure 12–2. A. Occlusal view of the arch of the alveolar process (*black arrows*) with a narrow alveolar process cleft (*yellow arrow*). **B.** Three-dimensional computed tomography (3D CT) scan of repaired left side alveolar process. Brackets denote alveolar process of maxilla. Arrow points to site of repaired alveolar cleft. Note asymmetry of pyriform rim. **C.** CT scan coronal view showing alveolar process (*red brackets*) supporting teeth.

The function of the alveolar process is to support the teeth and to provide a stable platform for biting and chewing. During infancy and early childhood, it is the location of the developing tooth buds. In the adult, it is the support for the erupted teeth with their roots attached to bone by a thin ligament. The alveolar process of the anterior maxilla is continuous superiorly with the pyriform rim, which is the component of the maxilla that makes up the anterior aspect of the nasal floor and provides skeletal support for the nasal soft tissue and the upper lip.

A cleft in the alveolar process extends from the crest of the ridge upward through the anterior aspect of the nasal floor, which includes the inferior aspect of the pyriform rim (Figure 12–3). It can be unilateral (Figure 12–4), bilateral (Figure 12–5), complete through the ridge, or partially through the ridge.

If it is completely through the ridge, a communicating passage exists between the oral and nasal cavities known as an oronasal fistula (Figure 12–6).

Some oronasal fistulas are wide, and others may be quite narrow. Some may be so narrow when the alveolar ridge segments abut each other that the opening of the passage may not be visible, and it may appear only as a groove in the gingiva (Figure 12–7).

In many cases, the bone defect through the pyriform rim and alveolar ridge extends posteriorly onto the hard palate (Figure 12–8).

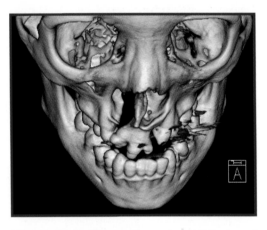

Figure 12–3. Three-dimensional CT scan of bilateral cleft, incomplete on left side extending into alveolar process but not through nasal floor, and complete on right side extending through right nasal floor.

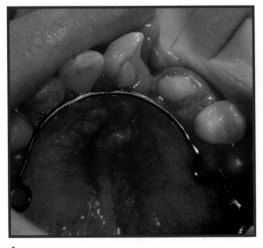

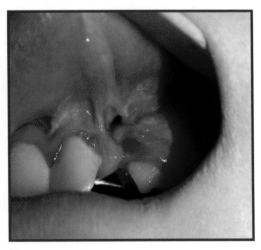

A   B

Figure 12–4. Palatal (**A**) and sublabial (**B**) views of left unilateral alveolar cleft.

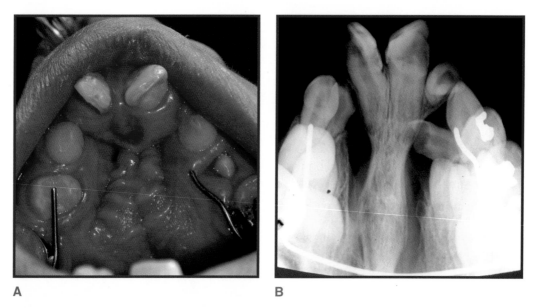

A

B

Figure 12–5. Palatal view (**A**) and occlusal x-ray (**B**) of bilateral alveolar clefts. The x-ray shows the premaxilla in continuity with nasal septum in bilateral cleft lip and palate. Note tooth erupting into cleft on left side.

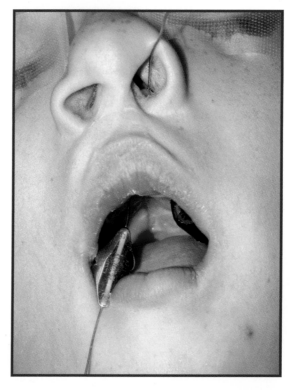

Figure 12–6. Left alveolar cleft with probe in the fistula tract passing through alveolar process into left nasal cavity.

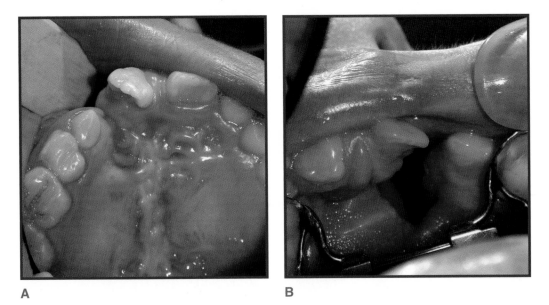

A   **B**

Figure 12–7. Occlusal views showing examples of a narrow right alveolar cleft (**A**) and a wide left alveolar cleft (**B**).

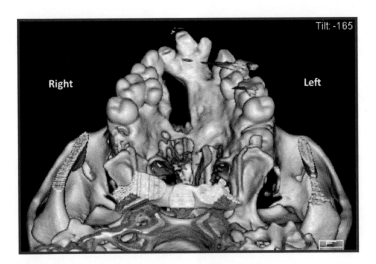

Figure 12–8. Three-dimensional CT scan showing complete right side alveolar cleft with bone defect extending through pyriform rim and posteriorly along the hard palate on the right side. On the left side, the bone defect of the cleft involves only the alveolar ridge.

The absence of bone deprives the maxillary arch of support, and this loss of integrity contributes to medial collapse of the alveolar segments resulting in a narrow maxilla (Figure 12–9).

This alters the dental occlusal relationship of the maxilla with the mandible resulting in posterior crossbite, either unilateral or bilateral (Figure 12–10).

Additionally, in the bilateral cleft, the premaxilla is attached to the remainder of the skull only by the thin nasal septum and is therefore mobile or unstable (see Figure 12–5)

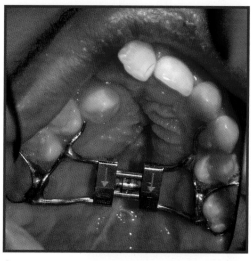
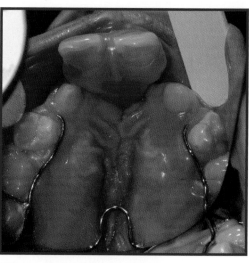

A   B

Figure 12–9. A. Narrow maxilla in a patient with right-side cleft lip and palate (note expansion appliance in place). **B.** A patient with bilateral cleft lip and palate.

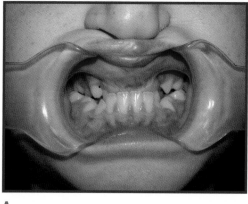
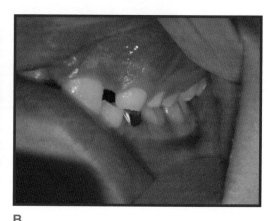

A   B

Figure 12–10. A. Bilateral posterior and anterior crossbite. **B.** Compare to patient without posterior crossbite.

INDICATIONS FOR SURGICAL REPAIR

A cleft through the alveolar ridge provides a potential pathway for food or liquid to pass into the nose during eating and may also provide a path for mucus to move from the nose into the mouth. Neither situation is hygienic and can lead to embarrassing situations if food or liquid exits the nose. Closing this pathway by repairing the alveolar ridge corrects this problem.

There are other effects of the cleft and fistula for which repair is indicated as well. When a cleft is present and bone is missing, there is insufficient support for the dentition. Repair or reconstruction of the alveolar ridge provides bone to support the teeth along the margin of the cleft and for tooth eruption (or orthodontic movement of teeth) into the alveolar ridge. The repair creates continuity of the alveolar ridge with a bone graft and thereby improves the stability of the alveolar segments. This stabilizing function of the repair is particularly important in patients with bilateral cleft lip and palate, a condition in which the premaxilla is often very mobile.

In patients with a wide alveolar cleft defect, there may be lack of support for the base of the nose. This can be corrected by restoring the bony integrity of the pyriform rim. This is usually accomplished at the time of the alveolar ridge reconstruction using bone graft.

Finally, the quality of speech can be influenced by air passing through the alveolar ridge fistula resulting in nasal emission. The range of effects on speech production may vary depending on the size, shape, and location of the fistula from almost no effect to significant nasal emission. Additionally, the position of the widest part of the cleft can affect speech. For example, if the oronasal opening is widest on the labial aspect of the alveolar ridge or in the sublabial vestibule, the upper lip may occlude the oronasal passage and prevent nasal air emission during speech. If, however, the oronasal passage is prominent on the palatal aspect of the alveolar ridge, anatomically approaching the anterior hard palate, it may be more likely to allow nasal air escape (or nasal emission) (Figure 12–11).

Although the alveolar fistula may be symptomatic for the presence of nasal emission, a fistula through the alveolar ridge is not usually associated with problems of resonance, and rarely is it a problem for articulation (Henningsson & Isberg, 1990). In some cases, the upper lip may prevent air loss through the fistula because of the pressure it naturally places on the alveolar ridge (Henningsson & Isberg, 1990). The upper lip usually covers any fistula on the labial surface of the alveolar process. In any case, closure of the alveolar ridge cleft, thereby separating the oral from the nasal cavity in this region, will eliminate this anatomic site as a source for speech impairment associated with inappropriate air escape.

REPAIR OF THE MAXILLARY ALVEOLAR CLEFT

In most centers, surgical repair of the alveolar ridge is usually done during the mixed dentition stage of development, when permanent teeth are erupting and primary teeth are still present. At this stage, the child is often able to cooperate with the necessary orthodontic preparation, which usually precedes the surgery to repair the alveolar ridge.

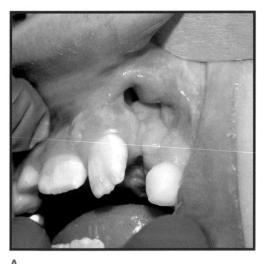
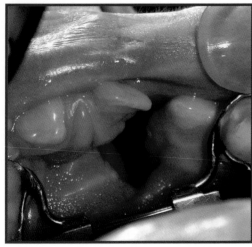

A   B

Figure 12–11. A. View of left side alveolar cleft with visible sublabial fistula but no significant opening on palatal aspect of alveolar process. **B.** Compare to left alveolar cleft with very wide opening on palatal aspect of alveolar ridge.

It is important to understand that by this age, children are aware of upcoming surgery and procedures and often have clear recollection of these events afterward. There are also effects on feeding, speech, other activities of daily living, and quality of life, so age-appropriate counseling and support should be included in their care.

The reason for doing the alveolar ridge repair during the mixed dentition stage of development is to assure that bone is present at the cleft site to allow a satisfactory environment for eruption of the permanent canine tooth, or a lateral incisor if one is present. Furthermore, the alveolar ridge fistula is usually not a major site of cleft associated speech errors, and hence, addressing it earlier for speech issues is usually not required. However, during early childhood prior to eruption of permanent teeth, if the oral-nasal fistula in the region of the alveolar ridge is symptomatic for food or fluid regurgita-tion or significant speech dysfunction, a soft tissue closure can be accomplished with mucosa and gingiva of the alveolar process at that time. Later, when dentally and skeletally more appropriate, a bone graft can be done to complete the alveolar ridge repair.

Repair of alveolar ridge defects in children with cleft lip and palate is usually done between ages 7 and 10 years and involves a two-phase process. As noted earlier, the width of the maxilla in children who have undergone the first two reconstructive stages of cleft repair, namely, repair of the cleft lip and repair of the cleft palate, is often deficient in transverse width and too narrow compared to the mandible. This results in a malocclusion known as crossbite. The first phase of treatment, therefore, involves orthodontic preparation in which the narrow maxilla is expanded to the proper width and the crossbite corrected (Figure 12–12).

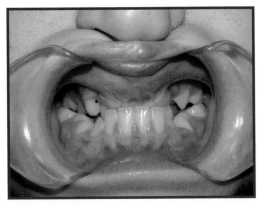 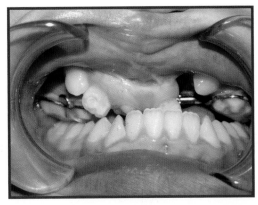

A **B**

Figure 12–12. Bilateral alveolar clefts, before expansion showing bilateral posterior crossbite (**A**) and after expansion (**B**).

The second phase involves surgery to eliminate the fistula by closing the soft tissue over a bone graft, thereby fusing the maxillary alveolar segments together. Alveolar bone grafting in conjunction with orthodontics is standard practice in the management of cleft lip and palate defects.

Orthodontic Preparation

Prior to proceeding with the bone graft procedure, the child undergoes expansion of the width of the maxilla using a device known as a palatal expander. The device is inserted by the child's dental specialist and can be activated with a spring within the device (Figure 12–13A) or by intermittently turning a jackscrew within the appliance (usually by the parents or caregivers) (Figure 12–13B).

The insertion of the appliance is most often done in the dental office without local anesthetic. This procedure can be uncomfortable or cause pain during insertion; however, once the appliance is in place, the discomfort is managed with over-the-counter analgesics and improves within a short time. During the activation of the expansion appliance, children may experience a sensation of pressure, but it is typically not painful and is well tolerated. Once the maxilla has been widened, the child is ready for the alveolar ridge repair with bone graft.

It is important for the SLP to note that during the process of expansion, two factors can lead to speech problems, which if not anticipated, may lead to parental concern regarding the "deterioration" in their child's speech. First, the expansion appliances can be somewhat bulky, and the additional hardware in the child's mouth may result in distorted speech, particularly the fricatives and tip-alveolar stops. These distortions are usually temporary as most children will adapt to the presence of the appliance and return to their baseline speech patterns present before the maxillary appliance was inserted. It has also been our observation that if the child does not adapt to the appliance and speech errors persist, once the appliance is removed the errors resolve.

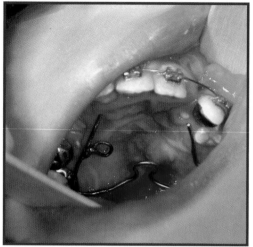
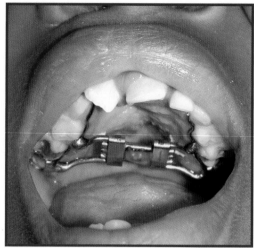

A   **B**

Figure 12–13. A. Palatal expander with spring. **B.** Palatal expander with jackscrew.

The second factor is less often anticipated and relates to widening of the oronasal fistula during the expansion process. Prior to maxillary widening, the gingiva on each side of the cleft may contact across the cleft gap and obstruct the passage of air through the fistula from the mouth into the nose. As the expansion appliance pushes the segments of the maxilla apart from each other, there may be minimal widening of the cleft gap (Figure 12–14A), or the oral-nasal opening may become wide and more patent, resulting in potential for increased nasal emission during speech (Figure 12–14B).

If this occurs, the family can be reassured that once the fistula is surgically closed, the newly created nasal emission will be eliminated. This applies only to the nasal emission via the alveolar ridge fistula, and not nasal emission related to soft palate or velopharyngeal function. Also, the parents should be reassured that the fistula is not caused by the expansion; it is just made more visible and will be closed at the time of surgery (Figure 12–14C).

Alveolar Cleft Repair: Surgical Technique

After orthodontic expansion, the next phase is the surgical procedure to close the oronasal fistula. This is usually done by making incisions in and around the cleft to create and elevate soft tissue flaps. These flaps are sutured together to create both a barrier between the mouth and the nose, and a pocket to receive the bone graft, which will bridge the bone gap in the maxillary alveolar ridge. The soft tissue walls of the pocket are the newly formed nasal floor, the gingival wall on the palatal surface of the alveolar process, and the labial surface of the alveolar process (Hall & Posnick, 1983).

The bone graft is usually autologous (i.e., harvested from the patient), but it can be allogeneic (bone donated from another individual and processed through a tissue bank in such a way as to reduce the risk of infection). Autologous bone grafts are usually harvested from the iliac crest

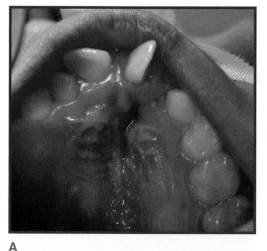

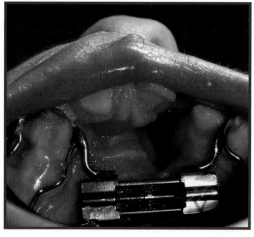

A

B

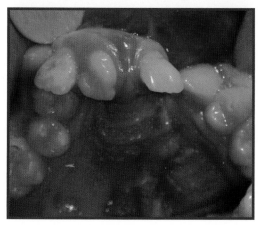

Figure 12–14. A. Palatal view of left alveolar cleft after expansion but minimal widening of fistula path. **B.** Palatal view after expansion showing significant widening of the cleft gap fistula path. **C.** Palatal view of repaired left alveolar cleft from patient shown in **B.**

C

(hip bone) where cancellous bone is taken from the marrow space (Figure 12–15).

Other sites for harvesting bone can be the cranial vault, rib, or tibia, although these sites are less often used than iliac crest (Boyne & Sands, 1972; Denny, Talisman, & Bonawitz, 1999; Murthy & Lehman, 2006).

The alveolar ridge repair with bone graft is done with the child under general anesthesia and may include an overnight stay in the hospital. As with many surgical procedures, postoperative pain can be significant and activity level reduced, both of which can have psychosocial con-

sequences for patients and their families. In addition to intravenous and oral analgesics, there is much that can be done to reduce postoperative pain and improve the child's experience including modification of bone harvesting techniques and use of long-acting local anesthetics administered during and after surgery. In the author's experience, and that of others, use of an analgesic pump to deliver local anesthetic to the bone graft donor site has reduced the hospital length of stay and improved comfort in the immediate postoperative period (Meara et al.,

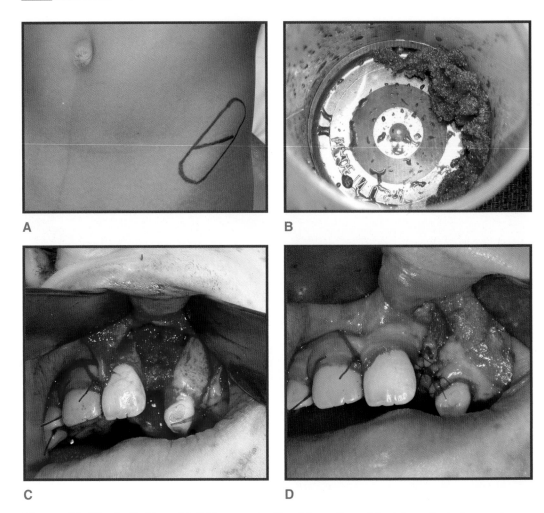

A
B
C
D

Figure 12–15. A. Outline of left iliac crest with oblique line at incision site to harvest cancellous bone. **B.** Harvested cancellous bone held in cup until ready to be used as graft. **C.** Cancellous bone placed into prepared bed within alveolar process extending from pyriform rim to alveolar crest. **D.** Gingival and mucosal soft tissue flaps sutured over bone graft.

2011; Muzaffar, Warren, & Baker, 2014). Most children are able to return to full activity, including sports, by 6 weeks after surgery.

There will also be dietary alterations in the early postoperative period to avoid injury to the surgical site. SLPs, with their known expertise in feeding and nutrition, may be called upon to assist and counsel patients and their families during this time.

Once the soft tissue and bone have healed, the patient may continue on with orthodontic treatment to align the teeth (Figure 12–16).

OUTCOME AND BENEFITS OF ALVEOLAR CLEFT REPAIR

There is ample evidence to suggest that alveolar bone grafting results in success-

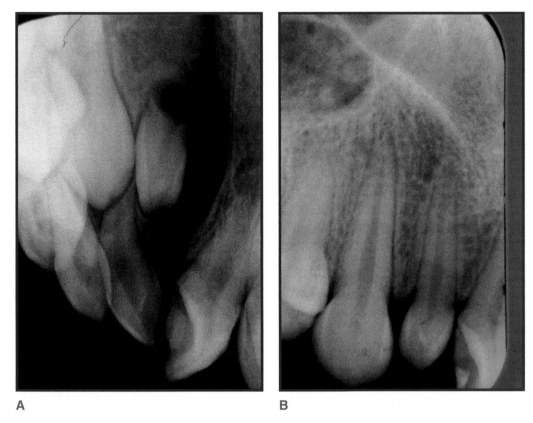

A   B

Figure 12–16. A. Periapical x-rays before (**A**) and after (**B**) bone graft. Note unerupted lateral incisor prior to graft has erupted with good bone support.

ful outcomes (Åbyholm, Bergland, & Semb, 1981; Enemark, Krantz-Simonsen, & Schramm, 1985; Murthy & Lehman, 2011; Sindet-Pederson & Enemark, 1985). The best results for structural repair of the alveolar process cleft are achieved when the bone graft is carried out before the canine has erupted, regardless of whether the patient has a unilateral or bilateral cleft palate.

From a dental/skeletal perspective, there are several benefits of alveolar bone grafting including maxillary arch continuity, stabilization of maxillary segments, nasal alar support (Jackson, Vanderword, McLennan, Christie, & McGreagor, 1982; Schultz, 1989), and provision of bone for dental implant if needed (Verdi, Lanzi, Cohen, & Powell, 1991). Closure of the fistula will also prevent nasal mucous from entering the mouth, which is of hygienic benefit, and prevent embarrassing oral-nasal regurgitation when eating.

Another benefit of alveolar cleft repair is the effect it may have on speech. Preoperative and postoperative data collection, including audio recording, can provide the SLP with baseline information and information about speech outcome following surgery. In patients with complex or multifactorial speech errors related to a cleft, knowledge of the anatomic pathology of the cleft and of its effect on speech after surgery provides the SLP with the tools to effectively manage speech production, counsel families and other team members, and understand prognosis. For example, nasal emission may be symptomatic of velopharyngeal inadequacy (VPI) or air escape through a fistula. The differentiation is important. If the oronasal fistula through an alveolar ridge defect is the sole site of nasal emission during speech, successful repair of the alveolar ridge defect will result in the decrease or elimination of nasal emission. It will not improve preexisting hypernasal speech caused by VPI. More importantly, if the nasal emission through a wide alveolar cleft fistula is mistaken for VPI, a patient may be inappropriately referred for VPI surgery, which would result in no speech benefit and possibly cause harm such as obstructive sleep apnea (see Chapter 11). In the interest of good patient care, the importance of clear communication between surgeon and SLP cannot be understated.

SURGICAL RISKS

There is a low level of risk of complications with alveolar bone grafting, a finding that is consistent across a number of studies (Bergland, Semb, & Åbyholm, 1986; Collins, James, & Mars, 1998; Kortebein, Nelson, & Sadove, 1991; Yi-Lin, James, & Mars, 1998). Reported complications include loss of the graft due to infection or inadequate soft tissue coverage, injury to the developing teeth or teeth adjacent to the cleft, recurrence of the fistula, and complications associated with the bone graft donor site.

POSTREPAIR ORTHODONTICS

Anterior teeth in the vicinity of a cleft are usually malaligned. Once the fistula is closed and the bone graft has fully healed, the orthodontist may begin to align the teeth with braces. In the author's experience, even though there is some discomfort with braces, alignment of once "crooked" anterior teeth is often very satisfying to patients and their parents (Figure 12–17).

Full correction of the malocclusion may not be possible at this age. Very often the orthodontist will complete what is necessary at this age, and begin a new phase of orthodontic care when the patient is older and closer to skeletal maturity. The final correction of the malocclusion may require a combination of orthodontic treatment and surgery to reposition the jaws. This will be discussed further in Chapter 13.

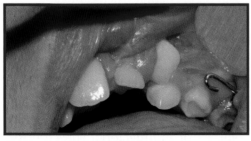
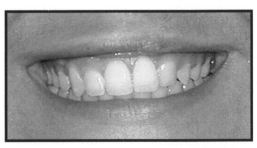

A   **B**

Figure 12–17. A. Dentition prior to bone graft and alignment of teeth. **B.** Same patient at conclusion of her orthodontic tooth alignment. (Orthodontic treatment provided by Dr. Constance Greeley, Wilmington, DE.)

CHAPTER SUMMARY

The alveolar cleft repair represents a significant milestone for patients born with cleft lip and palate. It completes the proper anatomic separation of the oral and nasal cavities by uniting the maxillary segments that were once separated by the cleft. In doing so, it provides structural, functional, and aesthetic benefits to patients. Thorough evaluation and treatment of the patient and of the effect of the cleft on speech, dentition, and the facial skeleton requires communication, close cooperation, and coordination of care among multiple disciplines, including the speech-language pathologist, surgeon, and dental specialist.

REFERENCES

Åbyholm, F. W., Bergland, O., & Semb, G. (1981). Secondary bone grafting of alveolar clefts. *Scandinavian Journal of Plastic and Reconstructive Surgery, 15,* 127–140.

Bergland, O., Semb, G., & Åbyholm, F. E. (1986). Elimination of the residual alveolar cleft by secondary bone grafting and subsequent orthodontic treatment. *Cleft Palate Journal, 23,* 175–205.

Boyne, P. J., & Sands, N. R. (1972). Secondary bone grafting of residual alveolar and palatal clefts. *Journal of Oral Surgery, 30,* 87–92.

Collins, M., James, D. R., & Mars, M. (1998). Alveolar bone grafting: A review of 115 patients. *European Journal of Orthodontics, 20,* 115–120.

Denny, A. D., Talisman, R. & Bonawitz, S. T. (1999). Secondary alveolar bone grafting using milled cranial bone graft: A retrospective study of a consecutive series of 100 patients. *Cleft Palate-Craniofacial Journal, 36,* 144–153.

Enemark, H., Krantz-Simonsen, E. K., & Schramm, J. E. (1985). Secondary bone grafting in unilateral cleft lip and palate patients: Indications and treatment procedure. *International Journal of Oral Surgery, 14,* 2–10.

Hall, H. D., & Posnick, J. C. (1983). Early results of secondary bone grafts in 106 alveolar clefts. *Journal of Oral and Maxillofacial Surgery, 41,* 289–294.

Henningsson, G., & Isberg, A. (1990). Oronasal fistulas and speech production. In J. Bardach & H. L. Morris (Eds.), *Multidisciplinary management of cleft lip and palate* (pp. 767–792). Philadelphia, PA: W.B. Saunders.

Jackson, I. T., Vandervord, J. G., McLennan, J., Christie, F. B., & McGregor, J. C. (1982). Bone grafting of the secondary cleft lip and palate deformity. *British Journal of Plastic Surgery, 35,* 343–353.

Kortebein, M. J., Nelson, C. L., & Sadove, A. M. (1991). Retrospective analysis of 135 secondary alveolar cleft grafts using iliac or calvarial bone. *Journal of Oral Maxillofacial Surgery, 49,* 493–498.

Meara, D. J., Livingston, N. R., Sittitavornwong, S., Ness, T., Boyce, J., Wang, D., & Waite, P. D. (2011). Continuous infusion of bupivacaine for pain control after anterior iliac crest bone grafting for alveolar cleft repair in children. *Cleft Palate-Craniofacial Journal, 48,* 690–694.

Murthy, A. S., & Lehman, J. A. Jr. (2006). Secondary alveolar bone grafting: An outcomes analysis. *Canadian Journal of Plastic Surgery, 14,* 172–174.

Muzaffar, R. A., Warren, A., & Baker, L. (2014). Use of the On-Q pain pump in alveolar bone grafting: Effect on hospital length of stay. *Cleft Palate-Craniofacial Journal,* doi:10.1597/14-174

Schulz, R. C. (1989). Cleft palate fistula repair. Improved results by the addition of bone. *Archives of Otolaryngology-Head and Neck Surgery, 115,* 65–67.

Sindet-Pedersen, S., & Enemark, H. (1985). Comparative study of secondary and late secondary bone-grafting in patients with residual cleft defects. Short-term evaluation. *International Journal of Oral Surgery, 14,* 389–398.

Verdi, F. J. Jr., Lanzi, G. L., Cohen, S. R., & Powell, R. (1991). Use of the Branemark implant in the cleft palate patient. *Cleft Palate-Craniofacial Journal, 28*, 301–303.

Wood, R. J., Grayson, B. H., & Cutting, C. B. (1997). Gingivoperiosteoplasty and midfacial growth. *Cleft Palate-Craniofacial Journal, 34*, 17–20.

Yi-Lin, J., James, D. R., & Mars, M. (1998). Bilateral alveolar bone grafting: A report of 55 consecutively-treated patients. *European Journal of Orthodontics, 20*, 299–307.

PART IV

Adolescents and Adults

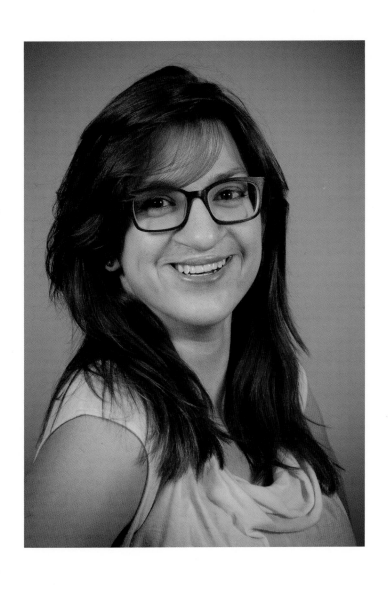

Adolescents and adults with repaired cleft lip and palate or other craniofacial conditions may face additional surgical procedures to correct discrepant relationships between the upper and lower jaws. This is called *orthognathic surgery*. In Chapter 13, Joseph Napoli and Linda Vallino review the relationship between malocclusion and speech production and describe the orthodontic and surgical techniques to correct jaw abnormalities. They review evidence to show that maxillary advancement by osteotomy has a positive impact on the articulation of sibilants and alveolar and bilabial stop consonants, and that changes occur fairly immediately following surgery.

In Chapter 14, the adult with cleft lip and palate is discussed relative to satisfaction with care, social relationships, marriage and children, education, and employment. Transition of care from a child-centered team approach to an adult-centered health care system is reviewed. We conclude that in most aspects, the adult with repaired cleft lip and palate is no different than his or her nonaffected peer, except, perhaps, for a few facial scars that are, if even visible, only skin deep.

13

Maxillary Advancement

Joseph A. Napoli and Linda D. Vallino

INTRODUCTION

Abnormalities of dental occlusion are prevalent in cleft lip and palate (CLP) and craniofacial disorders. These abnormalities may be inherent in the disorder itself or the result of treatment (iatrogenic) and can affect appearance and various functions, particularly mastication, speech, and breathing.

If the maxillary and mandibular teeth do not occlude properly, biting into foods or chewing may be difficult. Speech articulation and facial appearance can also be adversely affected by the size, shape, and position of the maxilla relative to the mandible (Witzel & Vallino, 1992) (Figure 13–1A). If the maxillary or mandibular deficiencies are severe enough, a person may also experience varying degrees of airway obstruction (Figure 13–1B).

Because the problems associated with jaw deformities in cleft lip and palate are complex, an interdisciplinary team approach to management is needed, including the services of dental specialists, surgeons, speech-language pathologists, audiologists, and psychologists. In this chapter, we will review the relationship between malocclusion and speech production and describe the orthodontic and surgical techniques to correct jaw abnormalities in adolescent and adult patients with craniofacial anomalies, concentrating on those with cleft lip and palate. Changes in articulation, resonance, velopharyngeal function, and hearing following surgery will be presented. Satisfaction with outcomes of surgery will be addressed. In the final section, a systematic approach for collecting data to evaluate clinical outcomes will be outlined.

ABNORMALITIES OF DENTAL OCCLUSION IN CLEFT AND CRANIOFACIAL CONDITIONS

Despite the obvious benefits of reconstruction, the surgical procedures commonly performed in childhood to repair cleft lip and palate can have unfavorable effects on midfacial growth, which in turn, affect appearance and function. As an outcome of these growth deficiencies, the hard palate is often narrow, and the

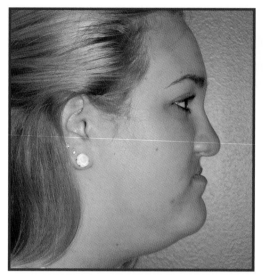 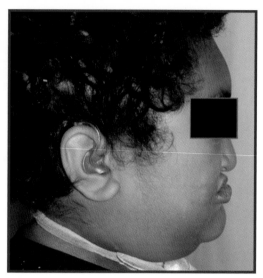

A   B

Figure 13–1. A. Young adult with unilateral cleft lip and palate and midface deficiency. **B.** Adolescent with Crouzon syndrome and airway obstruction in the process of undergoing Le Fort III advancement.

maxilla is hypoplastic or underdeveloped giving rise to a retruded midface, crossbite, and skeletal Class III malocclusion. Ross (1987) described the appearance as concave that becomes increasing more evident following pubertal growth (Lello, 2005) (Figures 13–2 and 13–3).

Maxillary retrusion in syndromic craniosynostosis may cause Class III open bite malocclusion (Figure 13–4).

Hypoplasia and malformation of the mandible as in the case of Treacher Collins syndrome may result in Class II open bite malocclusion (Figure 13–5).

In both cases, these problems may worsen with age and may be associated with upper airway obstruction.

Treatment of the dentofacial deformities associated with cleft lip and palate and craniofacial anomalies requires a combined orthodontic-surgical approach in order to improve facial aesthetics, mastication, airway, and speech.

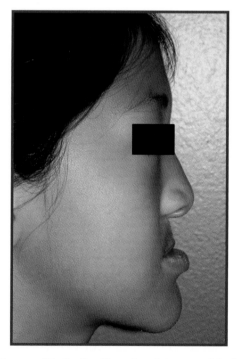

Figure 13–2. Profile of a 15-year-old girl with repaired unilateral cleft lip and palate showing maxillary deficiency.

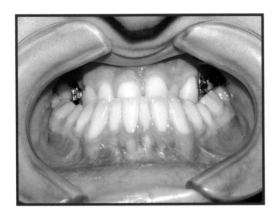

Figure 13–3. An 18-year-old with a history of repaired cleft palate only showing a narrow maxilla with bilateral posterior cross-bite and Class III malocclusion.

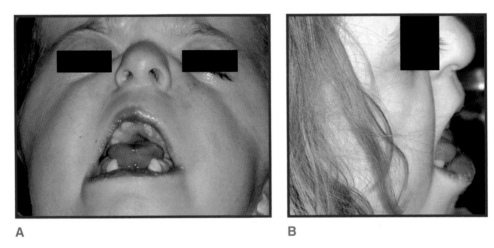

A

B

Figure 13–4. Frontal (**A**) and profile (**B**) view of patient with Apert syndrome with anterior open bite.

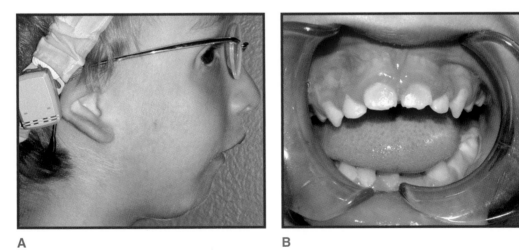

A

B

Figure 13–5. Profile (**A**) and anterior (**B**) view of occlusion in child with Treacher Collins syndrome and anterior open bite. This malocclusion will persist until treated with orthodontics and surgery during adolescence or young adulthood.

EFFECT OF MALOCCLUSION ON SPEECH

There is sufficient evidence to support the conclusion that skeletal Class II or Class III malocclusion with or without open bite associated with a cleft or craniofacial condition can result in aberrant speech production (Vallino, 1987; Vallino & Tompson, 1993). The relationship between these two features is not universal, as some people with malocclusion have normal speech, but there does indeed seem to be a relationship between the severity of the malocclusion and speech impairment. Although some individuals with malocclusion have normal speech, there seems to be structural limitations beyond which this may not be possible (Vallino, 1987).

Vallino (1987) studied articulation in 34 subjects who had skeletal malocclusion. Findings showed that the phonemes most frequently affected by malocclusion were the sibilants /s/ and /z/, followed by the affricates "sh," "ch," "zh" (as in measure), and "j,", and that those least frequently involved were the tip-alveolar stops /t, d, n/ and bilabial stops /p, b, m/. The majority of sibilant errors were made with the tongue tip distal to the mandibular incisors and the mandible depressed. Fewer sibilants were interdentalized. All errors produced on the bilabial consonants were produced using labiodental articulation in which the occlusion is made between the lower lip and upper incisors as opposed to both upper and lower lips. Errors on tip-alveolar stops were either dentalized, whereby the tongue tip was placed against the superior surface of the upper or lower teeth, or interdentalized.

The most prominent type of error produced on these sounds was a distortion that can be categorized as auditory, visual, or combined auditory and visual (Vallino & Tompson, 1993). An auditory distortion is one in which the sound is perceived as aberrant but looks acceptable to the listener, and a visual distortion is one in which the sound is perceived as correct but its production looks aberrant to the listener. Most distortions on sibilants were both auditory and visual. Errors made on bilabial stop consonants /p, b, m/ were generally visual.

In a person with a dentofacial deformity in which the underlying defect is skeletal, these articulation errors generally cannot be ameliorated using orthodontics or speech therapy alone. In these cases, surgery is often required to correct the skeletal anatomy, which in turn will alter the oral environment, making it conducive to accurate articulatory placement.

TREATMENT OF SKELETAL MALOCCLUSION

The most efficacious means for correcting the malocclusion in a person with cleft lip and palate and craniofacial anomalies is a combined orthodontic-surgical approach with each procedure planned to fit the needs of the individual. Treatment to correct skeletal occlusal defects is generally divided into three steps: presurgical orthodontics, surgery, and postoperative orthodontics. Presurgical orthodontics serves to align the teeth into their proper position within each of the dental arches (maxilla and mandible). During surgery, known as *orthognathic surgery*, the maxilla and mandible either separately or together, are moved to their proper relationships. Postsurgical orthodontics usually begins 6 to 8 weeks after surgery when the jaw is healed and allows for fine-tuning of tooth position.

Orthognathic Surgery

A jaw malrelationship may be due to abnormal size or position of the maxilla, the mandible, or both. Orthognathic ("ortho" meaning straight and "gnathic" relating to the jaws) surgery is a procedure to correct jaw deformities often resulting in improved facial aesthetics, mastication, and speech.

In patients with cleft lip and palate, the maxilla is most often the site of the abnormality. In these cases, the primary aim of surgery is to place the maxilla into a normal position relative to the rest of the face and in a proper occlusal relationship with the mandible. This most often requires advancement of the maxilla in a forward direction. Other directional movements and mandibular surgery may, however, also be required. Additionally, the maxilla may be moved as one unit (one piece Le Fort I osteotomy) or divided into segments with each segment moving in a different direction as needed to arrive at a corrected occlusal relationship (Le Fort I segmental osteotomy).

Orthognathic surgery is generally done at an age when skeletal maturity is reached and facial growth is complete or nearly complete. For females this is usually around 15 or 16 years of age and for males between 18 and 20 years. There are, however, situations when the procedures are carried out earlier. Preparing for orthognathic surgery in individuals with CLP involves a comprehensive assessment of dental and skeletal structures, orthodontic preparation, surgical planning, and a detailed speech assessment. It also involves an assessment of the patient's self image and psychosocial well-being.

As noted above, the most common procedure to correct midface retrusion and Class III malocclusion in the patient with CLP is maxillary advancement with or without mandibular set back. There are two basic approaches to advance the maxilla: conventional maxillary advancement (CMA) and maxillary advancement using distraction osteogenesis (MADO). The decision to perform one or the other depends on a number of factors including magnitude of movement.

Maxillary Advancement (Conventional)

Maxillary advancement is a commonly used procedure for correcting certain abnormalities in the relationship between the maxilla and mandible. In general, the maxilla can be advanced using one of three levels of osteotomy: Le Fort I, II, or III (Figure 13–6).

Le Fort I osteotomy is most commonly used in patients with CLP. Using this approach, the maxilla can be advanced, expanded, and lengthened to a more normal position with correction of the dental occlusion (Figure 13–7).

During this procedure, a horizontal incision is made through the bone above the roots of the teeth at or above the level of the nasal floor. This allows the maxilla to be mobilized. Once the maxilla is mobilized, it is placed into its new position and stabilized using small plates and screws inserted into the bone. If the new position results in a large bone gap, a bone graft is placed in the gap to promote bone healing (Figure 13–8).

In some patients, it may be technically difficult or impossible to obtain enough mobility of the maxilla to allow it to be placed in the proper position. This may be due to the presence of palatal scarring or pharyngeal flap. Relapse may also occur in some patients (Hochban, Ganb, &

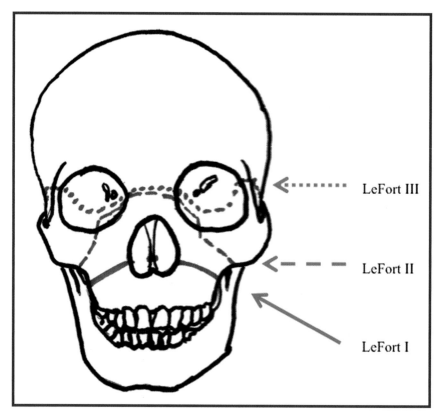

Figure 13–6. Approximate position for Le Fort I, II, and III osteotomies.

Austermann, 1993; Houston, James, Jones and Kavvadia, 1989; Poole, Robinson, & Nunn, 1986; Ward-Booth, Bhatia, & Moos, 1984; Willmar, 1974). Relapse refers to a complete or partial receding of the operated jaw to its preoperative position (Hochban et al., 1993). This may be caused by a number of factors including limited pliability of soft tissue, especially if scarring is present (Hochban et al., 1993) and muscle pull. Scar contracture during healing can result in pulling the maxilla back closer to its original position as well. Reports on the correlation between the amount of advancement made and the amount of relapse is equivocal (Arauio, Schen-

del, Wolford, & Epker, 1978; Eskenazi & Schendel, 1992; Houston et al., 1989; Posnick & Ewing, 1990). Although there may be a risk of relapse in all patients undergoing maxillary advancement, it is higher in patients with CLP (Epker & Wolford, 1976; Hochban et al., 1993; Proffit & Phillips, 1987; Welch, 1989).

Maxillary Advancement Using Distraction Osteogenesis

In patients with Class III malocclusion without CLP, conventional Le Fort I osteotomy for advancement most often produces stable results. However, in most people with CLP, maxillary hypoplasia is often

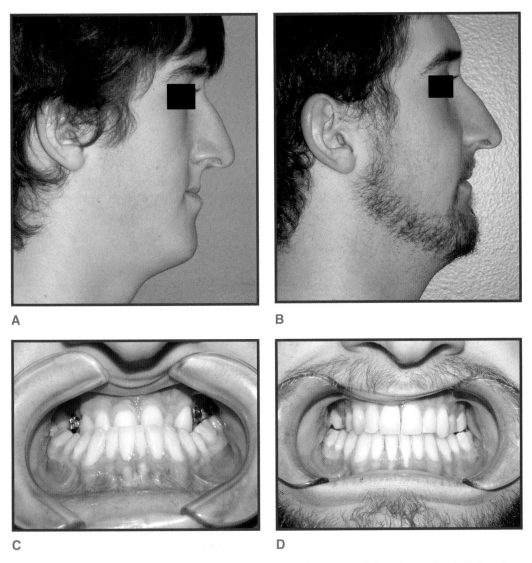

A

B

C

D

Figure 13–7. Profile and oral views of a 17-year-old young adult with repaired cleft palate only before (**A**, **C**) and after (**B**, **D**) maxillary advancement at Le Fort I level. (Orthodontic treatment provided by Dr. Constance Greeley, Wilmington, DE.)

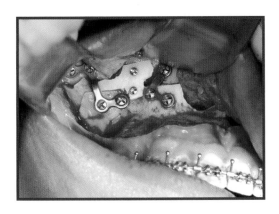

Figure 13–8. View of right side of surgical site showing two contoured plates held by bone screws and a bone graft spanning the gap at the osteotomy site in a patient with Goldenhar syndrome undergoing maxillary osteotomy at Le Fort I level.

363

much more significant than in those without a cleft condition, and the amount of advancement needed to correct the malocclusion may be greater than 10 mm (Cheung & Chua, 2006). Using conventional maxillary advancement, it may not always be possible to achieve this greater magnitude of movement needed to correct the occlusion. Additionally, there is a higher risk of relapse, and possibly velopharyngeal (VP) compromise.

Maxillary advancement using distraction osteogenesis (MADO) was introduced as an alternative option to advance the maxilla. The biological principle of distraction osteogenesis is that when a bone is cut and the segments gradually separated, new bone will form across the gap. This could then create a longer bone without the need for a bone graft. Dr. Gavriil Ilizarov pioneered the use of distraction osteogenesis to lengthen the long bones of the leg without the need for grafting (Ilizarov, 1989a, 1989b). McCarthy, Schreiber, Karp, Thorne, and Grayson (1992) reported on the use of distraction to lengthen the mandible in a child with hemifacial microsomia. Later, MADO was applied to advance the maxilla in children with CLP (Guyette, Polley, Figueroa, & Smith, 2001; Molina, Ortiz-Monesterio, de la Paz Aguilar, & Barrera, 1998). Since then, it has become popular in treating patients with maxillary and mandibular defects as well as other craniofacial skeletal deformities including those of the skull (Cedars, Linck, Chin, & Toth, 1999; Polley & Figueroa, 1997a, 1997b).

MADO involves creating an osteotomy of the maxilla similar to the conventional maxillary advancement. Distractors are attached to the facial skeleton and are gradually adjusted to advance the upper jawbone approximately 1mm each day

until the maxilla is in the desired position. The distraction devices fall into two general types: internal and external devices.

External devices for the maxilla consist of a head frame fixed to the skull and traction wires, which are usually fixed to the dental appliances (Figure 13–9). This type of device serves to move the maxilla forward by external traction forces transmitted to the bone by wires attached directly or indirectly to the teeth or to the bone.

The internal (or semi buried) type of devices are fixed directly to the bone and are covered by the oral soft tissue (Figure 13–10). The activation rod protrudes through the tissue to allow placement of the turning wrench. Internal devices serve to move the maxilla forward by internal pulling forces applied to the bone by the screws used to hold the distracters in place.

The distraction process is divided into three stages. Once the osteotomy is done and the distraction devices are placed, the patient enters the first stage known as the *latency period*. This may be as short as 1 or 2 days or as long as 1 week. During this time, the initial part of the healing across the osteotomy site takes place. Next is the activation stage during which time the distracters are set into function, by turning activation rods with a special wrench. Caregivers including family members are taught how to activate the distractors. The process takes several days to weeks as new bone fills in the gap created by the advancement. Figure 13–11 shows cephalometric x-rays of a young adult with CLP with the distractors before and after advancement. When the jaw is in the desired position, further advancement via the distractors is stopped, and the patient enters the third stage known as *consolidation*. During the consolidation stage, the newly formed soft bone

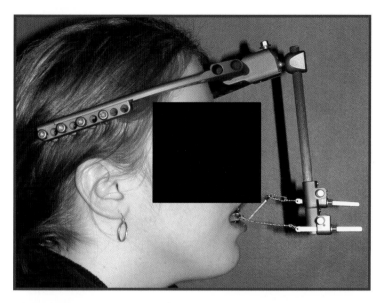

Figure 13–9. Head frame in place for external distraction to advance maxilla in patient with cleft lip and palate to correct mid-face deficiency and Class III malocclusion. Note traction wires extending to dental appliances.

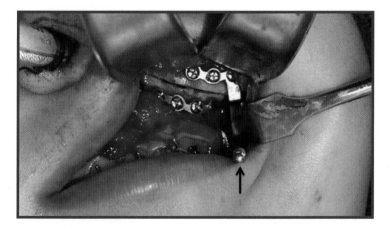

Figure 13–10. Intraoperative view of internal maxillary distractor shown on left side. The screws and plates will be covered by the mucosa, and the distractor activating rod will be exposed inside the mouth. Note the osteotomy at the Le Fort I level and the tip of the activating rod (*arrow*).

is allowed to mineralize and harden. Once the new bone has consolidated, the distractors are removed. Figure 13–12 shows the occlusion and face of the young adult shown in Figure 13–11 before and after surgery.

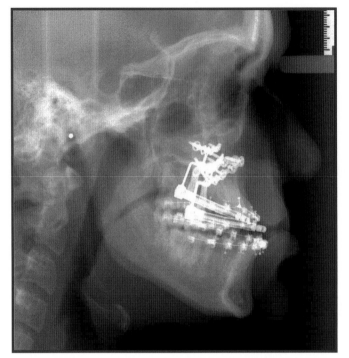

A

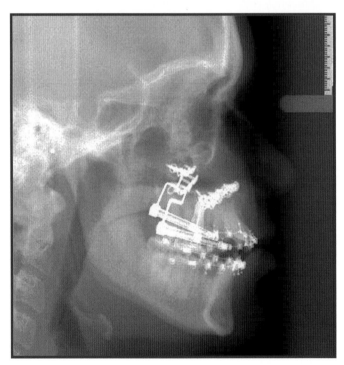

B

Figure 13–11. Lateral cephalometric x-rays showing internal maxillary distracters before (**A**) and after (**B**) distraction. Notice the change in the relative position between the maxillary and mandibular incisors.

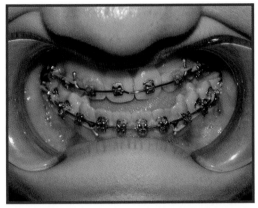

A

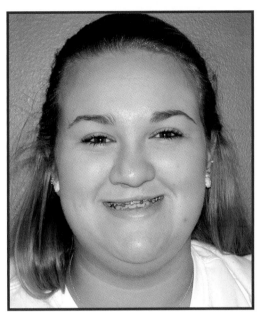

B

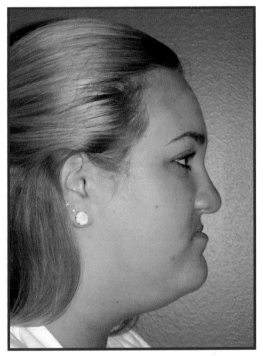

C

Figure 13–12. A–C. Preoperative occlusal and facial views of a young adult with unilateral cleft lip and palate. *continues*

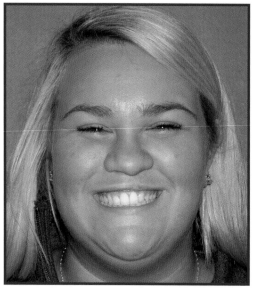
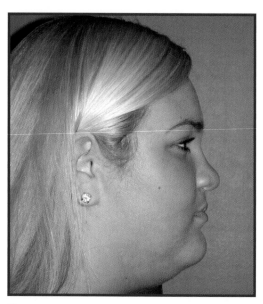

D

E

Figure 13–12. *continued* **D, E.** Postoperative frontal and profile view after maxillary advancement using distraction osteogenesis. This is the same patient shown in Figure 13–11. (Orthodontic treatment provided by Dr. Constance Greeley, Willmington, DE.)

With MADO, the maxilla can be advanced a greater distance than with conventional maxillary advancement. This is advantageous for persons with cleft lip and palate as well as those with craniosynostosis syndromes (e.g., Apert, Crouzon, Pfeiffer) who have significant maxillary hypoplasia requiring moderate to large movement of the maxilla or other parts of the midface. An additional advantage is reduced need for bone graft.

OUTCOMES OF MAXILLARY ADVANCEMENT

Maxillary advancement with or without mandibular setback corrects the occlusal relationship between the maxillary and mandibular teeth. The changes made in the skeletal structures also affect other functions. Relating to speech, com-

mon outcome measures used to evaluate the effect of orthognathic surgery are articulation, velopharyngeal function, nasal airway, and hearing.

Articulation

There have been several investigations of the effect of orthognathic surgery on articulation in individuals with and without CLP. More recently, Pereira, Sell, and Tuomainen (2013) conducted a systematic review to evaluate the impact of maxillary advancement on speech. A systematic review is a rigorous and efficient approach in identifying and summarizing the results of multiple original studies (Cook, Mulrow, & Haynes, 1997). Using a predefined set of criteria, these investigators identified relevant articles, evaluated the quality of the research, and assigned a level of evidence from strongest (Level I) to weakest (Level IV). Only seven studies met the inclusion criteria (Chanchareonsook, Whitehill, & Samman, 2007; Chua, Whitehill, Samman, & Cheung, 2010; Dalston & Vig, 1984, Kummer Strife, Grau, Creaghead, & Lee, 1989; Lee, Whitehill, Ciocca, & Samman, 2002; Trindade, Yamashita, Suguimoto, Mazzottini, & Trindade, 2003; Vallino, 1990). The evidence supports that maxillary advancement has a positive impact on the articulation of sibilants, bilabials, and alveolar sounds, and that the changes in articulation occur fairly immediately following surgery and continue to occur up to 1 year.

Vallino (1990) reported on the speech of 34 subjects before and after orthognathic surgery at 3-, 6-, 9-, and 12-month time intervals. Based on these data, a timetable for changes in articulation was developed. As shown in Figure 13–13, the greatest change in articulation occurred three months after surgery with a continual decrease in the number of errors between 3 and 12 months. Errors on bila-

bial consonants were completely eliminated by 3 months, tip alveolar consonants by 6 months, and affricates by 12 months. There was a tendency for errors to persist on /s/ and /z/ at 12 months but they did not occur with the frequency demonstrated before surgery.

The changes in articulation often occur spontaneously without any intervening speech therapy (Maegawa, Sells, & David, 1998; Vallino, 1990). Those in whom articulation errors persist after surgery may benefit from speech therapy.

Guyette, Polley, Figueroa, and Smith (2001) studied changes in articulation following maxillary distraction osteogenesis in 18 patients. Articulation improved in 67% of patients. Before surgery, the average number of errors was 21, and one year after surgery the average number or errors was 14.8 with a mean improvement of 6.2 errors. The sounds most improved were the sibilants and affricates.

Choi (2006) compared the changes in articulation in patients with cleft palate

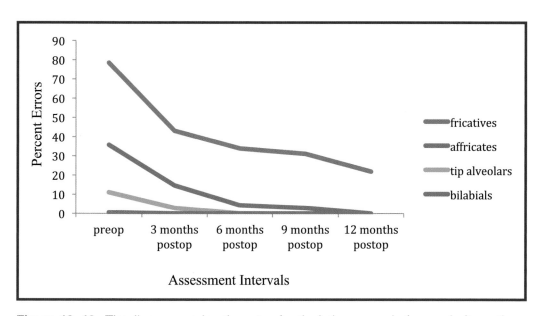

Figure 13–13. Timeline comparing the rate of articulation errors before and after orthognathic surgery shows a decrease in errors up to 12 months.

who were treated for maxillary hypoplasia using conventional maxillary osteotomy or distraction osteogenesis. There was no significant difference between conventional maxillary osteotomy and distraction on the articulation performance of the patients studied.

Velopharyngeal Function and Resonance

During maxillary advancement, the soft palate moves anteriorly causing changes in the size of the velopharyngeal orifice and nasopharyngeal area (Schendel, Oeschlaeger, Wolford, & Epker, 1979). These changes can potentially cause velopharyngeal inadequacy (VPI) and changes in resonance. Although this may be a particular concern in the patient with CLP, the evidence from systematic reviews is mixed regarding whether or not maxillary advancement actually causes VPI—some individuals will develop postoperative VPI and hypernasality, and others will not (Chanchareonsook, Samman, & Whitehill, 2006; Pereira et al., 2013).

Chanchareonsook et al. (2007) compared the effect of treatment of maxillary hypoplasia in patients with cleft palate by conventional maxillary osteotomy (n = 10) to that by MADO (n = 11) on hypernasality, nasal emission, nasalance, and velopharyngeal (VP) status. Subjects were assessed before and 3 months after surgery using a protocol that consisted of both perceptual and instrumental procedures (nasoendoscopy, nasometry, and video and audio recordings). The main finding was that there was no significant difference between the two groups on any of these four outcome measures. Regardless of the procedure, some subjects experienced mild deterioration in VP function, others experienced improve-

ment, still others experienced no noticeable change. These authors noted that the results should be interpreted with caution because of the small number of subjects and the short follow-up time. On the other hand, the strength of this study is that outcome data were collected in an equivalent manner that facilitated comparisons between surgical groups.

Regardless of the procedure used to advance the maxilla, it is important for clinicians to know that the nasopharyngeal depth increases as a result, and this can potentially have a negative effect on VP function in the person with cleft palate. If VP function is borderline or the VP mechanism is shown to sometimes but not always close (Morris, 1972, 1984), it is reasonable to believe that a person might be predisposed to developing VPI and hypernasal speech after surgery.

Attempts have been made to identify aspects of speech and VP function that might predict postoperative VPI in patients with CLP (McComb et al., 2011; Phillips, Klaiman, Delorey, & MacDonald, 2005), but these studies are retrospective in nature and do not account for individual anatomical and physiologic variation that makes such predictions difficult. Suffice it to say, cleft palate is considered a risk factor for VPI following maxillary surgery, but not all individuals with cleft palate will develop VPI after advancement. With this understanding, any patient with cleft palate who is preparing to undergo maxillary advancement should be counseled appropriately.

Sometimes the negative effect on VP function after maxillary advancement is temporary and resolves. However, in their study of the effect of maxillary osteotomy on speech in patients with and without cleft lip and palate, Pereira et al. (2013) reported that surgery may have an adverse effect on VP function for speech and that changes seen as early as 3 months postoperatively can persist at 12 months postoperatively. Although we would not be inclined to surgically treat VPI 3 months after maxillary advancement, if symptoms persist after 1 year, management to improve VP function would be considered (see Chapter 11).

Nasal Airway

Increased nasal airway resistance is common in individuals with CLP caused by conditions such as deviated septum and reduced nasal airway size (Warren, Duany, & Fisher, 1969; Zajac, 2008). These conditions may be attributed to the inherent anatomical deformities associated with a cleft or as a consequence of surgical procedures to repair the cleft defect. Using pressure-flow methods, Turvey, Hall, and Warren (1984) reported that superior repositioning of the maxilla using Le Fort I osteotomy resulted in decreased nasal resistance, even though this procedure reduces nasal cavity volume. Based on rhinomanometric results, Guenther, Sather, and Kern (1984) also found reduced nasal resistance after maxillary advancement.

Hearing

There is evidence to suggest that hearing sensitivity, middle ear pressure, and eustachian tube function can be altered after maxillary advancement (Baddour et al., 1981; Barker, 1987; Bayram, Deniz, Aydin, & Uckan, 2012; DeRuyter & Diefendorf, 1980; Vallino, 1990; Yaghmaei et al., 2009). Advancement of the maxilla puts increased tension on the levator veli palatini and tensor veli palatini muscles.

This, coupled with edema of the soft tissues in the nearby nasopharyngeal area from prolonged nasotracheal intubation during surgery, can prevent the eustachian tube from opening effectively (Barker, 1987; Bayram, et al., 2012; Götzfried & Thumfart, 1988). These conditions create negative middle ear pressure, which could potentially lead to the development of middle ear effusion and mild conductive hearing loss (Baker, 1987; Baddour et al., 1981; DeRuyter & Diefendorf, 1980; Götzfried & Thumfart, 1988; Yaghmaei et al., 2009).

Fortunately, the changes in hearing sensitivity and middle ear status after surgery are usually transitory and resolve spontaneously to the preoperative level (DeRuyter & Diefendorf, 1980; Wong, Samman, & Whitehill, 2002). The gradual recovery of eustachian tube function may begin as early as 48 hours after surgery with complete resolution of the problem within 4 weeks (Baddour et al., 1981) but may take as long as 3 months after surgery (DeRuyter & Diefendorf, 1980). The ability to adjust to middle ear changes is dependent on good auditory function before surgery, and this may not be easily attained in a person with cleft palate and craniofacial anomalies who is predisposed to middle ear disease. These findings underscore the need for an audiologic assessment before maxillary advancement that includes studies of middle ear function and monitoring after surgery. Any person who continues to experience long-term auditory dysfunction should receive attention and treatment.

Satisfaction With Surgical Outcomes Following Maxillary Advancement

Satisfaction with function and appearance is also an important outcome measure in evaluating the effect of orthognathic surgery because it has a potential impact on a person's quality of life (QOL). In this era of patient-centered care, QOL (see Chapter 14) is receiving increasing attention and is now being included as a key outcome in studies of surgery to treat dentofacial anomalies in individuals with CLP.

Anderson et al. (2012) compared ratings of satisfaction in patients with CLP who had undergone either CMA or MADO. After treatment, patients were asked to complete a questionnaire about their satisfaction with facial aesthetics and aspects of function. At the end of treatment, patients in both groups reported satisfaction with their appearance, the perception of relatives and other people's reaction to the changes, and general well-being. They also reported feeling less discomfort with social activities. There was no significant difference between the two groups. However, the patients treated using MADO expressed more dissatisfaction with the duration of treatment than those who were treated using CMA. The authors attributed this dissatisfaction to the period of activation and the long consolidation phase where the patient is wearing the appliance.

Expanding upon their earlier work (Cheung, Loh, & Ho, 2006), Chua, Ho, and Cheung (2012) compared levels of social anxiety and distress, self-esteem, and satisfaction with life in patients with CLP who underwent maxillary advancement using CMA or MADO. Patients were assessed before and 2 to 8 weeks after surgery, and at 3, 6, 12, and 24-month intervals thereafter. Patients in the MADO group reported lower self-esteem and stress up to 3 months after surgery compared to the CMA group, but by the end of 2 years, they reported a significantly higher satisfaction with their lives than those in the CMA group. The authors related this lower self-esteem

in the MADO group to the visibility and need for adjustment of the distractors in MADO and having to keep them in place for up to 3 months after surgery. For those patients in the CMA group who were more satisfied during the early postoperative period, the authors suggested that it was likely due to the opportunity for them to see the changes in their facial appearance and occlusion immediately after surgery, whereas those treated with MADO needed to wait a bit longer to see their outcome.

In summary, the functional and aesthetic outcomes following maxillary surgery are positive. Nonetheless, the stress of the adolescent and young adult undergoing major surgery, hospitalization, and prolonged postoperative management can be great, and it can also create stress for his or her caregiver (Belluci & Kapp-Simon, 2007). Efforts should be made to provide psychosocial support for the effects of treatment, including changes in appearance, and effect on self-image, as well as the usual rigors associated with surgery. This is critical when considering that much of this work is done during adolescence and young adulthood when school and peer relationships play a very large role in their lives.

LE FORT III OSTEOTOMY (TOTAL MIDFACE OSTEOTOMY)

Le Fort III osteotomy or total midface advancement is a procedure undertaken to correct the functional and aesthetic problems in individuals with midface deficiency associated with craniofacial dysostosis who commonly exhibit dental malocclusion, upper airway obstruction, and hyponasal resonance (e.g., Apert, Crouzon, and Pfeiffer syndromes) (Nout et al., 2008). This procedure involves total mobilization and advancement of the midface and has been extensively described in the literature.

Similar to maxillary advancement at the Le Fort I level, the surgical procedures can include conventional Le Fort III osteotomy or midface distraction (distraction osteogenesis). As with the Le Fort I maxillary advancement, the distraction devices can be external or internal (semi-buried).

Effects of Midface Advancement on Articulation and Resonance

In contrast to the number of studies about the effects of maxillary advancement on speech and velopharyngeal function; there are few about the effects of midface advancement on these parameters in patients with syndromic craniosynostosis (craniofacial dysostosis) (Bordbar, Blumenow, Duncan, & Richardson, 2012; Pereira, Sell, Ponniah, Evans, & Dunaway, 2008; Witherow et al., 2008). Findings from these studies show that the articulation often improves after surgery and in others there is no change at all; it seldom worsens (Bordbar et al., 2012; Pereira et al., 2012). With respect to resonance, hyponasality may be improved, remain unchanged, or the degree of hyponasality may be reduced. Patients with cleft palate, particularly those with Apert syndrome, who are not hypernasal before surgery may become hypernasal after surgery, though it is possible that in some few cases this may occur even in the absence of a cleft (Bordbar et al., 2012). Importantly, there seems to be no significant difference between conventional midface osteotomy and distraction on speech and velopharyngeal function.

Another positive outcome of midface advancement in those with craniosynostosis is the correction of airway obstruction.

In fact, an improved airway may permit decannulation of patients who prior to midface advancement were tracheotomy dependent (Witherow et al., 2008).

Satisfaction With Outcome Following Midface Advancement

The reasons for undergoing midface advancement in the infant or young child are somewhat different than for the adult. For the young child, the primary reasons for having the surgery are functional (e.g., airway obstruction, increased intracranial pressure), whereas in the adult facial aesthetics are included. As part of their study of 20 patients with craniofacial dysostosis and severe midface hypoplasia who underwent monobloc midface advancement (Le Fort III), Witherow et al. (2008) included a psychological interview about the parents' and patient's perception about function and overall satisfaction with appearance. Without exception, the parents of the younger children indicated that they were pleased with their child's postoperative functional outcome; improved facial appearance was seen as an additional benefit. In the older group, overall measures of confidence and self-esteem were better after surgery. Although the results from the older patients were variable, overall measures of confidence and self-esteem were better than before surgery.

ASSESSMENT AND MEASURING OUTCOMES

The optimal means by which to evaluate the effect of orthognathic surgery is to collect data using a systematic, purposeful, and reliable protocol in order to capture the comprehensive information about speech, velopharyngeal function, nasal airway, and hearing relative to the type of malocclusion and treatment. The preoperative assessment provides the clinician with baseline data about these parameters against which to measure the degree and quality of change that may occur after surgery and to monitor progress over time. Without baseline data, it is difficult to demonstrate any change as a function of the intervention. The postoperative assessment provides a mechanism by which clinicians can evaluate change that may occur as a consequence of surgery and, if necessary, determine the need for additional treatment (e.g., speech therapy to correct residual articulation errors or surgical procedures to correct VPI).

The assessment protocol should be composed of a combination of perceptual and instrumental techniques and include a variety of outcome measures such as articulation, resonance, intelligibility, and hearing (Chanchareonsook et al., 2007; Pereira, Sell, Ponniah, Evans, & Dunaway, 2008; Vallino, 1990) (Chapters 6 and 9). The evaluation should be conducted before surgery and 3 to 6 months, 1 year, 2 years, and 4 years after surgery. There is much information about short-term benefits of maxillary advancement on speech and velopharyngeal function, but we lack sufficient follow-up, and there is much to be gained by studying the effects of treatment several years later. Limited follow-up precludes definitive conclusions about the procedure outcomes relative to speech, relapse, and overall satisfaction (Witzel & Vallino, 1992).

QOL measures to assess the impact of the condition and treatment should be included in the protocol. Examples of patient-reported outcomes include but are not limited to satisfaction with function and facial appearance, social functioning, course of treatment, and overall well-being.

Among the number of surveys available, the SF-36 Health Survey is a popular quality of life measure that measures subjective health status on eight dimensions: physical function, role limitations, social function, mental health, energy/vitality, pain, health perceptions, and change in health (Ware & Sherbourne, 1992).

CHAPTER SUMMARY

Although midface deficiency is a common inherent feature of some craniofacial anomalies, its presence in patients with cleft lip and palate can be iatrogenic. There is a relationship between the skeletal, dental, and the speech abnormalities in patients with midface deficiency, whether it is an inherent feature or one of iatrogenic origin. Technological advancements in treatment, namely, distraction osteogenesis, have allowed for excellent correction of the structural abnormalities with improved facial appearance and functional occlusal relationship. The effect of treatment on speech, though mixed, is very often one of improvement. Overall, patients appear to be satisfied with both functional and aesthetic outcomes. Patient and caregiver support is an essential component in the overall management in those undergoing maxillary surgery.

Standardized pretreatment and posttreatment assessment is key in evaluating the effects of treatment over time. Including QOL measures, such as treatment satisfaction and social functioning, is consistent with the drive toward quality care and continual improvement.

REFERENCES

Anderson, K., Norhölt, S. E., Küseler, A., Jensen, J. & Pedersen, T. K. (2012). A retrospective study of cleft lip and palate patients before and after maxillary distraction or traditional advancement of the maxilla. *Journal of Oral and Maxillofacial Research 3*(2), e3. Retrieved from http://www.ejomr.org/JOMR/archives/2012/2/e3/v3n2e3ht.pdf doi:10.5037/jomr.2012.3203

Arauio, A., Schendel, S. A., Wolford, L. M., & Epker, B. N. (1973). Total maxillary advancement with and without bone grafting. *Journal Oral Surgery, 16/17,* 335–337.

Baddour, H. M., Watson, M. A., Erwin, B. J., Clark, M. J., Holt, A. R., Steed, D. L., & Tilson, H. B. (1981). Tympanometric changes after total maxillary osteotomy. *Journal of Oral Surgery, 39,* 336–339.

Barker, G. R. (1987). Auditory tube function and audiogram changes following corrective orthognathic maxillary and mandibular surgery in cleft and non-cleft patients. *Scandinavian Journal Plastic Reconstructive Surgery, 21,* 133–138.

Bayram, B., Deniz, K., Aydin, E., & Uckan, S. (2001). Is auditory function affected after Le Fort I osteotomy? *International Journal of Oral Maxillofacial Surgery, 41,* 709–712.

Bellucci, C. C., & Kapp-Simon, K. S. (2007). Psychological considerations in orthognathic surgery. *Clinics in Plastic Surgery, 34*(3), e11–e16.

Bordbar, P., Blumenow, W., Duncan, C., & Richardson, D. (2012). Resonance and speech articulation after midface advancement in craniofacial dysostosis. *Journal of Craniofacial Surgery, 23,* e100–e103.

Cedars, M. G., Linck, D. L. 2nd, Chin, M., & Toth, B. A. (1999). Advancement of the midface using distraction techniques. *Journal of Plastic and Reconstructive Surgery, 103*(2), 429–441.

Chanchareonsook, N., Samman, N., & Whitehill, T. L. (2006). The effect of craniomaxillofacial osteotomies and distraction osteogenesis on speech and velopharyngeal status: A critical review. *Cleft Palate-Craniofacial Journal, 43,* 477–487.

Chanchareonsook, N., Whitehill, T.L., & Samman, N. (2007). Speech outcome and velopharyngeal function in cleft palate: comparison of LeFort I maxillary osteotomy

and distraction osteogenesis-early results. *Cleft Palate Craniofacial Journal, 44,* 23–32.

Cheung, L. K., & Chua, H. D. (2006). A meta-analysis of cleft maxillary osteotomy and distraction osteogenesis. *International Journal of Oral and Maxillofacial Surgery, 35,* 14–24.

Cheung, L. K., Loh, J. S., & Ho, S. M. (2006). The early psychological adjustment of cleft patients after maxillary distraction osteogenesis and conventional orthognathic surgery: a preliminary study. *Journal of Oral and Maxillofacial Surgery, 64,* 1743–1750.

Choi, O. V. (2006). *Traditional osteotomy versus distraction osteogenesis: Articulation changes in Cantonese patients with cleft palate* (Bachelor of science dissertation). The University of Hong Kong. Retrieved from http://hub.hku.hk/bitstream/10722/50053/1/ft.pdf?accept=1

Chua, H. D. P., Ho, S. M. Y., & Cheung, L. K. (2012). The comparison of psychological adjustment of patients with cleft lip and palate after maxillary distraction osteogenesis and conventional orthognathic surgery. *Oral Surgery Oral Medicine Oral Pathology Oral Radiology, 114*(Suppl. 5), S5–S10.

Chua, H. D., Whitehill, T. L., Samman, N., & Cheung, L. K. (2010). Maxillary distraction versus orthognathic surgery in cleft lip and palate patients: Effects of speech and velopharyngeal function. *International Journal of Oral and Maxillofacial Surgery, 39,* 633–640.

Cook, D. J., Mulrow, C. D., & Haynes, R. B. (1997). Systematic reviews: Synthesis of best evidence for clinical decisions. *Annals of Internal Medicine, 126,* 376–380.

Dalston, R. M., & Vig, P. S. (1984). Effects of orthognathic surgery on speech: A prospective study. *American Journal of Orthodontics, 86,* 291–298.

DeRuyter, F., & Diefendorf, A. O. (1980). Hearing sensitivity and measurements of middle ear and Eustachian tube function after maxillary osteotomy with advancement surgery. *Journal of Oral Surgery, 38,* 343–347.

Epker, B. N., & Wolford, L. M. (1976). Middle-third facial osteotomies: Their use in the correction of congenital dentofacial and craniofacial deformities. *Journal of Oral Maxillofacial Surgery, 34,* 324–342.

Götzfried, H. F., & Thumfart, W. R. (1988). Pre- and postoperative middle ear function and muscle activity of the soft palate after total maxillary osteotomy in cleft patients. *Journal Craniomaxillofacial Surgery, 16,* 64–68.

Guenther, T. A., Sather, A. H., & Kern, E. B. (1984). The effect of Le Fort I maxillary impaction on nasal airway resistance. *American Journal of Orthodontics, 85,* 308–315.

Guyette, T. W., Polley, J. W., Figueroa, A., & Smith, B. E. (2001). Changes in speech following maxillary distraction osteogenesis. *Cleft Palate-Craniofacial Journal, 38,* 199–205.

Havestam, C., & Lohmander, A. (Eds.). (2011). *Cleft palate speech: Assessment and intervention.* West Susssex, UK: Wiley-Blackwell.

Hochban, W., Ganb, C., & Austermann, K. H. (1993). Long-term results after maxillary advancement in patient with clefts. *Cleft Palate-Craniofacial Journal, 30,* 237–243.

Houston, W. J. B., James, D. R., Jones, E., & Kavvadia, S. (1989). Le Fort I maxillary osteotomies in cleft palate cases. *Journal of Craniomaxillofacial Surgery, 17,* 9–15.

Ilizarov, G. A. (1989a). The tension-stress effect on the genesis and growth of tissues. Part I. The influence of stability of fixation and soft-tissue preservation. *Clinical Orthopaedics and Related Research, 238,* 249–281.

Ilizarov, G. A. (1989b). The tension-stress effect on the genesis and growth of tissues. Part II. The influence of the rate and frequency of distraction. *Clinical Orthopaedics and Related Research, 239,* 263–285.

Kummer, A. W., Strife, J. L, Grau, H. H., Creaghead, N. A., & Lee, L. (1989). The effects of Le Fort I osteotomy with maxillary movement on articulation, resonance, and velopharyngeal function. *Cleft Palate Journal, 26,* 193–199.

Lee, A. S., Whitehill, T. L., Ciocca, V., & Samman, N. (2002). Acoustic and perceptual analysis of the sibilant sound /s/ before and after orthognathic surgery. *Journal of Oral Maxillofacial Surgery, 60,* 364–372.

Lello, G. E. (2005). Orthognathic surgery. In A. C. H. Watson, D. A. Sell, & P. Grunwell (Eds.), *Management of cleft lip and palate* (pp. 338–351). London, UK: Whurr.

Maegawa, J., Sells, R. K., & David, D. J. (1998). Speech changes after maxillary advancement in 40 cleft lip and palate patients. *Journal of Craniofacial Surgery, 9,* 177–182.

McCarthy, J. G., Schreiber, J., Karp, N., Thorne, C. H., & Grayson, B. H. (1992). Lengthening the human mandible by gradual distraction. *Journal of Plastic and Reconstructive Surgery, 89,* 1–8.

McComb, R. W., Marrinan, E. M., LaBrie, R. A., Mulliken, J. B., & Padwa, B. L. (2011). Predicting VPI in cleft patients after maxillary advancement. *Journal of Oral Maxillofacial Surgery, 69,* 226–2232.

Molina, F., Ortiz-Monesterio, F., de la Paz Aguilar, M., & Barrera, J. (1998). Maxillary distraction: Aesthetic and functional benefits in cleft lip-palate and prognathic patients during mixed dentition. *Plastic and Reconstructive Surgery, 101*(4), 951–963.

Morris, H. L. (1972). Cleft palate. In A. J. Watson (Ed.), *Communicative disorders.* Springfield, IL: Thomas.

Morris, H. L. (1984). Marginal velopharyngeal competence. In H. Wintiz (Ed.), *For clinicians by clinicians, articulation disorders.* Baltimore, MD: University Park Press.

Nout, E., Cesteleyn, L. L. M., van der Wal, K. G. H., van Adrichem, L. N. A., Mathijssen, I. M. J., & Wolvius, E. B. (2008). Advancement of the midface, from conventional Le Fort III osteotomy to Le Fort III distraction: Review of the literature. *International Journal of Oral Maxillofacial Surgery, 37,* 781–789.

Pereira, V., Sell, D., Ponniah, A., Evans, R., & Dunaway, D. (2008). Midface osteotomy versus distraction: The effect on speech, nasality, and velopharyngeal function in craniofacial dysostosis. *Cleft Palate-Craniofacial Journal, 45,* 353–363.

Pereira, V. J., Sell, D., & Tuomainen, J. (2013). The impact of maxillary osteotomy on speech outcomes in cleft lip and palate: An evidence-based approach to evaluating the literature. *Cleft Palate-Craniofacial Journal, 50,* 25–39.

Phillips, J. H., Klaiman, P., Delorey, R., & Mac-Donald, D. B. (2005). Predictors of velopharyngeal insufficiency in cleft orthognathic surgery. *Journal of Plastic and Reconstructive Surgery, 115*, 681–686.

Polley, J. W., & Figueroa, A. A. (1997a). Management of severe maxillary deficiency in childhood and adolescence through distraction osteogenesis with an external, adjustable, rigid distraction device. *Journal of Craniofacial Surgery, 8*, 181–185.

Polley, J. W., & Figueroa, A. A. (1997b). Distraction osteogenesis: Its application in severe mandibular deformities in hemifacial microsomia. *Journal of Craniofacial Surgery, 8*, 422–430.

Poole, M. D., Robinson, P. P., & Nunn, M. E. (1986). Maxillary advancement in cleft palate patients. *Journal of Maxillofacial Surgery, 14*, 123–127.

Posnick, J. C., & Ewing, M. P. (1990). Skeletal stability after Le Fort I maxillary advancement in patients with unilateral cleft lip and palate. *Journal of Plastic and Reconstructive Surgery, 85*, 706–710.

Proffit, W. R., & Phillips, C. (1987). Stability following superior repositioning of the maxilla by LeFort1-osteotomy. *American Journal of Orthodontics and Dentofacial Orthopedics, 92*, 151–161.

Rosen, H. M. (1986). Miniplate fixation of the LeFort I-osteotomy. *Plastic and Reconstructive Surgery, 78*, 748–754.

Ross, R. B. (1987). Treatment variables affecting facial growth in complete unilateral cleft lip and palate. Part 7: An overview of treatment and facial growth. *Cleft Palate Journal, 24*(1), 71–77.

Schendel, S. A., Oeschlaeger, M., Wolford, L. M., & Epker, B. N. (1979). Velopharyngeal anatomy and maxillary advancement. *Journal of Maxillofacial Surgery, 7*, 116–124.

Trindade, I. E., Yamashita, R. P., Suguimoto, R. M, Mazzottini, R., & Trindade, A. J. Jr. (2003). Effects of orthognathic surgery on speech and breathing of subjects with cleft lip and palate: Acoustic and aerodynamic assessment. *Cleft Palate-Craniofacial Journal, 40*, 54–64.

Turvey, T. A., Hall, D. J., & Warren, D. W. (1984). Alterations in nasal airway resistance following superior repositioning of the maxilla. *American Journal of Orthodontics, 85*, 109–114.

Vallino, L. D. (1987). *Speech, velopharyngeal function, and hearing before and after orthognathic surgery* (Doctoral dissertation). University of Pittsburgh, Pittsburgh, PA.

Vallino, L. D. (1990). Speech, velopharyngeal function, and hearing before and after orthognathic surgery. *Journal of Oral Maxillofacial Surgery, 48*, 1274–1281.

Vallino, L. D., & Tompson, B. (1993). Perceptual characteristics of consonant errors associated with malocclusion. *Journal of Oral Maxillofacial Surgery, 51*, 850–856.

Ward-Booth, R. P., Bhatia, S. N., & Moos, K. F. (1984). A cephalometric analysis of the LeFort I-osteotomy in the adult cleft patient. *Journal Maxillofacial Surgery, 12*, 208–212.

Ware, J. E., Jr., & Sherbourne, C. D. (1992). The MOS 36-item short-form health survey (SF-36). I. Conceptual framework and item selection. *Medical Care, 30*, 473–483.

Warren, D. W., Duany, L. F., & Fisher, N. D. (1969). Nasal pathway resistance in normal and cleft lip and palate subjects. *Cleft Palate Journal, 6*, 134–140.

Welch, T. B. (1989). Stability in the correction of dentofacial deformities: A comprehensive review. *Journal of Oral Maxillofacial Surgery, 47*, 1142–1149.

Willmar, L. (1974). On LeFort I-osteotomy; a follow-up study of 106 operated patients with maxillofacial deformity. *Scandinavian Journal of Plastic and Reconstructive Surgery, 12*(Suppl), 1–68.

Witherow, H., Dunaway, D., Evans, R., Nischal, K. K., Shipster, C., Pereira, V., Hearst, D., . . . Hayward, R. (2008). Functional outcomes in monobloc distraction using the rigid external device. *Plastic and Reconstructive Surgery, 121*, 1311–1322.

Witzel, M. A., & Vallino, L. D. (1992). Speech problems in patients with dentofacial or craniofacial deformities. In W. H. Bell (Ed.), *Modern practice of orthognathic and reconstructive surgery* (Vol. 2, pp. 1686–1735). Philadelphia, PA: Saunders.

Wong, L. L. N., Samman, N., & Whitehill, T. L. (2002). Are hearing and middle ear statuses at risk for Chinese patients undergoing orthognathic surgery? *Clinics in Otolaryngology, 27*, 480–484.

Yaghmaei, M., Ghoujeghi, A., Sadeghinejad, D., Aberoumand, M., Seifi, A., & Saffar-shahroudi, A. (2009). Auditory changes in patients undergoing orthognathic surgery. *Oral and Maxillofacial Surgery, 38*, 1148–1153.

Zajac, D. J. (2008). Speech aerodynamics. In A. W. Kummer (Ed.), *Cleft palate and craniofacial anomalies: Effect on speech and resonance* (pp. 415–445). Clifton Park, NY: Delmar Cengage Learning.

14

The Adult With Cleft Lip and Palate

INTRODUCTION

Children born with cleft lip and palate grow up to be adults with cleft lip and palate. By the time a child reaches adulthood, he or she will have undergone surgery to repair the cleft lip and palate (CLP) and alveolar bone cleft, correct a lip and nose deformity, insert ventilation tubes, improve occlusion, and may even have undergone surgery to improve velopharyngeal function. He or she will have endured years of orthodontic treatment, and may have had a few years of speech therapy. By the time the person with CLP reaches adulthood, he or she will have gone to school, made friends, and dated. He or she will have obtained employment, married, and may have even started a family.

For at least 18 to 20 years, the person with CLP will have been involved with an interdisciplinary team that coordinated and managed virtually all aspects of his or her treatment, the goal of which was to normalize structure and function. Now, as the person is older, he or she will begin the transition from child-centered multidisciplinary care to adult-centered care.

When reviewing outcomes in the adult with CLP, conventional measures have targeted the effect of the condition (e.g., hypernasal speech) and the effect of treatment (e.g., changes in articulation after maxillary advancement). Clinician reported outcomes are valuable but, they do not reflect all facets a person considers important in his or her life. There is every reason to believe, and few would argue, that the presence of a cleft and the effect of treatment have an impact on a person's quality of life (QOL), and this impact is not necessarily the same for every person. There are factors beyond the presence of a cleft that can influence how a person's life will be affected (Havstam & Lohmander, 2011). They include satisfaction with care, social relationships, marriage and children, education, and employment—indices of QOL that are said to contribute to a person's well-being (Han, Park, Kim, Kim, & Park, 2014; OECD Better Life Index, 2015). The International Classification of Functioning, Disability, and Health (The World Health Organization (WHO), 2001) provides a framework for considering the totality of this complex disorder that takes into consideration the cleft diagnosis and what CLP means for the person's overall QOL.

Over the past 15 years, there has been a paradigm shift in evaluating health care outcomes from a focus on clinical outcomes to patient reported outcomes. There is a growing amount of research using QOL as a measure of health outcome. This chapter centers on the adult with CLP. We begin this chapter with an overview of QOL and related concepts and ICF framework. It is beyond the scope of this chapter to complete an exhaustive examination of the psychosocial aspects of the cleft. Rather, we will focus on several indices of QOL—satisfaction of care, relationships, education, and employment—for which the impact of the cleft is explored. We will discuss transition of care from a child-centered team program to an adult-centered health care system.

OVERVIEW OF QOL AND ICF

QOL is a broad multidimensional concept that conveys an "overall sense of well being" (Centers for Disease Control (CDC), 2000, p. 7). WHO (2001) defines QOL as "the perception of individuals of their position in life in the context of the culture and value systems in which they live and in relation to their goals, expectations, standards and concerns." Health-related quality of life (HRQOL) is an extension of QOL that includes a person's perceived physical, social, and mental health functioning (CDC, 2000). It focuses on the impact that health status

(e.g., CLP) has on QOL and relates to a person's ability to function in a variety of roles throughout his or her life and being able to achieve satisfaction with them. The emphasis placed on both QOL and HRQOL is the self-reported impact of a disorder not the cause (Havstam & Lohmander, 2011). These measures are useful in monitoring and tracking the effects of treatment based on the person's perspective, facilitating shared decision making, and monitoring the quality of care.

The most widely recognized conceptual framework for describing the impact or consequences of a disorder is the World Health Organization International Classification of Functioning, Disability, and Health (ICF) (WHO, 1980). Recognizing that a cleft is just not a cleft, this model integrates the biological, psychological, and social (biopsychosocial) aspects of the condition with a person's lived experience with the disorder. The interrelated elements of the ICF are illustrated in Figure 14–1 and defined in Table 14–1.

As shown in Figure 14–1, the ICF is structured into two domains, each with two components. The first domain is functioning and disability and includes (a) body functions and structures and (b) activities and participation. The second domain is contextual factors and includes (c) environmental factors and (d) personal factors. Although these two additional factors are often considered to be outside the domain of health, they can have an impact on a person's life (Huber, Sillick, & Skarakis-Doyle, 2010; WHO, 2001). The categories, activities and participation and personal experiences are particularly relevant to CLP.

Figure 14–2 illustrates how the WHO framework might be applicable to an adult with CLP.

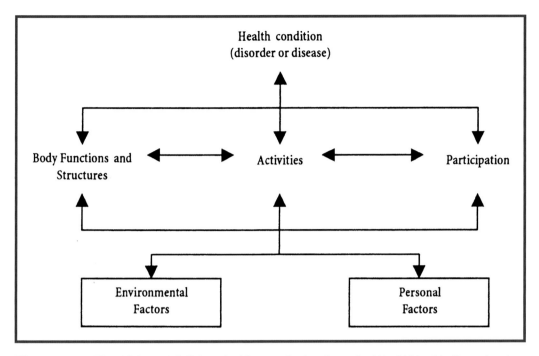

Figure 14–1. The ICF model. Printed with permission from the World Health Organization.

Table 14–1. Definitions of the Major Components of ICF

Body Functions are physiological functions of body systems (including psychological functions).

Body Structures are anatomical parts of the body such as organs, limbs and their components.

Impairments are problems in body function or structure such as a significant deviation or loss.

Activity is the execution of a task or action by an individual.

Participation is involvement in a life situation.

Activity Limitations are difficulties an individual may have in executing activities.

Participation Restrictions are problems an individual may experience in involvement in life situations.

Environmental Factors make up the physical, socal and attitudinal environment in which people live and conduct their lives.

Source: ICF: WHO (2001). Printed with permission from the World Health Organization.

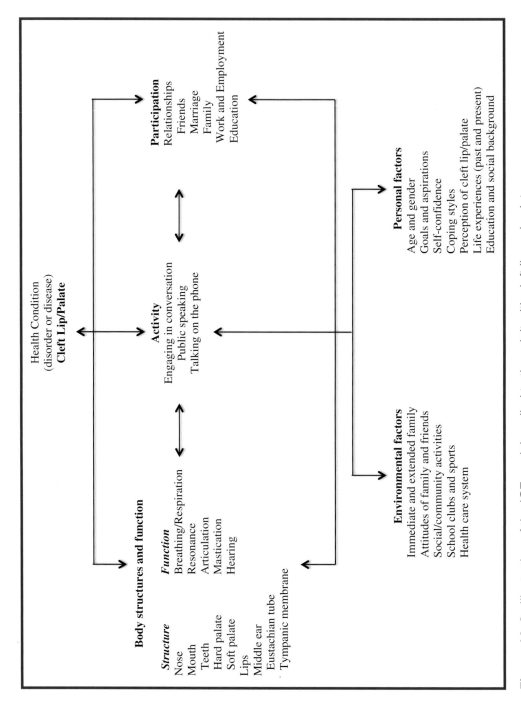

Figure 14–2. Illustration of the ICF model applied to the adult with cleft lip and palate.

Although once considered two separate perspectives, clinicians and researchers are appreciating the integration of QOL and HRQOL into the ICF framework (Cruice, 2008; Huber et al., 2010). As will be shown in the following section, this holistic approach is ideally suited for the adult with CLP.

REPORTS OF HEALTH-RELATED QUALITY OF LIFE (HRQOL)

HRQOL has been used to evaluate the impact of CLP in adults, providing a multidimensional perspective that encompasses the person's physical, psychological, and social functioning. It has been the main focus in several studies.

Using a questionnaire, Marcussen, Akerlind, and Paulin (2001) compared ratings of QOL in general (i.e., global life, life meaning, bodily health, family life, active life, private economy), HRQOL, and well-being (e.g., basic mood, loneliness, sociability, attitude toward self) of adults with repaired CLP to adults without clefts. The overall QOL was rather high in both groups. However, further analysis showed that adults with CLP rated their QOL significantly lower than their noncleft counterparts in the areas of life meaning, family life, and private economy. Other factors in this group that could have contributed to the lower QOL were a lower educational level, higher frequency of unemployment, and residence in a small or rural area. On the other hand, there were no differences between the groups with respect to basic mood, self-concept in social interactions, and view of the future. The impact of the CLP on HRQOL was pronounced in the areas concerning global life, disturbed life, social contacts, and family life. Women with

CLP rated these factors lower than men with CLP. The findings of this study are consistent with other reports of restricted social experiences in adults with CLP (Bjørnsson & Agustsdottir, 1987; Ramstad et al., 1995). Marcusson et al. pointed out that adults with CLP appear to be fully aware that their condition influences the essential aspects of their lives, but their QOL was only marginally lower than adults without a cleft. They concluded that adults with CLP show a fairly good life adjustment.

Mani, Carlsson, and Marcusson (2010) used the SF-36 questionnaire (described in Chapter 13) to assess the effect of gender and age on HRQOL in adults with unilateral CLP and without CLP. Age groups were categorized as younger (20–32 years old) and older (33–47 years old). As a group, the adults with CLP had lower SF-36 values on the Mental Health Scale when compared to the norm population. There were no differences between the adults with CLP and those without CLP on social function, physical role function, emotional role function, vitality, bodily pain, and general health scales. However, the presence of a cleft notably affected HRQOL differently depending on gender and age. Men were more negatively affected than females in the emotional role aspects, whereas women were more negatively affected on the physical aspects. When compared to the older age group, younger adults were more negatively affected in the areas of social function, physical role function, and emotional role function. The authors summed up their findings by saying that although overall HRQOL of adults with CLP is similar to that of adults without CLP, the presence of a cleft does affect some aspects of HRQOL depending on gender and age.

The average age in most studies of adults with cleft generally falls somewhere between the mid-20s and mid-40s. Seeing the lack of research in the over 50-year age group, Hamlet and Harcourt (2015) interviewed six adults between the ages of 57 and 82 about their experiences of living with a CLP. The authors underscored that these adults grew up and lived at a time when medical and surgical care was much different than it is today, and so we must keep this in mind as we learn about their experiences. Their findings showed that in some ways, the presence of a CLP had an effect on the lives of some of these people, particularly when it came to the time of building romantic relationships and making a decision to have children. Even though the adults developed an increased acceptance of their cleft over time and aging appearance, they spoke of feeling somewhat isolated. They described how societal attitudes toward visible differences, despite having changed throughout the years, did not necessarily make things easier for them. The participants made clear the importance of having good dentition but reported that they had to find a way to navigate the system in order to access care, and indicated the desire for more information, support, and advice in this area. Hamlet and Harcourt emphasized that as we manage the older adult with CLP, we need to consider their special needs and ensure that appropriate care and support are provided.

In summary, overall HRQOL is quite good in the adult with CLP. However, for some people, having a CLP is perceived as affecting certain aspects of their lives. The impact of the cleft can be different depending upon gender, age, and generation. Research in the area continues to grow.

SATISFACTION WITH THE TREATMENT

Satisfaction With Appearance

Despite successful results of treatment during childhood, adults with CLP will invariably have some continued cleft-related concerns, the most common being satisfaction with appearance. Aspects of appearance that are most dissatisfying to adults are lip and nasal deformities, facial profile, overall facial appearance, and dental appearance (Bardach et al., 1992; Clifford, Crocker, & Pope, 1972; Chuo et al., 2008; Libby, Schneiderman, McCann, & Kane, 2015; Marcusson, Paulin, & Östrup, 2002).

Marcusson, Paulin, and Östrup (2002) compared 68 adults with repaired CLP to adults without clefts regarding satisfaction with appearance and psychosocial function. Outcome measures included self-reports of body image, QOL, HRQOL, somatization, and depression. Both groups indicated a high satisfaction with body image except for facial appearance. Adults with CLP expressed dissatisfaction with the appearance of their nose, lip, profile, and overall facial appearance. Women with CLP rated their mouth and profile significantly worse than men. Almost half of them wanted additional surgery to correct lip deformities and profile.

The general QOL was judged to be good in both groups and the general HRQOL was partially influenced by the cleft. Satisfaction with appearance was correlated with a better QOL and HRQOL in both groups and a lower level of somatization in the group with CLP. Dissatisfaction with facial appearance was a predictor of depression regardless of whether a cleft was present. The authors concluded that even though adults with CLP were not satisfied with their facial appearance, they seemed to be psychologically well-adjusted to the condition.

Sinko et al. (2005) used the SF-36 to evaluate aesthetic, functional, and QOL outcomes in 70 adults with CLP, ranging in age from 18 to 30 years. Two-thirds of the participants were fully satisfied with their treatment, whereas one third were moderately satisfied. No one was completely dissatisfied. When interviewed, more than half of the adults asked for further treatment to correct lip and nose deformities. Women indicated a desire for additional treatment to improve facial appearance twice as often as men (62.5% versus 34.8%). Regarding HRQOL, adults with CLP showed significantly lower scores only on two subscales, social functioning and emotional role, and a trend toward lower scores on the vitality subscale compared to adults without clefts. Adults who wanted additional surgery to correct their lip and nasal deformities reported a lower HRQOL than those who did not want additional corrective surgery. Based on these findings, Sinko et al. (2005) suggested that if the patient expectations are realistic, surgery to improve QOL should be done, and if the wishes of the patient cannot be fulfilled, referral to a psychologist is recommended.

Satisfaction with Speech

Thirty years ago, Heller, Tidmarsh, and Pless (1981) reported that adults with CLP expressed a persistent dissatisfaction with speech and hearing. Such a perception appears to have changed since then. The current evidence suggests that the majority of adults are satisfied with their speech and that this satisfaction increases as a person gets older (Broder,

Smith, & Strauss, 1992). Libby and colleagues (2015) surveyed adults with CLP about their continuing medical and dental needs and reported that speech, hearing, and swallowing were, in fact, the three greatest areas of satisfaction. The study by Heller et al. (1981) was conducted 35 years ago, and it is reasonable to consider that improvements in surgery over time have since led to better speech outcomes.

SOCIAL FUNCTIONING

Studies conducted more than 25 years ago suggested that the cleft has a discernable impact on the social life of adults with CLP (McWilliams & Paradise, 1973; Peter, Chinsky & Fisher, 1975a). The most recent work by Stock, Feragen, and Rumsey (2015) provide a more positive outcome. Based on telephone interviews with adults with clefts, these authors found that most are socially well adjusted and become involved in long-term romantic relationships. This is not to say that some of the respondents expressed concerns about social anxiety and discomfort, but it is reassuring to know that most adults with cleft lip and palate report positive social outcomes.

MARRIAGE AND CHILDREN

Marriage

Past studies of marital status in adults with cleft lip and palate report that these adults are less likely to marry or marry at an older age than their siblings or noncleft peers (Bjørnsson & Agustsdottir, 1987; McWilliams & Paradise, 1973; Peter & Chinsky, 1974a; Ramstad, Ottem, & Shaw, 1995).

Recent studies of marriage in individuals with CLP reveal something different. Marcusson, Akerlind, and Paulin (2001) compared information collected from adults with CLP about marriage and children to a group of adults without a CLP. Their findings showed no difference in marital status or having children between adults with CLP and their peers. In their interview of 20 adults with cleft palate, Patel and Ross (2003) reported that 60% of the respondents indicated that the cleft did not have an impact on marital life, 30% stated that the cleft had influenced it somewhat, and 10% reported that the anomaly influenced marital life greatly. They further noted that none of the adults who were married or in a relationship reported that their CLP affected their relationship with their partner.

Having Children

Both past and current studies have shown that women with clefts are less likely to have children (Peter & Chinsky, 1974a; Ramstad et al., 1995; Yttri, Christensen, Knudsen, & Bille, 2011). Using population-based data obtained from national registries in Denmark, Yttri et al. (2011) reported that when women with oral clefts had children, they did so at a later age, and that the number of children they had was similar to their noncleft counterparts within the general population.

Stock and Rumsey (2015) conducted an interesting study in which they interviewed 24 parents who had a CLP to find out that if having a cleft affected their decision to start a family. Of these parents, 8 children were born with CLP and 16 were not. From these interviews, five themes emerged: issues surrounding heritability, reactions to their child's diagnosis, factors affecting parental adjustment, impact of own experiences on parenting styles, and impact of becoming a parent on their own outlook. Over half of the parents were unaware that CLP was a heritable condition, and yet most said that knowing the risk of having an affected child would not have influenced their decision to have children. Reactions to their child's diagnosis varied. Although some parents felt sad for their child or responsible for the cleft, they did not believe that a diagnosis of CLP was a significant problem for their child. Parents who had other children with a cleft said they were shocked when they received the news of having another child with a cleft because they were told that it was most unlikely to happen again. A number of parents wanted to help their child avoid some of the negative experiences they had when growing up. Several indicated that having a child with a cleft had changed the way they viewed themselves. They had second thoughts about pursuing further surgery to improve appearance because their children knew them and accepted them. Yet other parents found that having a child with cleft gave them reason to seek additional treatment. Stock and Rumsey (2015) concluded that young adults with CLP understand what it means to grow up with this birth defect and that this experience may have an impact on whether or not they start a family and how they might manage if they have a child with a cleft. These investigators emphasize that each person responds to this challenge differently and caution the reader about making assumptions that the experiences are uniform. We would agree.

Andrews-Casal et al. (1998) surveyed families to assess whether or not the presence of a family history of CLP had an impact on family planning, timing of cleft surgery, and parental stress.

They compared families who had a child with a CLP and positive family history of a cleft (familial group) with families who had a child with a cleft and negative family history of cleft (isolated group). Their findings showed that although the familial group perceived their recurrence risk as high and those in isolated groups perceived their recurrence risk as low, the reproductive plans for neither group changed because their child was born with a cleft. There was also no discernible difference in parental stress levels because their child was affected. Lastly, having or not having a family history of cleft did not influence the timing of cleft lip and palate repair. Parents deferred to their physician's recommendation about the timing of their child's cleft repair.

EDUCATION

As of this writing, there still remain limited data on education and academic achievement in adults with CLP. Some studies suggest that individuals born with CLP are less likely to attain the same educational achievements (Demb & Reuss, 1967; McWilliams & Paradise, 1973; Persson, Becker, & Svensson, 2012; Peter & Chinsky, 1974b). Others found few differences in educational attainment (Clifford et al., 1972; Ramstad et al., 1995). Recently, in their interviews with 52 adults having CLP, Stock and Rumsey (2015) reported that most participants believed that having a cleft did not make a difference in their educational experience, that it did not hold them back. Although some adults reported that they had to work harder in school and some indicated having academic challenges, they were able to work through this with the support of a tutor. Stock and Rumsey recognize the paucity of data on education and support continued investigation into the factors that contribute to academic achievement in individuals with CLP.

EMPLOYMENT

Researchers (Peter, Chinsky, & Fisher, 1975b; Van Demark & Van Demark, 1970) reported that the presence of a cleft did not influence the selection of employment, a finding similar to that by Peter et al., 1975). The studies by McWilliams and Paradise (1973) and Peter et al. (1975b) found no difference between occupational levels of adults with a cleft, their fathers, and nearest-aged sibling. Years later, Patel and Ross (2003) interviewed adults about employment and concluded that having a cleft did not appear to influence their ability to find a job.

Based on interviews, Stock and Rumsey (2015) also reported that adults with cleft palate felt that having a cleft did not negatively affect their vocational achievement. As a matter of fact, 90% of the participants were employed. Cited reasons for those who were not employed included retirement, disability, or a mental health issue. There were few participants who perceived that they had to work harder to prove themselves capable, or that they were concerned about the stigma associated with a cleft when looking for employment. As a result of their findings, Stock and Rumsey suggested that a lack of awareness of CLP in the general population may be more of a factor in entering the workplace than having the cleft.

TRANSITION OF CARE AND MULTIDISCIPLINARY TEAM

For many years, the care provided by the multidisciplinary team provides the person with CLP with a positive experience that enhances their QOL. However, adulthood often marks the transition from child-centered interdisciplinary care to adult-centered care. Some adults may be fortunate enough to transition easily from a pediatric cleft palate team to an interdisciplinary adult cleft palate team who can manage their specific needs, but for the majority of adults this service may not be easily accessible. In a telephone interview exploring the possible support needs of adults with CLP in the United Kingdom (UK), Stock, Feragen, and Rumsey (2014) reported that the participants stressed the importance of being able to access information, treatment, and support after discharge from the cleft team. As an outcome of this study, many cleft teams in the UK were reorganizing their cleft teams using a life span approach to care that will offer adults with clefts multidisciplinary team management well past 20 years of age (Stock et al., 2014). There are few adult cleft palate teams in the United States. For the majority of adults with CLP, continuation with team care after 21 years is generally not available. As of this writing, there is very little known about the process of transition of care for adults with CLP, and for their caregivers as well. There are no known models of care.

Without the accessibility of an interdisciplinary team, the adult now must rely on his or her own resources to obtain the care needed. This is challenging when the number and nature of problems associated with a cleft require the services of several specialists for whom the adult must independently seek out, arrange for appointments, and be able to pay for it.

Once the transition of care is initiated, it is likely that the adult will come upon a number of barriers that reduce the quality of care and perhaps even the quality of life. One barrier is the community practitioner's limited knowledge about

and inexperience with CLP (Damiano et al., 2010). Another barrier is the practitioner's lack of accessible resources to make appropriate referrals for care. For example, finding a dentist who is able to or willing to provide services to a person with cleft related dental problems.

The adult too may have difficulty in continuing his or her health care needs once he or she ages out of medical coverage. He or she may lack adequate finances or medical insurance to pay for the necessary care. Then, too, because of reimbursement limitations, there may be some unwillingness for a practitioner to accept care for the adult patient (White, 2002). Unlike the team, where the social worker or support service worker can seek out sources of support, the person must try to obtain funding for their services on their own. However, if these barriers can be addressed, it is very possible that a model of transition of care can be successful in the management of the adult with CLP, but given the current economic and health care climate it may not be possible in the near future.

These challenges make a strong case for multidisciplinary team services to be provided past 21 years of age in order to offer the necessary services to enable the adult with CLP to meet his or her maximum potential. Importantly, a multidisciplinary team is the standard of care in meeting the complex needs of the individual with CLP. Team care begins at infancy, and it seems very reasonable for it to continue into adulthood.

CHAPTER SUMMARY

The overall quality of life in most adults with cleft lip and palate is good. Certainly these adults are aware of the impact of the cleft on appearance and other aspects of their lives, but the evidence supports that they have adjusted fairly well to this birth defect. Based on the evidence, it appears that having a CLP is not the sole factor in determining a person's QOL or HRQOL. There are other factors that influence his or her life. The ICF model with its integration of QOL provides an opportunity to examine the impact of CLP on a person's activities and participation in life. Lastly, there will be challenges for the young adult with CLP who transitions from the child multidisciplinary team to adult-centered care. Best care for these individuals is the adult multidisciplinary team.

REFERENCES

Andrews-Casal, M., Johnston, D., Fletcher, J., Mulliken, J. B., Stal, S., & Hecht, J. T. (1998). Cleft lip with or without cleft palate: Effect of family history on reproductive planning, surgical timing, and parental stress. *Cleft Palate-Craniofacial Journal, 35,* 52–57.

Bardach, J., Morris, H., Olin, W., Gray, S., Jones, D., Kelly, K., . . . Semb, G. (1992). Results of multidisciplinary management of bilateral cleft lip and palate at the Iowa Cleft Palate Center. *Plastic and Reconstructive Surgery, 89,* 419–432.

Bjørnsson, A., & Agustsdottir, S. A. (1987). A psychosocial study of Icelandic individuals with cleft lip or cleft lip and palate. *Cleft Palate Journal, 24,* 152–157.

Broder, H. L., Smith, F. B., & Strauss, R. P. (1992). Habilitation of patients with clefts: Parent and child ratings of satisfaction with appearance and speech. *Cleft Palate-Craniofacial Journal, 29,* 262–267.

Centers for Disease Control and Prevention. (2000). *Measuring healthy days.* Atlanta, GA: Author. Retrieved from http://www.cdc.gov/hrQOL/pdfs/mhd.pdf

Chuo, C. B., Searle, Y., Jeremy, A., Richard, B. M., Sharp, I., & Slator, R. (2008). The continuing multidisciplinary needs of adult patients with cleft lip and/or palate. *Cleft Palate-Craniofacial Journal, 45,* 633–638.

Clifford, E., Crocker, E. C., & Pope, B. A. (1972). Psychological findings in the adulthood of 98 cleft lip-palate children. *Plastic and Reconstructive Surgery, 50,* 234–237.

Cruice, M. (2008). The contribution and impact of the International Classification of Functioning, Disability, and Health on quality of life in communication. *International Journal of Speech Language Pathology, 10,* 38–49.

Demb, N., & Reuss, A. L. (1967). High school dropout rates for cleft palate patients. *Cleft Palate Journal, 4,* 327–333.

Damiano, P. C., Tyler, M. C, Romitti, P. A., Druschel, C., Austin, A. A., Burnett, W., & Robbins, J. M. (2010). Primary care physician experience with children with oral clefts in three states. *Birth Defects Research (Part A), 88,* 1050–1056.

Hamlet, C., & Harcourt, D. (2015). Older adults' experiences of living with cleft lip and palate. A qualitative study exploring aging and appearance. *Cleft Palate-Craniofacial Journal, 52,* e32–e40.

Han, K-T., Park, E-C., Kim, J-H., Kim, S. J. & Park, S. (2014). Is marital status associated with quality of life? *Health and Quality of Life Outcomes, 12,* 109. doi:10.1186/s12955-014-0109-0

Havstam, C., & Lohmander, A. (2011). Communicative participation. In *Cleft palate speech: Assessment and intervention* (pp. 305–315). West Sussex, UK: Wiley.

Heller, A., Tidmarsh, W., & Pless, I. B. (1981). The psychosocial functioning of young adults born with cleft lip or palate. *Clinical Pediatrics, 20,* 459–465.

Huber, J. G., Sillick, J., & Skarakis-Doyle, E. (2010). Personal perception and personal factors: Incorporating health-related quality of life into the International Classification of Functioning, Disability and Health. *Disability and Rehabilitation, 32,* 1955–1965.

Libby, M., Schneiderman, E., McCann, A., & Kane, A. (2015). *Continuing medical and dental needs of adults with cleft lip and/or palate: A needs assessment.* Presented at the 72nd Annual Meeting of the American Cleft Palate-

Craniofacial Association, Palm Springs, CA. April 23.

Mani, M., Carlsson, M., & Marcusson, A. (2010). Quality of life varies with gender and age among adults treated for unilateral cleft lip and palate. *Cleft Palate-Craniofacial Journal, 47*, 491–498.

Marcusson, A., Akerlind, I., & Paulin, G. (2001). Quality of life in adults with repaired complete cleft lip and palate. *Cleft Palate-Craniofacial Journal, 38*, 379–385.

Marcusson, A., Paulin, G., & Östrup, L. (2002). Facial appearance in adults who had cleft lip and palate treated in childhood. *Scandinavian Journal of Plastic and Reconstructive Surgery and Hand Surgery, 36*, 16–23.

McWilliams, B.J. & Paradise, J.P. (1973). Educational, occupational, and marital status of cleft palate adults. *Cleft Palate Journal, 10*, 223–229.

OECD Better Life Index. (2015). *Organisation for economic co-operation and development.* Retrieved October 19, 2015, from http://www.oecdbetterlifeindex.org/about/better-life-initiative/

Patel, Z., & Ross, E. (2003). Reflections on the cleft experience by South African adults: Use of qualitative methodology. *Cleft Palate-Craniofacial Journal, 40*, 471–480.

Persson, M., Becker, M., & Svensson, H. (2012). Academic achievement in individuals with cleft. A population-based register study. *Cleft Palate-Craniofacial Journal, 49*, 153–159.

Peter, J. P., & Chinsky, R. R. (1974a). Sociological aspects of cleft palate adults: I. Marriage. *Cleft Palate Journal, 11*, 295–309.

Peter, J. P., & Chinsky, R. R. (1974b). Sociological aspects of cleft palate adults: II. Education. *Cleft Palate Journal, 11*, 443–449.

Peter, J. P., Chinsky, R. R., & Fisher, M. J. (1975b). Sociological aspects of cleft palate adults: III. Vocational and economic aspects. *Cleft Palate Journal, 12*, 193–199.

Peter, J. P., Chinsky, R. R., & Fisher, M. J. (1975a). Sociological aspects of cleft palate adults: IV. Social integration. *Cleft Palate Journal, 12*, 304–310.

Ramstad, T., Ottem, E., & Shaw, W. C. (1995). Psychosocial adjustment in Norwegian adults who had undergone standardized treatment of complete cleft lip and palate. *Scandinavian Journal of Plastic and Reconstructive Surgery and Hand Surgery, 29*, 251–257.

Sinko, K., Jagsch, R., Prechti, V., Watzinger, F., Hollmann, K., & Baumann, A. (2005). Evaluation of esthetic, functional, and quality-of-life outcome in adult cleft lip and palate patients. *Cleft Palate-Craniofacial Journal, 42*, 355–361.

Stock, N. M., Feragen, K. B., & Rumsey, N. (2014). "It doesn't all just stop at 18": Psychological adjustment and support needs of adults born with cleft lip and/or palate. *Cleft Palate-Craniofacial Journal, 52*, 543–554.

Stock, N. M., Feragen, K. B., & Rumsey, N. (2015). Adults' narratives of growing up with a cleft lip and/or palate: Factors associated with psychological adjustment. *Cleft Palate-Craniofacial Journal.* doi: http://dx.doi.org/10.1597/14-269

Stock, N. M., & Rumsey, N. (2015). Starting a family: The experience of parents with cleft lip and/or palate. *Cleft Palate-Craniofacial Journal, 52*, 425–436. doi:10.1597/14-178

Van Demark, D., & Van Demark, A. (1970). Speech and socio-vocational aspects of individuals with cleft palate. *Cleft Palate Journal, 1970*, 284–299.

White, P. H. (2002). Access to health care: Health insurance considerations for young adults with special health care needs/disabilities. Pediatrics, 110, 1328–1335.

World Health Organization. (1980). *International Classification of Impairments, Disabilities, and Handicaps: A manual of classification relating to the consequences of disease.* Geneva, Switzerland: Author.

World Health Organization. (2001). *The International Classification of Functioning, Disability and Health (ICF).* Geneva, Switzerland: Author.

Yttri, J. E., Christensen, K., Knudsen, L. B., & Bille, C. (2011). Reproductive patterns among Danish women with oral clefts. *Cleft Palate-Craniofacial Journal, 48*, 601–607.

Glossary of Terms

Acquired hearing loss. A hearing loss that can occur after birth as a result of a medical condition or injury.

Active intraoral appliance. A presurgical orthopedic appliance designed to actively move and align cleft segments, often called a Latham-type appliance.

Adenoids. Lymphatic tissue located along the posterior wall of the nasopharynx, may assist with velopharyngeal closure in children.

Ala nasi. Curved, lateral portion of the nose.

Alelle. Genes on specific location on the chromosome that may have a slightly varied form.

Allogeneic bone graft. Bone donated from another person processed through a tissue bank.

Alveolar bone graft. A surgical procedure to repair or reconstruct the alveolar cleft in order to provide bone support to the teeth and continuity of the alveolar ridge. Called *primary* alveolar bone graft if done early, usually 12 months of age; called *secondary* alveolar bone graft if done in late childhood, usually 7 to 9 years of age.

Alveolar cleft. A bony defect in the alveolar ridge.

Alveolar ridge. A ridge of the maxilla or mandible that contains the bony support for the teeth.

Anophthalmia. Absence of an eye.

Anotia. Total absence of the pinna.

Anterior crossbite. An abnormal relationship between the maxillary and mandibular teeth when they occlude with the mandibular teeth anterior or buccal to the maxillary teeth; abnormal labiolingual tooth relationship, often occurs with Class III malocclusion.

Anterior faucial pillars. Muscular folds that extend from the velum to the sides of the tongue, contains the palatoglossus muscle.

Anterior nasal fricative. A learned, maladaptive articulation that is characterized by complete occlusion of the oral cavity and shunting of all airflow through the nose. Can sound similar to obligatory audible nasal air emission.

Association. A nonrandom occurrence of a pattern of multiple congenital anomalies in two or more individuals that are not known to be a syndrome or sequence.

Atresia. Abnormal development or nondevelopment of a passage or canal (e.g., external auditory canal).

Audible nasal air emission. Turbulent nasal air escape generated at the internal nasal valve during production of obstruent consonants, primarily voiceless. An obligatory symptom that can be simulated by forcefully exhaling through the nose.

Auditory brainstem response (ABR). A physiologic assessment of hearing used to estimate hearing threshold sensitivity. Electrodes are placed on the scalp and brain wave activity in response to sound is recorded.

Auditory distortion. A speech sound that is perceived as aberrant but looks acceptable to the listener.

Autologous bone graft. Bone harvested from the patient.

Bone conduction hearing aid. A type of hearing aid consisting of a bone vibrator that is connected to a headband and sits on the mastoid process through which sound vibrations are transmitted.

Bone-anchored hearing aid (BAHA). Implantable bone conduction hearing aid device.

Brachycephaly. A skull shape that is short from front to back caused by premature fusion of the coronal sutures.

Canonical babbling. Reduplicated vocalizations with consonants that sound adult-like, may begin by 4 to 6 months of age.

Centromere. A constriction that joins the two identical halves (chromatids) of the chromosomes.

Cheiloplasty. Surgery to repair cleft lip.

Chromosome. Very long strands of DNA that contain hundreds and thousands of genes; the normal human chromosome has 46 chromosomes consisting of 23 pairs, one half of each pair from the mother and the other half from the father. The 23 pairs of chromosomes include 22 autosome pairs (numbered 1 to 22 according to size) and one pair are sex chromosomes, termed X and Y (XX = female, XY = male).

Class I malocclusion. Normal molar relationship but with misalignment of the teeth, crowding, overbite, or other types of dental anomalies.

Class II malocclusion. The maxillary first molar aligns with or is anterior to the mandibular first molar; the buccal groove of the mandibular first molar is distal to the mesiobuccal cusp of the maxillary first molar.

Class III malocclusion. The maxillary first molar is more posterior to the mandibular first molar than normal; the buccal groove of the mandibular first molar is mesial to the mesiobuccal cusp of the maxillary first molar.

Cleft muscle of Veau. Abnormal attachment of the levator veli palatini and palatopharyngeus muscles onto the posterior hard palate.

Cholesteatoma. An invasive tumor resulting from abnormal skin growth in the middle ear behind the eardrum.

Coloboma. Notch of the upper eyelid.

Compensatory articulations. Learned maladaptive articulations such as glottal stops, pharyngeal stops, and pharyngeal fricatives that valve expiratory airflow before the velopharyngeal port.

Compression pressure. Positive pressure generated by the tongue against the nipple during feeding to express milk from the nipple.

Congenital. A condition present at birth.

Congenital hearing loss. A hearing loss that is present at birth.

Continuous positive airway pressure (CPAP) therapy. A therapeutic approach to treat velopharyngeal inadequacy through the application of CPAP while speaking to strengthen velar muscles through resistance training.

Conventional air conduction hearing aid. A type of hearing aid in which sound is captured by a microphone, amplified, and transmitted through an earmold in the ear canal.

Craniofacial. The soft tissues and bones of the skull and face.

Craniofacial anomaly. An abnormality of the head (skull) and face.

Craniosynostosis. Premature closure of the cranial sutures causing an abnormal head shape.

Crossbite. A type of malocclusion in which a tooth (or teeth) has a more buccal or lingual position relative to the opposing teeth; may be anterior or posterior.

Cul-de-sac resonance. A muffled quality that is due to obstruction at some point in the vocal tract, either oral-pharyngeal or nasal.

Cytogenetics. The branch of science that studies the number and structure of chromosomes and their relationship to a disease or disease process.

Decannulation. Removal of the tracheostomy tube.

Deformation. Abnormal shape, form, or position of a body structure usually caused by extrinsic mechanical force acting upon the structure.

Dental malocclusion. Improper alignment of the maxillary and mandibular teeth.

Dentofacial. Teeth, alveolar process, and face.

Deoxyribonucleic acid (DNA). The hereditary material of all organisms; a double-stranded molecule that resembles a twisted ladder (double helix).

Disruption. Defect caused by extrinsic breakdown of a normally developing tissue.

Dominant inheritance. A trait that is inherited as result of one mutant gene from one affected parent; the other parent who is unaffected has a copy of the normal gene.

Double-opposing Z-plasty. A surgical procedure developed by Furlow that uses Z-shaped incisions to lengthen and repair a palatal cleft, including submucous cleft palate. It is also used as a secondary procedure to treat velopharyngeal inadequacy in older children.

Dysmorphogenesis. The process of abnormal structure development or formation.

Dysmorphology. The study of congenital malformations.

Dysplasia. A structural anomaly resulting from a breakdown in the organization of tissues from which normal structures are formed.

Ear tubes. See *ventilation tubes*.

Ectopic tooth. A normal tooth that erupts in the wrong place.

Enhanced Milieu Training. A model of early intervention that applies behavioral principles to prompt and support functional language use in routine daily activities in a naturalistic environment.

Epiblast. One of two distinct cell layers in the early embryo, the other is the hypoblast.

Epibulbar dermoid. A cyst on the eyeball (often a feature of OAVS).

Eustachian tube. A tube extending from the middle ear to the nasopharynx that functions to ventilate the middle ear space, protect the middle ear from nasopharyngeal reflux, and drain fluids from the middle ear space; also called *auditory tube*.

Exophthalmos. Abnormal protrusion of the eyeball.

Expressivity. The range of clinical features that a person with the disorder can present.

Feeding plate. An artificial palate used to cover a palatal cleft during feeding.

Fistula. Abnormal connection or a hole between two structures.

Flow coefficient k. A mathematical constant used to correct for turbulent airflow during pressure-flow assessment. Warren derived a value of 0.65 based upon models of the upper airway.

Fluorescence in situ hybridization (FISH). A cytogenetic technique that studies specific regions of a chromosome using a probe to localize a microdeletion that cannot be detected by standard chromosome analysis.

Focused stimulation. A naturalistic intervention that emphasizes modeling and responsive interaction with use of modeling and little direct prompting of the child's language production.

Forme fruste. A microform of cleft lip.

Gastrulation. A process of cell migration in the early embryo that leads to the formation of three distinct cell layers: the ectoderm, mesoderm, and endoderm.

Genetics. The study of genes and heredity.

Genome. The genetic material that contains all the information needed to build an organism.

Genotype. A person's genetic makeup; a set of genes in the DNA that is responsible for a particular trait.

Gingivoperiosteoplasty (GPP). A surgical procedure that closes the alveolar cleft(s) by elevating flaps of gingival tissue and periosteum, typically done at time of lip repair.

Glossopexy. A surgical procedure designed to relieve obstruction of the upper airway due to glossoptosis. The anterior tip of the tongue is sutured to the inner surface of the lower lip; also known as *tongue-lip adhesion*.

Glossoptosis. Posterior displacement of the tongue resulting in upper airway obstruction, common in Pierre Robin sequence.

Grommets. See *ventilation tubes*.

Health-related quality of life (HRQoL). A multidimensional concept that encompasses overall quality of life. It refers to the ability to function within a variety of roles and deriving satisfaction from them. The emphasis is on the self-reported impact of the disorder.

Heterogenous. A feature where gene mutations at different loci can cause the same clinical disorder.

Heterozygous. Having different alleles at the same location (locus) on a pair of homologous chromosomes.

Homologous. Having the same position or structure; homologous chromosomes are a pair of chromosomes, one from the mother and one from the father whose copies are similar in size and shape and contain the same genes in the same location.

Homozygous. Having identical alleles on a pair of homologous chromosomes.

Hypernasality. Excessive resonance of the nasal cavity during production of vowels and voiced oral consonants.

Hypertelorism. Abnormal distance between the two eyes.

Hypoblast. A layer of cells that lies below the epiblast in the early embryo.

Hyponasality. Lack of normal nasal resonance during production of nasal consonants and vowels adjacent to nasal consonants.

Hypoplasia. An underdeveloped structure. Mandibular or maxillary hypoplasia refers to an underdeveloped lower or upper jaw.

Iatrogenic. An illness or condition caused by medical treatment.

Incisive foramen. A small opening in the hard palate behind the premaxilla that passes nerves and blood vessels to the oral mucosa of the hard palate.

Internal nasal valve. The smallest cross-sectional area of the nasal cavity, bounded by the upper lateral cartilage, the medial wall of the septum, and the anterior part of the inferior turbinate.

International Classification of Functioning, Disability, and Health (ICF). A conceptual framework for describing the impact of a disorder that integrates the biological, psychological, and social aspects of a condition.

Intravelar veloplasty. Surgical repair of a velar muscles to reconstruct the levator sling.

Karyotype. A pictorial representation of a pattern of chromosomes.

Lateral cephalogram. A standardized skull radiograph that shows the occlusal relationship of the jaws and soft tissue dimensions of the face.

Lateral maxillary prominence. Area on the first pharyngeal arch that will contribute to formation of the upper lip and secondary palate.

Le Fort I osteotomy. Surgical procedure that involves separating the maxilla and the palate from the skull above the roots of the upper teeth and repositioning as a single unit.

Le Fort II osteotomy. Surgical procedure that involves a cut into the nasomaxillary projection without altering the orbital volume or zygomatic arch.

Le Fort III osteotomy. Surgical procedure that involves a cut in the bones of the frontotemporal skull, cheekbones, orbital rims, nasion, and alveolar arch.

Levator veli palatini. Primary muscle that elevates and retracts the velum.

Lip adhesion. A surgical procedure done prior to definitive lip repair designed to reduce the width of the cleft deformity.

Malformation. An abnormal shape or form.

Malocclusion. Improper relationship between the maxillary (upper) and mandibular (lower) dental or skeletal arches so that the teeth do not come together normally.

Mandibular lengthening by distraction osteogenesis (MLDO). A surgical procedure involving osteotomies (bone cuts) on both sides of the mandible and insertion of hardware to gradually lengthen the mandible over time.

Maxillary retrusion. The maxilla (upper jaw) is small relative to the mandible (lower jaw); also called *maxillary hypoplasia.*

Median palatine suture. Fusion line of the two palatal shelves, also called *intermaxillary suture.*

Metathetic dimension. A perceptual stimulus that varies according to quality and is considered substitutive, an example is pitch.

Microarray-based comparative genomic hybridization (array CGH). A cytogenetic technique that studies the entire genome for abnormalities caused by deletions and duplications of segments of DNA.

Microphthalmia. Abnormally small eye.

Microtia. Underdevelopment of the pinna or auricle. The severity may range from a malformed pinna to one that is completely absent; see *anotia.*

Middle ear effusion. Buildup of fluid in the middle ear space caused by eustachian tube dysfunction.

Mid-dorsum palatal stop. A learned maladaptive articulation characterized by palatal contact with the middle of the tongue, usually used to replace alveolar stops.

Midface hypoplasia. The underdevelopment of the maxilla resulting in a concave appearance; also known as *midface retrusion.*

Morphogenesis. A biological process that causes a tissue, structure, or organ to develop its shape.

Multifactorial inheritance. A trait that is inherited as a result of a combination of factors, genetic and environmental.

Multiview videofluoroscopy. A radiographic procedure that allows dynamic assessment of the velopharyngeal mechanism during speech production. Lateral, frontal, and base views of the velopharyngeal sphincter are usually obtained.

Musculus uvulae. Velar muscle that adds bulk and may assist with closure. Only completely intrinsic muscle of the velum.

Mutation. Any change in the nucleotide sequence of DNA that alters an individual gene resulting in extra gene material (insertion) or loss of genetic material (deletion) or a chromosome structure or number.

Myringotomy. A surgical incision made into the eardrum to relieve pressure caused by a buildup of fluid, or to drain middle ear fluid; usually accompanied by insertion of ventilation tubes.

Nasalance. An acoustic measure of the intensity of a nasal microphone signal relative to the combined oral and nasal microphones signals, expressed in percentage.

Nasal columella. Skin and underlying tissue that separates the nose into two nostrils.

Nasal grimace. Constriction of the nares that may accompany either obligatory audible nasal air emission and anterior nasal fricatives. When part of obligatory nasal air emission, it may increase oral air pressure. When part of anterior nasal fricatives, it may increase frication noise.

Nasal ram pressure. A local, airflow velocity measure obtained by inserting the prongs of an oxygen-delivery cannula into the nostrils.

Nasal turbinates. Mucous-lined bones of the nasal cavity, also called *conchae.*

Nasal turbulence. A type of obligatory audible nasal air emission characterized by turbulent airflow generated by a small velopharyngeal opening, often accompanied by tissue flutter.

Nasal valve appliance. A device used to treat velopharyngeal inadequacy. Two one-way valves are fitted into the nostrils to prevent nasal air emission.

Nasion. Bony part of the nose between the eyes.

Nasoalveolar molding appliance (NAM). A type of passive presurgical orthopedic appliance designed to align cleft segments and shape the collapsed nostril(s).

Neural crest cells. Multipotent migratory cells in the embryo that give rise to structures of the face and brain.

Normal occlusion. The mesiobuccal cusp of the maxillary first molar is aligned with the buccal groove of the mandibular first molar; the teeth are aligned, and there is normal overbite and overjet; also called *neutocclusion* and *Class I*.

Obturator nipple. A nipple with a hood that functions to cover a palatal cleft during bottle feeding.

Occlusion. The relationship between the maxillary (upper) and mandibular (lower) teeth when the jaw is closed.

Olfactory placodes. Neural ectodermal cells that line the nasal pits of the embryo and eventually form the olfactory nerve.

Open bite. A condition in which there is lack of occlusion between the maxillary and mandibular teeth; failure of the upper and lower teeth to meet.

Oronasal fistula. See *palatal fistula.*

Orthognathic surgery. Surgery to correct skeletal anomalies involving the maxilla or mandible.

Ossicles. Three bones of the middle ear, malleus, incus, and stapes; also called *auditory ossicles.*

Osteotomy. A surgical procedure in which a bone is cut and made to be shorter or longer or changed in alignment.

Otitis media with effusion (OME). A collection of non-infected fluid in the middle ear space behind the eardrum.

Otoacoustic emissions (OAEs). Sounds emitted by the cochlea when stimulated by an auditory signal.

Otoscopy. A procedure used to visualize the tympanic membrane and external auditory canal.

Palatal expander. A fixed orthodontic appliance that is used to expand the width of the maxilla; it is activated by turning a screw in the center of the appliance to gradually separate the mid-palatal sutures to make the maxilla wider.

Palatal fistula. A hole or an opening in the palate that causes direct communication between the oral and nasal cavities; a breakdown at the site of a cleft palate repair; also called an *oronasal fistula.*

Palatal lift appliance. A prosthetic device used to treat velopharyngeal inadequacy. An extension from the appliance physically lifts and holds the velum against the posterior pharyngeal wall.

Palatoglossus. Velar muscle that elevates the posterior tongue, may also lower the velum.

Palatopharyngeus. Velar muscle with vertical fibers that narrows the lateral pharyngeal walls, also elevates the larynx and may lower the velum.

Passavant's ridge. A shelf-like muscular projection from the posterior pharyngeal wall during phonation, may assist with velopharyngeal closure.

Passive intraoral appliance. A presurgical orthopedic appliance designed to passively guide growth to align cleft segments.

Penetrance. The proportion of people who have the genetic mutation and actually exhibit any of the clinical features of the disorder; complete penetrance (100%) means that everyone who has the gene shows the clinical trait; incomplete penetrance means only some people with a gene for a specific disorder will exhibit the trait.

Pharyngeal arches. A series of outgrowths of embryologic cells during the fourth week of gestation. The first pharyngeal arch gives rise to the mandible and maxilla. The second pharyngeal arch gives rise to the hyoid bone and various structures of the ear.

Pharyngeal constrictors. Inferior, medial, and superior muscles that form the muscular tube of the pharyngeal wall. Superior constrictor assists with velopharyngeal closure.

Pharyngeal plexus. A network of branches of the glossopharyngeal, vagus, and accessory cranial nerves.

Phenotype. The observable or physical characteristics produced by the genotype.

Philtrum. Midline depression from the nose to the upper lip, bounded laterally by the philtral ridges.

Phoneme-specific nasal emission. A speech-sound disorder characterized by the use of learned nasal fricatives in the presence of adequate velopharyngeal function. Can occur in children with or without cleft palate.

Pneumotachometer. An airflow meter used during pressure-flow testing to obtain rates of oral and nasal airflow. It is usually heated to prevent condensation during speech and breathing.

Posterior choanal atresia. Congenital blockage of the posterior nasal airway leading to respiratory distress and failure in the newborn.

Posterior crossbite. The posterior teeth occlude in an abnormal buccolingual relationship with the opposite teeth.

Posterior faucial pillars. Muscular folds that extend from the sides of the velum into the lateral pharyngeal walls, contains the palatopharyngeus muscle.

Posterior nasal fricative. A learned, maladaptive articulation characterized by complete occlusion of the oral cavity and shunting of all airflow through a partially closed velopharyngeal port, often accompanied by tissue flutter. Can sound similar to obligatory nasal turbulence.

Posterior pharyngeal flap. A surgical procedure to treat velopharyngeal inadequacy. A myomucosal flap is released from the posterior pharyngeal wall and its free end is attached to the velum.

Posterior pharyngeal wall augmentation. A surgical procedure to treat velopharyngeal inadequacy. Various materials (e.g.,

autogenous fat) are injected into the posterior pharyngeal wall.

Preauricular pit. A dimple or dent located anywhere near the front of the ear; also known as *preauricular fistula*.

Preauricular tag. A mound of tissue or pedunculated tissue typically located in front of the ear or tragus.

Premaxilla. Bony part of the hard palate that is anterior to the incisive foramen, contains the incisor teeth.

Pressure-equalizing (PE) tubes. See *ventilation tubes*.

Presurgical orthopedics. Any of a variety of procedures used to reduce the extent of a cleft and align segments prior to lip repair.

Primary palate. Structures anterior to the incisive foramen, includes the premaxilla and the lip.

Proptosis. Protrusion of the eyeball (globe) with respect to the eye socket (orbit).

Prothetic dimension. A perceptual stimulus that varies according to quantity or magnitude and is considered additive; loudness is an example.

Pseudo-prognathism. The tendency of the lower jaw to appear protruded relative to the upper jaw due to restricted growth of the upper jaw.

Quad helix. A fixed orthodontic appliance used to expand the maxillary arch; bands are cemented to the molars to keep the appliance in place while four active helix springs widen the arch.

Quality of life (QoL). A broad multidimensional concept that reflects a person's physical, psychological, and social well-being.

Recessive inheritance. A trait that is inherited when both parents have the same gene mutation.

Relative prognathism. A situation in which the lower jaw appears too far forward due to the maxilla being too far back.

Retracted eardrum. A condition whereby the eardrum is pulled inward by negative middle ear pressure created within the middle ear space, caused by eustachian tube dysfunction.

Rooting reflex. A reflex elicited by tactile stimulation of the corners of the infant's mouth. The infant will turn the head toward the stimulation and open the mouth.

Rotation-advancement lip repair. A surgical technique developed by Millard involving the release and rotation of a tissue flap to recreate the Cupid's bow while advancing contralateral tissue to close the flap area.

Rule of 10s. Criteria promoted in the 1960s for timing of cleft lip repair, based on age (at least 10 weeks), weight (at least 10 pounds), and general health (at least 10 g hemoglobin) of the infant.

Scaphocephaly. A skull shape that is long and narrow caused by premature fusion of the sagittal suture.

Secondary palate. Structures posterior to the incisive foramen, includes the hard and soft palate.

Sequence. A pattern of multiple anomalies occurring as a result of a single known or presumed prior anomaly or mechanical factor causing a cascade of secondary anomalies.

Sex-linked (X-linked) inheritance. A trait resulting from a gene mutation on the sex (X) chromosome.

SF-36. Short form (SF) quality of life measure of functional health and well-being.

Skeletal malocclusion. Improper relationship between the maxilla and mandible; may result in retrognathia, maxillary hypoplasia or deficiency, or open bite.

Speech-bulb appliance. A prosthetic device used to treat velopharyngeal inadequacy. An obturator bulb extends from the appliance into the velopharyngeal space.

Speech-bulb reduction therapy. Gradual reduction in the size of an obturator bulb over time to stimulate velopharyngeal movement.

Sphincter pharyngoplasty. A surgical procedure used to treat velopharyngeal inadequacy. Two myomucosal flaps are released from the posterior faucal pillars and attached in the midline on the posterior pharyngeal wall.

Submucous cleft. A cleft of the secondary palate that involves separation of muscle and, at times, bone but without overlying tissue involvement.

Sucking reflex. Rhythmic movements of the tongue elicited by tactile stimulation of the hard palate. Observed as early as 15 to 18 weeks' gestation.

Supernumerary teeth. Extra teeth.

Stenosis. Abnormal narrowing of passage or structure (e.g., auditory canal).

Stomodeum. A depression of tissue in the embryo that will eventually become the mouth.

Syndactyly. A condition in which two or more digits of the fingers or toes are fused together.

Syndrome. A recognizable pattern of multiple anomalies that occur together and are thought to be pathogenetically related and have a known or suspected cause. Individuals with a syndrome will look alike even though they are unrelated.

Tensor veli palatini. Velar muscle that opens the eustachian tubes.

Teratogen. An agent that interferes with the development of the fetus (e.g., drugs, infection, environmental chemicals).

Tracheostomy. A surgical procedure that creates an opening into the trachea to allow direct access to the airway; done to relieve upper airway obstruction.

Tracheotomy. An incision into the trachea to relieve airway obstruction.

Two-flap palatoplasty. A surgical procedure developed by Bardach to repair cleft palate. Lateral tissue flaps are released and moved to the midline to repair the cleft.

Tympanometry. Objective measure of middle ear function.

Tympanosclerosis. Calcification of tissue in the middle ear, a condition that can lead to conductive hearing loss.

Uvula. A pedunculus structure at the end of the velum. Often bifid when part of submucous cleft palate.

Velar bounce. Slight up and down movement of the closed velum during speech due to contractions of the levator veli palatini muscle.

Velopharyngeal inadequacy. The inability to adequately separate the oral and nasal cavities during production of oral speech segments.

Ventilation tubes. Tiny tubes surgically inserted into the eardrum to ventilate the middle ear and prevent the accumulation of fluid behind the eardrum; also called *ear tubes, pressure-equalizing (PE) tubes, tympanostomy tubes,* and *grommets.*

Vermilion zone. The pigmented portion of the lips.

Video nasoendoscopy. Insertion of a flexible fiberoptic endoscope through the nasal cavity to record movement of velopharyngeal structures during speech.

Visual distortion. A speech sound that is perceived as correct but looks aberrant to the listener.

Vomer. A thin, plowshare-shaped bone that forms the posterior and inferior parts of the nasal septum.

Zona pellucida. An anatomical feature of submucous cleft palate. The velum appears short, translucent, or V-shaped.

Zygoma. The prominence of the cheek bone.

Index

Note: Page numbers in **bold** reference non-text material.